中华传统经典养生术

（汉英对照）

(Chinese- English) Traditional and Classical Chinese Health Cultivation

Chief Producer　Li Jie	总策划　李　洁
Chief Compilers　Li Jie　Xu Feng　Xiao Bin　Zhao Xiaoting	总主编　李　洁　许　峰　肖　斌　赵晓霆
Chief Translator　Han Chouping	总主译　韩丑萍
English Language Reviewer　Charles Savona Ventura	英译主审　查尔斯·萨沃纳·文图拉

《诸病源候论》导引术

Zhu Bing Yuan Hou Lun Dao Yin Shu

(Explanations for the Daoyin Exercises in *Zhu Bing Yuan Hou Lun*)

编著　赵晓霆　陆　颖　陈超洋
Compilers　Zhao Xiaoting　Lu Ying　Chen Chaoyang

翻译　张凯维　潘　霖
Translators　Zhang Kaiwei　Pan Lin

上海科学技术出版社
Shanghai Scientific & Technical Publishers

图书在版编目（ＣＩＰ）数据

《诸病源候论》导引术 : 汉英对照 / 赵晓霆，陆颖，陈超洋编著；张凯维，潘霖翻译. -- 上海 : 上海科学技术出版社，2024.1
（中华传统经典养生术）
ISBN 978-7-5478-6392-3

Ⅰ. ①诸… Ⅱ. ①赵… ②陆… ③陈… ④张… ⑤潘… Ⅲ. ①《诸病源候总论》—汉、英 Ⅳ. ①R228

中国国家版本馆CIP数据核字(2023)第207397号

《诸病源候论》导引术

编著 赵晓霆 陆 颖 陈超洋

上海世纪出版(集团)有限公司
上海 科 学 技 术 出 版 社 出版、发行
(上海市闵行区号景路159弄A座9F-10F)
邮政编码201101 www.sstp.cn
上海新华印刷有限公司印刷
开本 787×1092 1/16 印张 32.25
字数 300千字
2024年1月第1版 2024年1月第1次印刷
ISBN 978-7-5478-6392-3 / R·2873
定价: 180.00元

本书如有缺页、错装或坏损等严重质量问题，请向印刷厂联系调换

内容提要

Synopsis

《诸病源候论》又称《诸病源候总论》《巢氏病源》，由隋朝医官巢元方等编撰。该书总结了隋以前的医学成就，对临床各科病证进行了搜求、征集、编纂，并予系统地分类，叙述了各种疾病的病因、病理、证候等。诸证之末多附导引，但不记载治疗方药，是中国最早的论述以内科为主、各科疾病病因和证候的专著。《诸病源候论》从宋代开始被尊奉为中医"七经"之一，全书共载"导引术"289条、213种具体方法。《诸病源候论》的问世，标志着气功导引在医学上的应用已进入成熟的阶段。

中医导引术，不仅仅有外在姿势，也需要配合内在的呼吸，精神的净化与升华。导引术的进一步的深入研究，更应当注重动作、呼吸，存思内在规律、效应，以及运用的原则。本书以"天人感应"为基本理论，讨论了人与社会环境、自然地理生态环境、天体运行、万物运化的规律、万化本源之间的关系与互动。以此提出：导引之术，是研究生命本质和生命在不同的时空下种种变化的功法。故而导引术教学实践要符合事物内在（阴阳）属性，全局整体性观念，以及万事万物不断变化的规律。

本书围绕调身、调息、调心三大基础操作，紧扣"可操作性""辨证施功""天人感应的理论"三个方面，以中医养生"顺应自然，法于阴阳，和于数术"为原则，遵循脏腑气血运行规律，并结合作者多年中医养生术临床与教学的实践经验，对289条导引术操作进行复原，详细地说明每个动作的基本操作、练习要领、注意事项、临床应用；介绍导引方在四种常见慢性疾病中的具体运用。

本书图文并茂、汉英双解，可为系统地研究导引术打下基础，为更好地将传统经典养生术运用于疾病康复与预防提供借鉴，同时也有利于传统经典文化走向世界。本书附练功视频，可供中医临床工作者、中医学生、中医养生爱好者、慢性病患者，以及太极健康爱好者和传播者选用。

Zhu Bing Yuan Hou Lun (Treatise on the Origins and Manifestations of Various Diseases), also known as *Chao Shi Bing Yuan* (The Origin of Disease According to Chao), was compiled by Chao Yuanfang and other medical officials during the Sui Dynasty (581 AD–618 AD). This book summarized the medical achievements before the Sui Dynasty, also collected and categorized various clinical diseases, and described the etiology, pathology, symptoms and signs of these diseases. It is the earliest monograph in China on the etiology and syndrome of the diseases that mainly fall under internal medicine. Most syndromes are followed by daoyin treatment methods instead of medicines. *Zhu Bing Yuan Hou Lun* has been regarded as one of the TCM classics since the Song Dynasty (960 AD–1279 AD). It contains 289 provisions of daoyin, totally 213 specific methods. The publication of *Zhu Bing Yuan Hou Lun* marked the maturity of the application of qigong daoyin in the field of medicine.

The practice of daoyin not only involves physical movements but also requires the coordination of breathing and mind. For in-depth research, it is significant to emphasize the integration of body movements, breathing, mind, intrinsic principles and effects. Based on the theory of man-nature correspondence, this book (*Explanations for the Daoyin Exercises in Zhu Bing Yuan Hou Lun*) introduces the relationship and interaction between individuals and the social environment, natural environment and celestial movements. Therefore, it is suggested that daoyin exercises involve the study of the essence of life and the various changes that life undergoes in different temporal and spatial contexts. Daoyin exercises should align with the inherent properties of phenomena (yin and yang), embrace a holistic perspective, and adhere to the principles of constant change in all things and phenomena.

This book revolves around the three fundamental practices of body regulation, breathing regulation and mind regulation. It adheres to the three aspects of "practicability", "practice based on pattern identification" and "man-nature correspondence." Following the principles of TCM methods for health preservation and the rules governing the circulation of qi and blood, and drawing upon the author's extensive practical experience in clinical settings and teaching of TCM health preservation, the book provides detailed explanations for the 289 daoyin exercises. It covers their basic operations, exercise essentials, precautions and clinical applications. Furthermore, it introduces their specific applications in four common chronic diseases, namely, sequelae of apoplexy, lung distention, depression and consumptive conditions.

This book is richly illustrated and provides bilingual (Chinese-English) content. It lays a solid foundation for the systematic study of daoyin, enabling the effective application of traditional health preservation techniques in disease rehabilitation and prevention. Furthermore, it contributes to the going out of traditional Chinese culture. This book includes video demonstrations. It is suitable for clinical practitioners of TCM, TCM students, enthusiasts of TCM health preservation, individuals with chronic diseases, and Taiji Health enthusiasts.

顾问委员会
Advisory Committee Members

主任

徐建光　陈凯先　严世芸　胡鸿毅

Directors

Xu Jianguang　Chen Kaixian　Yan Shiyun　Hu Hongyi

副主任

王拥军　舒　静　郑林赟　林　勋

Vice Directors

Wang Yongjun　Shu Jing　Zheng Linyun　Lin Xun

学术顾问

林中鹏　林　欣　俞尔科　潘华信　潘华敏
姚玮莉　王　彤　王庆华　刘　华　聂爱国

Academic Advisers

Lin Zhongpeng　　Lin Xin　　Yu Erke　　Pan Huaxin
Pan Huamin　　Yao Weili　　Wang Tong　　Wang Qinghua
Liu Hua　　Nie Aiguo

编纂委员会
Compilation Committee Members

总策划

李　洁

Chief Producer

Li Jie

总主编

李　洁　许　峰　肖　斌　赵晓霆

Chief Compilers

Li Jie　Xu Feng　Xiao Bin　Zhao Xiaoting

副总主编

沈晓东　孙　磊　陆　颖

Vice Chief Compilers

Shen Xiaodong　Sun Lei　Lu Ying

总主译

韩丑萍

Chief Translator

Han Chouping

副主译

翁　玮　张凯维　潘　霖

Vice Chief Translators

Weng Wei　Zhang Kaiwei　Pan Lin

项目资助

Acknowledgements

· 上海市进一步加快中医药传承创新发展三年行动计划（2021—2023 年）"中医药健康素养提升工程"［项目编号：ZY（2021–2023）–0105］

· 健康上海行动专项项目（2022—2024 年）"名家推广中医传统功法，冠军带动全民健身活动"［项目编号：JKSHZX–2022–04］

· The Three-Year Action Plan for Inheritance, Innovation and Development of Traditional Chinese Medicine in Shanghai (2021–2023) on Improvement of Traditional Chinese Medicine Health Literacy under grant No. ZY(2021–2023)–0105

· Healthy Shanghai Action Project (2022–2024) on Masters Promoting Traditional Chinese Medicine Exercises and Champions Leading Public Fitness Activities under grant No. JKSHZX–2022–04

序

Foreword

　　中华传统养生术源远流长，在数千年的发展演化过程中，汲取儒、道、释等与人的生命活动和治病养生有关的文化营养，形成了独特的理论体系和身心锻炼技法。有些技术和方法甚至在砭、针、灸、药之前，是中华民族最早修身养性、祛病延年的重要组成部分。

　　出土文献马王堆《导引图》、张家山《引书》、战国《行气玉佩铭》等为中华导引术提供了珍贵的考古史料，存世文献《庄子》《吕氏春秋》《黄帝内经》等也有相关理论和方法的记载。此后，导引学术思想不断丰富、发展和创新，20世纪50年代又以"气功"之名呈现于世，闻名海内外。

　　中华传统导引术和中医养生学是中华民族健康维护的原点，蕴含了中华文明的生生之理。"天人合一"的整体观和辩证观是中华文明的精髓和核心。《道德经》曰：人法地，地法天，天法道，道法自然。整体观既是中国传统哲学的基石，也是中医学和养生学的重要理论基础。中医学认为人体是一个有机的整体，脏腑、经络、精气神等都是有机整体，同时人与社会和自然也是一个整体，相互融合不可分割。

　　上海市气功研究所在建所三十年之际，提出构建现代气功"气以臻道"学术思想，得到学界广泛响应。研究所总结多年来教学培训经验，汇集成第一批凡八种养生术——易筋经、古音六字诀、逍遥功、八段锦、天柱导引功、松柔功、六合功和放松功，以汉英对照方式出版发行，得到国内外同道的青睐和赞誉。

　　世界卫生组织（WHO）提出健康新概念："健康不仅为疾病或羸弱之消除，而系体格、精神与社会之完全健康状态。"随着当代世界面临的传染病、慢性疾病、老龄化和精神卫生等健康问题的前所未有的挑战，WHO提出要寻找低成本干预措施，延缓发展态势，减轻经济负担。WHO提出的战略目标之一，就是通过把传统和补充医学服务纳入卫生保健服务供给和自我卫生保健之中，来促进全民健康覆盖。

2016年在WHO指导下，上海中医药大学、上海市中医药研究院成立太极健康中心。该中心秉承以中华传统文化"太极"为标志，以WHO倡导的生理、心理健康及良好社会适应性的健康新理念为目标，以传统中医养生、保健、导引、按蹻、食疗、药膳、心理为技术手段，结合中华太极文化深厚底蕴，整体构建"太极健康"的自我疗愈模式，并推广于世界各地各民族中。李洁教授及其同仁在第一批"中华传统经典养生术"基础上，精选传统导引术以及与日常生活密切相关的站、行、坐、卧方式，汇集第二批凡五种养生术——《诸病源候论》导引术、站桩功、行步功、卧功、神气五行操等，再次以汉英对照形式出版发行。

我深信这套丛书的出版会对传承中华传统文化，发挥中医药整体观和治未病特色、提升全民中医药健康素养起到良好的促进作用。我深切期待着他们能够再接再厉，不断创新，让中华优秀文化和传统养生术惠及世界各地更多民众。

胡鸿毅

2022年8月

Traditional Chinese health preservation has a long-standing history. Its well-established theoretical system has evolved over thousands of years by integrating Confucianism, Taoism, Buddhism and cultural understanding on human health and disease. As an essential part in promoting health and longevity, some practice methods were long before the emergence of *Bian*-stone, acupuncture, moxibustion and Chinese herbs.

These ancient practice methods have been proved by unearth books including the *Dao Yin Tu* (Daoyin Diagram) in Mawangdui, *Yin Shu* (Book on Daoyin) in Zhangjiashan and *Xing Qi Yu Pei Ming* (Jade Inscriptions on Qi Cultivation) from the Warring States Period, along with the later books such as *Zhuang Zi* (Zhuangzi), *Lü Shi Chun Qiu* (Spring and Autumn of Master Lü), and *Huang Di Nei Jing* (Yellow Emperor's Internal Classic). The academic idea on Daoyin has been further enriched and developed. In 1950s, the Daoyin became known as Qigong.

Traditional Chinese Daoyin and health preservation are essential to the health and wellness of Chinese people and contain the philosophical wisdom of Chinese civilization, which highlights the holistic and dialectic view on man-nature unity. The *Daodejing* states, "Men emulate earth; earth emulates heaven; heaven emulates the Dao; and the Dao emulates spontaneity." The holistic view is both the corner stone of traditional Chinese philosophy and theoretical foundation of Chinese medicine and health preservation. Chinese medicine believes that the human body is an organic whole, including the zang-fu organs, meridians, essence, qi and spirit. In addition, man is inseparable to society and nature.

On the occasion of celebrating the 30th anniversary, Shanghai Qigong Research Institute put forward the academic idea of "Qi-Dao harmony" and compiled a set of eight books (in Chinese and English) on health preservation exercise—*Yi Jin Jing* (Sinew-Transformation Classic), *Gu Yin Liu Zi Jue* (Six Healing Sounds), *Xiao Yao Gong* (Free and Easy Exercise), *Ba Duan Jin*, *Tian Zhu Dao Yin Gong*, *Song Rou Gong* (Soft and Relaxed Exercise), *Liu He Gong* (Six-Unity Exercise) and *Fang Song Gong* (Relaxation Exercise).

The World Health Organization (WHO) defines health as "a state of complete physical, mental, and social well-being and not merely the absence of disease or infirmity." To address the unprecedented health challenges of infectious diseases, chronic diseases, aging and mental health issues, the WHO is seeking low-cost interventions to reduce economic burden. One of the WHO's strategic goals is to promote universal health coverage by integrating traditional and complementary medicine services into health service delivery and self-care.

In 2016, the Taiji Health Center was established within the Shanghai University of Traditional Chinese Medicine and Shanghai Academy of Traditional Chinese Medicine. The Center focuses on Taiji, aims to help achieve health as "a state of complete physical, mental, and social well-being", and thus constructs a self-healing Taiji health model by combining ancient health preservation, Daoyin, massage, food therapy, herbal diet and mental regulation. Professor Li Jie and her colleagues compiled another five books (in Chinese and English) on health preservation: *Zhu Bing Yuan Hou Lun Dao Yin* Shu (Explanations for the Daoyin Exercises in *Zhu Bing Yuan Hou Lun*), *Zhan Zhuang Gong* (Post Standing Exercise), *Xing Bu Gong* (Qigong Exercise in Walking), *Wo Gong* (Qigong Exercise in Lying Position) and *Shen Qi Wu Xing Cao* (Exercise of Five Elements).

I firmly believe that the publication of this book series will benefit the inheritance of traditional Chinese culture and promote the public health and wellness. I deeply hope that they will continue to dedicate and make efforts to introduce excellent Chinese culture and traditional health preservation exercise to more people around the world.

Hu Hongyi
August, 2022

前 言
Preface

中华文化源远流长,历经数千年发展。中华传统养生术是其重要的组成部分,是中华民族的瑰宝,是修身治学的根本大道,是中华民族最早用以防治疾病、养生保健的重要方法之一,为人民健康做出了巨大贡献。

2015年,上海市气功研究所向海内外气功学界发出倡言——构建现代气功"气以臻道"的学术思想,同年编纂出版"中华传统经典养生术"丛书一套八种,取得良好的社会反响,在海外也取得了广泛的影响。2016年,在世界卫生组织传统医学、补充医学与整合医学部指导下,上海中医药大学成立太极健康中心,以中华传统文化之"太极"为标志,以WHO倡导的身体、心理、社会适应性和道德的完好状态为健康目标,以传统中医养生、气功、导引、按跷、食疗、药膳、心理为技术手段,结合中华太极文化的深厚底蕴,构建"太极健康"自我疗愈模式,推广和提升世界各族人民的健康与福祉。

中华传统经典养生术是"太极健康"自我身心锻炼的重要技术方法,我们在第一批出版基础上,精选编纂第二批"中华传统经典养生术"一套五种功法,涉及人的行、立、坐、卧各种姿势的锻炼方法。希望在已经到来的全球化、人口老龄化时代中,探索出一种集自我保健、疗愈与康复于一体的新型健康促进模式,构建"太极健康"的理念与平台,为当代人的身心健康服务。

上海市气功研究所
2022年夏

Traditional Chinese culture has a long-standing and well-established history of thousands of years. As an important part of it, traditional Chinese health cultivation is a treasure of the Chinese nation and the fundamental way to cultivate one's body and mind. It is also one of the earliest important methods used for disease prevention and treatment as well as life cultivation, thus making great contributions to people's health.

In 2015, Shanghai Qigong Research Institute advocated the concept of "*Qi-Dao Harmony*" for its academic advance. The *(Chinese-English) Traditional and Classical Chinese Health Cultivation* series of eight books published in the same year has achieved positive social feedback and extensive influence overseas. In 2016, under the guidance of the WHO Traditional, Complementary and Integrative Medicine (TCI) Unit, Shanghai University of Traditional Chinese Medicine (SHUTCM) established the Taiji Health Center. The center aims for the health concept advocated by WHO, which is a state of complete physical, mental and social well-being as well as moral integrity. With the traditional Chinese concept "Taiji" as its symbol, the center combines with the profound Chinese Taiji culture. It also takes traditional Chinese medicine (TCM) as the technical means, including TCM health cultivation, Daoyin, massage, dietary therapy, medicated diet, mental therapy, and so on. We hope to build a self-healing model of "Taiji Health" for the health and well-being of people all over the world.

Traditional and classical Chinese health cultivation exercises are important methods of "Taiji Health" mind-body exercises. On the basis of the first series, we have selected and compiled five kinds of exercises in the second series of *Traditional and Classical Chinese Health Cultivation*, involving exercise methods in different positions of walking, standing, sitting and lying. In this age of globalization and population aging, we try to explore a new health promotion model integrating self-care, self-healing and self-recovery, and construct the concept and platform of "Taiji Health", in order to improve the physical and mental health of contemporary people.

Shanghai Qigong Research Institute
Summer 2022

编写说明

Words from the Compilers

近年来,随着太极健康在海内外各地的逐渐传播,运用传统太极哲学、太极文化来指导人们的身心康养,促进当代人健康理念的提升以及与之相伴的各种太极健康技法,如气功、导引、太极拳、养生术等,越来越受到人们的广泛关注。中华传统养生术根植于中华传统哲学、中医学和养生学,充分发挥主动锻炼、身心调节的优势,已经越来越引起世人的广泛关注。

2016年以来,中国、希腊、西班牙、法国、日本等地先后涌现了各类太极健康机构,传播相关的太极健康理念与技法。但总体而言,海内外市场上还是缺乏太极健康的相关书籍出版,尤其没有成套、成系列的科普作品,更缺乏汉英对照的专业著作。

上海中医药大学太极健康中心、上海市气功研究所研究人员在前期研究工作基础上,继编纂出版第一批"中华传统经典养生术"取得良好反响后,此次精选编纂第二批一套五种。从历史源流、功法理论、特色要领、图解动作、分解说明与具体运用等方面进行编纂,由上海中医药大学中医英语专业人员进行翻译,并邀请专家进行中文审稿,邀请马耳他大学中医中心主任Charles Savona Ventura博士审定英文翻译。

本套丛书沿袭第一批图文并茂、视频摄像的形式,同时配以二维码,以便读者扫码观看,方便学习与传播,尤其适合海外太极健康爱好者用汉英双语来学习。

编者

As the concept of Taiji health has spread at home and abroad in recent years, people pay more attention to the traditional Taiji philosophy and Taiji culture due to their guidance on health, as well as various Taiji health techniques such as qigong, Daoyin, Taijiquan, health preservation, etc. Rooted in the traditional Chinese philosophy, traditional Chinese medicine and health preservation, traditional and classical Chinese health cultivation exercises have given full play to the advantages of active exercise and mind-body improvement, and have attracted increasing attention across the world.

Since 2016, Taiji health organizations have sprung up in China, Greece, Spain, France, Japan and other places to spread Taiji health concepts and techniques. However, there are few books related to Taiji health in domestic and overseas markets, especially popular science book series. There are even fewer bilingual Chinese-English versions of these books.

Based on their previous studies and the positive feedback of the first series, research staff at the Taiji Health Center of Shanghai University of Traditional Chinese Medicine (SHUTCM) and Shanghai Qigong Research Institute compiled five traditional and classical Chinese health cultivation exercise methods as the second series. These books cover the history, theoretical foundation, characteristics and key principles, illustrated movements and application of the five exercises. Then these contents have been translated by professional translators at SHUTCM. The Chinese version was reviewed by an expert team, while the English version was reviewed by Dr. Charles Savona Ventura, the director for the Center of Traditional Chinese Medicine at the University of Malta.

In addition to illustrations and videos, QR codes are also available for readers, which is convenient especially for overseas Taiji health fans to learn.

Compilers

目 录

Contents

《诸病源候论》导引术 • *Zhu Bing Yuan Hou Lun Dao Yin Shu* (Explanations for the Daoyin Exercises in *Zhu Bing Yuan Hou Lun*)

History

源流

《诸病源候论》又称《诸病源候总论》《巢氏病源》。由隋朝医官巢元方等编撰,成书于隋代大业六年(610年)。该书总结了隋以前的医学成就,对临床各科病证进行了搜求、征集、编纂,并予系统地分类。全书共50卷,分为67门、1 739病候,叙述了各种疾病的病因、病理、证候等。诸证之末多附导引术,但不记载治疗方药,是中国最早论述以内科为主各科疾病病因和证候的专著。

Zhu Bing Yuan Hou Lun, also known as Chao Shi Bing Yuan, was compiled by Chao Yuanfang and other medical officials in 610 AD. This book summarized the medical achievements before the Sui Dynasty, also collected and categorized various clinical diseases, and described the etiology, pathology, symptoms and signs of these diseases. The book consists of 50 volumes including 67 categories and 1 739 syndromes. Most syndromes are followed by daoyin treatment methods instead of medicines. It is the earliest monograph in China on the etiology and syndrome of the diseases that mainly fall under internal medicine.

《诸病源候论》内容丰富,包括内、外、妇、儿、五官、口齿、骨伤等多科病证,对一些传染病、寄生虫病、外科手术等方面,有不少精辟论述,对后世医学影响较大。

The book is rich in content, covering such branches of medical conditions as internal medicine, external medicine, gynecology, pediatrics, ophthalmology, dentistry, and orthopedics. It also provides insightful discussions on some infectious diseases, parasitic diseases and surgical procedures, thus making a significant impact on future medicine.

巢元方约生活于隋唐年间,籍贯、生卒年均不详,一说为西华人。巢元方在隋大业年间(605—615年)医事活动频繁,任太医博士,业绩卓著。然而《隋书》无巢氏传记,仅宋代《开河记》有一段关于巢氏的记载。说隋大业五年八月,开凿运河总管麻叔谋,患了"风逆"证,不能行动,头晕恶心,每天只好卧床。巢元方为他诊病后,认为是风邪侵入腠理造成的,病的部位在胸臆之中,便叫他用嫩肥羊蒸熟,掺上药粉同食,麻依法服后,很快就好了。从此便常服此方以自养。巢元方在治疗过程中,灵活掌握,可以做到药食同疗的地步,可见医术很高。而这种小方治大病、食药相合的治疗方法,足以见得医者的强闻博识,聪颖敏锐。

Chao Yuanfang lived during the Sui and Tang Dynasties (581 AD–907 AD). His birthplace and the exact years of his birth and death are unknown, but some sources suggest he was from Shanxi province, north China. He was highly active in the field of medicine between 605 AD and 615 AD. He held the position of Imperial Physician, and his achievements were remarkable. However, there is no biography of him in *Sui Shu* (Book of Sui). Only the Song Dynasty's *Kai He Ji* (The Story of Canal Construction) contains a passage with some records about him—In August 609 AD, Ma Shumou, the general manager in charge of canal construction, suffered from a contraction of pathogenic wind, with the manifestations of inability to move, dizziness and nausea, and had to stay in bed every day. After diagnosis, Chao held that this condition was caused by the attack of pathogenic wind into the interstices and the disease was located in the chest. He just prescribed steamed tender mutton with some medicinal powders. Ma soon recovered after taking this prescription. Since then, Ma had often taken it to maintain his health. Chao integrated food therapy with medicines to deal with Ma's condition, proving that he was a skilled doctor.

最早辑录《诸病源候论》的是《隋书·经籍志》，其中记载《诸病源候论》五卷。《外台秘要》《太平圣惠方》等医著的病因、病理分析，大多依据此书。日本医家丹波康赖撰《医心方》，成于公元982年（相当于北宋太宗时），其中于每门之前引录《病源论》（即《诸病源候论》）的"病候"内容，全书30卷中，有24卷直引《诸病源候论》540余处，640余条。可见，在北宋之初，《诸病源候论》已流传至日本。可惜由于唐宋之间连年战乱，北宋以前的传本均佚。

Sui Shu is the first book to excerpt the contents from *Zhu Bing Yuan Hou Lun* (five volumes). The etiological and pathological analysis in *Wai Tai Mi Yao* (Arcane Essentials from the Imperial Library) and *Tai Ping Sheng Hui Fang* (Formulas from Benevolent Sages Compiled during the Taiping Era) are mostly based on *Zhu Bing Yuan Hou Lun*. In addition, in his book *Ishinpō* (compiled in 982), the Japanese physician Tanba Yasunori also cited the contents of *Zhu Bing Yuan Hou Lun*. It indicates that during the beginning of the Northern Song Dynasty (960 AD–1127 AD), *Zhu Bing Yuan Hou Lun* was introduced to Japan. Regrettably, due to the constant conflicts during the Tang and Song Dynasties, the versions of this book before the Northern Song Dynasty have been lost.

《诸病源候论》在北宋时期受到极大重视，北宋政府把它同《素问》《难经》《脉经》《千金翼方》《龙树论》等一起作为"医学"（宋代医学教育的专门机构）必读教材，同时规定，试补"医学"考试，也要从此书中选题。

Zhu Bing Yuan Hou Lun enjoyed a high position in the Northern Song Dynasty. Together with *Su Wen* (Basic Questions), *Nan Jing* (The Classic of Difficult Issues), *Mai Jing* (The Pulse Classic), *Qian Jin Yi Fang* (Supplement to 'Important Formulas Worth a Thousand Gold Pieces') and *Long Shu Lun* (The Secret Transmission of Long-mu's Ophthalmology), the government took it as a compulsory textbook and examination content for medical students.

《诸病源候论》在中医病因、病机方面具有了系统的、全面的认识，对后世中医学的发展产生了巨大而深远的影响，在基础理论文献领域，填补了一项空白。

Zhu Bing Yuan Hou Lun has a systematic and comprehensive illustration on the etiology and pathogenesis of varying diseases, thus greatly influencing the TCM development in later generations.

其内容不仅学科齐全，而且对病与证的病因、病机、病候以至于病变类型等各个方面，均具有较为详尽地论述。如唐代王焘的《外台秘要方》、宋代王怀隐等编著的《太平圣惠方》、刘昉的《幼幼新书》、明代朱橚主编的《普济方》以及日本医家丹波康赖编撰的《医心方》等医学名著中有关病因、病机的内容，大多依据《诸病源候论》，或以此书作为重要的参考文献，故《四库全书总目》称誉此书为"证治之津梁"。《诸病源候论》最不同于前人之处在于，全书基本不涉及方药，只在每论末尾写上"其汤、熨、针、石，别有正方，补养宣导，今附于后"一笔带过。相反，全书共载"导引术"289条。《诸病源候论》的问世，标志着气功导引在医学上的应用已进入成熟的阶段。

Not only does it cover a comprehensive range of diseases, but it also provides detailed discussions on every aspect of disease and syndrome, including etiology, pathogenesis, symptoms and pathological changes. In such renowned medical works as *Wai Tai Mi Yao* (Arcane Essentials from the Imperial Library) compiled in the Tang Dynasty, *Tai Ping Sheng Hui Fang* (Formulas from Benevolent Sages Compiled during the Taiping Era) compiled in the Song Dynasty, *You You Xin Shu* (A New Book of Pediatrics) compiled in the Song Dynasty, *Pu Ji Fang* (General Aid Prescriptions) compiled in the Ming Dynasty, and *Ishinpō* compiled by the Japanese physician Tamba Yasuyori, contents related to etiology and pathogenesis are largely based on *Zhu Bing Yuan Hou Lun* or use this book as an important reference. Hence, in *Si Ku Quan Shu Zong Mu* (Catalogue of the Complete Library in Four Chapters), *Zhu Bing Yuan Hou Lun* is praised as the "bridge to diagnosis and treatment". The most distinctive feature of this book is that it does not give any formulas to the illustrated diseases but 289 daoyin exercises. The publication of *Zhu Bing Yuan Hou Lun* marked the maturity of the application of qigong daoyin in the field of medicine.

Theoretical Foundation

理论基础

导引的基本概念

Basic Concepts of Daoyin

"导引"亦作"道引"。导气令和,引体令柔的意思。导引术起源于上古,原为古代的一种养生术,早在春秋战国时期就已非常流行,为当时医家所重视,认为它有调荣卫、消水谷、除风邪、益血气、疗百病以至延年益寿的功效。

Daoyin consists of the two characters 导 (dao) and 引 (yin) in Chinese. Dao means to guide qi to harmonize the body and yin means to stretch the body to make it soft. Daoyin adopts varying breathing patterns and body movements to promote qi and blood circulation and thus helps maintain health. This practice is often combined with qi ingestion and meditation techniques. Daoyin originated in ancient times as a health preservation practice. It was very popular as early as the Spring and Autumn and Warring States periods (770 BC–221 BC), and was highly valued by medical practitioners at that time. They believed daoyin could regulate the functions of the body, promote digestion, dispel pathogenic wind, nourish blood and qi, treat various diseases and prolong life.

长沙马王堆汉墓(西汉初期诸侯家族墓地)出土的帛画,是现存全世界最早的导引图谱。每图式为一人像,男、女、老、幼均有,或著衣,或裸背,均为工笔彩绘。其术式除个别人像作器械运动外,多为徒手操练。三国时期的华佗把导引术式归纳总结为五种方法,名为"五禽戏",即虎戏、鹿戏、熊戏、猿戏、鸟戏,比较全面地概括了导引疗法的特点，且简便易行，对后世医疗和保健都起了推进作用。

The silk painting unearthed from the Mawangdui Han tomb in Changsha (a burial site of the early Western Han Dynasty nobility) is the earliest surviving daoyin chart across the world. Each movement is demonstrated by a human figure, ranging from young to old, and both male and female. Some are clothed, while others are depicted with their backs exposed. These illustrations were all created using the meticulous brushwork technique of traditional Chinese painting. Apart from a few people depicted with equipment exercises, most of the figures are practicing daoyin without any tools. During the Three Kingdoms period (220 AD–280 AD), Hua Tuo summarized daoyin into five methods, known as *Wu Qin Xi* (Frolics of the Five Animals), a series of exercises based on movements of the tiger, deer, bear, ape, and crane. This system comprehensively summarizes the features of daoyin therapy and is easy to practice, which has promoted its application in medical treatment and health preservation in later generations.

《诸病源候论》是我国历史上第一部专述病源和证候的书，全书基本不涉及方药，只在每论末尾写上"其汤、熨、针、石，别有正方，补养宣导，今附于后"一笔带过。相反，全书共载导引术289条。"辨证施功"是本书的最大特色，全书所介绍的导引术都根据不同证候选用。例如治"大便不通"："龟行气，伏衣被中，覆口、鼻、头、面，正卧，息息九道，微鼻出气。"标明"肝病候"条目下的方法是"肝脏病者，愁忧不乐，悲思嗔怒，头眩眼痛，'呵'气出而愈"。

Zhu Bing Yuan Hou Lun is the first book in China that specialized in the study of disease origins and symptoms. The book hardly mentioned any prescriptions, and only added a brief note at the end of each chapter saying, "There are proper prescriptions, acupuncture, moxibustion, and stone treatment, which will be added later." The book contains a total of 289 entries on daoyin. Daoyin exercise based on pattern identification is the most distinctive feature of *Zhu Bing Yuan Hou Lun*. The daoyin exercises introduced in the book are all selected according to corresponding symptoms and conditions. For example, to treat constipation: "Assume the posture of a turtle, lie on the back covered by clothes, cover the mouth, nose, head, and face, and breathe slowly and deeply 9 times, with a little breath from the nose." To treat liver disorders: "Those with liver disorders are worried, unhappy, sad, angry, and dizzy, and experience eye pain. They can be relieved by pronouncing the sound 'he'."

导引的主要形式与方法
Main Forms and Methods of Daoyin

1. 调形
1. Body Regulation

调整姿势，以利祛邪扶正，调和气血。《诸病源候论》："一足踏地，足不动，一足向侧相，转身欹势，并手尽急回。左右迭互二七。去脊风冷，偏枯不通润。"一脚踏地不动，另一脚向旁侧打开，成丁字步。身体旋转侧身，一手从上往下，使两手并拢，尽力做到最大幅度，然后两手快速收回，左右互换各做14次。可以去除脊柱中的风冷，半身偏枯，气血不畅通、不滋润的病症。

Adjusting postures can help dispel pathogenic factors, support healthy qi, and harmonize qi and blood. *Zhu Bing Yuan Hou Lun* states: "Place one foot firmly on the ground while opening the other to the side to form a T-shape stance. Turn the body sideways, and move one hand from top to bottom to bring the hands together with a full range of motion. Then, retract both hands quickly, and perform the same procedure on the other side. Repeat 14 times on each side. This exercise can help remove pathogenic cold and wind in the spine, and also alleviate hemiplegia, and unsmooth circulation as well as malnourishment of qi and blood."

2. 吐纳

2. Breathing Regulation

古代亦称服气，主要分为自然呼吸、不息、闭气、发音呼吸等。通过呼吸，沟通物我、内外、天地与脏腑气机。试以发音呼吸为例：有六字诀、"哼，哈"二音、"嘿"字壮气法等。发音呼吸方法有助于沟通气机。例如在普通的生活中，有经验的妈妈给婴儿把尿，发"嘘"音帮助婴儿小便顺畅。在练功中特殊的发音能调和脏腑、人与人、天地与人之间的精神往来。中医就有五音与五行、五脏相配的道理。如《灵枢·脉度》曰："肾气通于耳，肾和则耳能闻五音矣。"五音，即宫、商、角、徵、羽，是我国古代五声音阶的名称。《素问·阴阳应象大论》之五音："角谓木音，调而直也。徵谓火音，和而美也。宫为土音，大而和也。商谓金音，轻而劲也。羽谓水音，沉而深也。"在《医门法律》这本医著中，记有："《内经》本宫、商、角、徵、羽五音，呼、笑、歌、哭、呻五声，以参求五脏表里虚实之病。"又如《史记》所言："故音乐者，所以动荡血脉，通流精神，而和正心也。故宫动脾而和正圣，商动肺而和正义，角动肝而和正仁，徵动心而和正体，羽动

肾而和正智。"其所言"五音内动五脏"之义，正与《内经》所
论同。

In ancient times, breathing exercises were also referred to as qi ingestion. Breathing is mainly divided into natural breathing, non-stop breathing, breath-holding, and sound breathing. Through breathing, one can connect the physical and spiritual, the internal and external, the heaven and earth, and the internal organs' qi movements. Taking sound breathing as an example, it helps to harmonize qi movements. In everyday life, experienced mothers help their babies urinate smoothly by making a "xu" sound. In qigong practice, special sounds can be used to harmonize the internal organs, as well as the connection between individuals, and between individuals and the universe. In TCM, there is a theory that correlates the five tones with the five elements and the five zang organs. For example, *Ling Shu Mai Du* (Chapter 17 of the Spiritual Pivot) states: "Since kidney qi flows to the ears, when kidney qi is in normal functions, the ears can hear the five tones." The five tones are *jué* (mi), *zhǐ* (sol), *gōng* (do), *shāng* (re), and *yǔ* (la). In *Su Wen Yin Yang Ying Xiang Da Lun* (Chapter 5 of the Basic Questions), the five tones are described as follows: "*Jué* refers to the sound of wood, which is tuned and straight. *Zhǐ* refers to the sound of fire, which is harmonious and beautiful. *Gōng* refers to the sound of earth, which is large and harmonious. *Shāng* refers to the sound of metal, which is light and strong. *Yǔ* refers to the sound of water, which is deep and profound." The medical book *Yi Men Fa Lv* (Medical Laws) records that "In *Huang Di Nei Jing* (Yellow Emperor's Internal Classic), the five musical notes are associated with cheer, laughter, singing, crying, and groaning, respectively. These associations are used to diagnose the deficiency or excess of the five zang organs." As stated in *Shi Ji* (Records of the Grand Historian), "Music serves to promote the circulation of blood and qi, and calm down the mind. The tone *gōng* corresponds to the spleen, *shāng* corresponds to the lung, *jué* corresponds to the liver, *zhǐ* corresponds to the heart, and *yǔ* corresponds to the kidney." The meaning of "the five tones corresponding to the five zang organs" mentioned in *Shi Ji* is consistent with that discussed in *Huang Di Nei Jing*.

3. 存思
3. Mind Regulation

一名"存想"，简称"存"，道教修炼方术之一。要求闭合双眼或微闭双眼，存想内观某一物体或神真的形貌、活动状态等，以期达到集中思想，去除杂念，进入心物合一境界。存思对象很广泛，包括存思天象（日、月、五星，云雾）、景物（气、炎火）、人体（五脏、丹田）及神真（身内神和身外神）等。单存思身内、身外诸神者名"存神"。存思有助于寂然入静，感而遂通。《诸病源候论》："治百病……存视五脏，各如其形色；又存胃中，令鲜明洁白如素。为之倦极，汗出乃止，以粉粉身，摩捋形体。汗不出而倦者，亦可止，明日复为之。"治百病……内视五脏，看到五脏的形色，再内视胃中，令神光充盈，鲜活明晰洁白如丝绢。做到疲倦至极并且出汗就可以停止了，用粉轻扑于身上，按摩身体。汗未出但感到疲倦的，也可以停止。待第二天再做。

It is one of the Taoist cultivation practices. For mind regulation, close or partially close the eyes and visualize the form and activity of a certain object or deity in order to achieve focused thinking, eliminate distracting thoughts, and enter a state of unity between mind and body. The objects of focus are wide-ranging, including celestial bodies (the sun, moon, stars and clouds), natural scenery (qi and flames), human body (the five zang organs and *Dantian*), and divine beings (deities inside and outside the body). Mind regulation is helpful in achieving inner peace and spiritual insight. According to *Zhu Bing Yuan Hou Lun*, "To treat various diseases...look at the five zang organs to observe their forms and colors. Then look at the stomach, and make it bright, lively, clear and white as silk. Continue until exhaustion and sweating are present, then stop, lightly apply powders to the body, and massage the body. If exhaustion is felt but sweating has not yet occurred, stop and repeat the practice the following day."

导引是我国古代医学上主要治疗方法的一种。从医疗意义来说，它是充分发挥、调动内在因素、积极地防病治病。从预防意义上看，它可以锻炼身体，增强体质，保持朝气，焕发精神。导引，从本质上说就是通过外形动作，吐纳呼吸，存思这些方法，更好地发挥人的天赋与本能，即"天人感应"，终极是回到自然，回到本源，天地人一体。

Daoyin is one of the main treatment methods in ancient Chinese medicine. From a medical perspective, it is a way to fully tap into and activate internal factors to proactively prevent and treat diseases. From a preventative perspective, it can exercise the body, enhance physical fitness, maintain vitality, and invigorate the spirit. Essentially, daoyin allows people to better utilize their innate abilities and instincts through body movements, breathing exercises, and meditation. It involves a connection between man and nature, ultimately leading to a return to one's natural state and origin, with the integration of the heaven, earth, and human beings.

"天人感应"的理论在导引中的运用

Man-Nature Correspondence in Daoyin

1. "天人感应"的理论基础

1. Theoretical Foundation

天地时空和人是互相感应、互为反应、互为映照的。《灵枢·邪客》："此人与天地相应者也。"《庄子》："天地与我并生，万物与我为一。"这是从整体角度来看。《老子》："人法地，地法天，天法道，道法自然。"反映了局部统一于整体。天地万物，一以贯之。

The heaven, earth, and humans are interrelated, which was recorded in numerous ancient Chinese classics. For example, *Ling Shu Xie Ke* (Chapter 71 of the Spiritual Pivot) says, "Humans correspond to the heaven and the earth." *Zhuang Zi* says, "The heaven and the earth coexist with me, and all things unite with me as one." This is a holistic perspective. *Lao Zi* says, "Man follows the earth, the earth follows the heaven, the heaven follows *Dao*, and *Dao* follows nature." This reflects the unity of the part and the whole. The universe, time and space, and all things in it are interconnected.

个体生命发展受五方面影响：① 社会环境；② 自然地理生态环境；③ 天体运行；④ 万物运化的规律；⑤ 万化本源。分述如下。

The development of individual life is influenced by the following five factors: social environment, natural geographic and ecological environment, celestial movements, the laws of transformation and movement of all things, and the origins of all transformations.

（1）社会环境
(1) Social Environment

社会环境则包括社会政治环境、经济环境、文化环境和心理环境等。具体可以分为原生态家庭、后天教育、成长后工作生活环境；如果从人际关系来看，可分为亲人、邻里、老师、朋友、工作伙伴、生活伴侣等。

Specifically, the social environment includes social, political, economic, cultural, and psychological environments. It can be further divided into family, education, work and living environments after growth. From the perspective of interpersonal relationships, it can be divided into families, neighbors, teachers, friends, colleagues, and life partners.

对于绝大多数人来说，后天接受什么样的教育，至为关键。

For the vast majority of people, the education they receive after birth is crucial.

（2）自然地理生态环境
(2) Natural Geographic and Ecological Environment

所谓一方水土养一方人，从大的方面讲涉及地质、地貌、水文、气候、生态等。

As the saying goes, "Each place has its own way of supporting its own inhabitants." We can talk about a place from its geological, topographical, hydrological, climatic, and ecological features.

周围的环境、自然的变化，不仅影响人的身体、生命，还影响人的思维和精神活动。例如在传统文化中"负阴抱阳"的居住环境：基址背后有主峰来龙山，也称靠背山，来龙山后面要有龙脉为连绵高山群峰为屏障，并与大山形势相连通；基址前要有月牙形池塘或河流婉转经过；水的前面又有远山近丘的朝案对景呼应；基址恰好处于这个山水环抱的中央，内有千顷良田，山林葱郁，河水清明，安详和谐。上述这种"负阴抱阳"的人居环境就是理想的居住环境模式。基址背后的山峦屏挡冬季北来的寒风；东西面低岭岗阜缓坡避免淹涝之灾和保持水土、绿化植被；南面有流水经过可以接纳夏季南来的凉风，又能解决生活饮水和灌溉问题，又利于舟楫之便，有了污水还可以排出；南面向阳，明堂开阔，具有充足的日照，这样形成了良好的生态环境。和谐、舒适的环境使人精力充沛、神清气爽、思维活跃、判断精准。

The environment and natural changes around us not only affect our bodies and health, but also impact our thinking and mental activities. In this regard, ancient Chinese advocated the living environment of "embracing yang and bearing yin". Behind the house, there should be the main peak of mountains, and behind the mountains, there should be higher mountains serving as barriers. In front of the house, there should be a crescent-shaped pond or river, with distant higher mountains and nearby mountains echoing in front of the water. The house is embraced by mountains and water, with lush forests, clear river water, and a serene and harmonious ambiance. The living environment described above is an ideal model for residential settings. The mountain ranges behind the house can block the cold north wind in winter; low hills, gentle slopes, and ridges on the east and west sides can avoid floods, and maintain water and soil; the south has flowing water that can take in the cool breeze in summer, solve drinking water and irrigation problems, and facilitate boat transportation. Facing south, the main hall is open and has sufficient sunshine, creating a good ecological environment. A harmonious and comfortable environment can make people energetic, clear-minded, and accurate in judgment.

（3）天体运行
(3) Celestial Movements

简而言之，月亮、木星、太阳……星辰太空对人的影响。《灵枢·岁露论》："人与天地相参也，与日月相应也。"昼夜变化，四季交替，我们身在其中，太习以为常了。大自然日月星辰的运动节律，也就是人体和生物体内生理和病理时间节律的根源。

In short, we talk about the influence of such celestial bodies as the sun, moon and stars on human beings. *Ling Shu Sui Lu Lun* (Chapter 79 of the Spiritual Pivot) states, "Humans are closely related to the heaven and the earth, and correspond to the sun and the moon." We have become so accustomed to the changes of day and night and the alternation of the four seasons that we take them for granted. The rhythmic movements of the sun, moon, and stars in nature are the origin of the physiological and pathological time rhythms within the human body and other organisms.

昼夜变化对人身心的影响：有些病人发烧，上午轻，下午重；而有些精神抑郁症的病人，常常是晨重夜轻，早上一醒，身体酸懒疼痛，心情郁闷，到了晚上，太阳落山后，身心渐渐轻松。其实，我们的呼吸、血压、心率、内分泌活动、消化机能，都有昼夜节律。

The effects of day-night changes on human physical and mental health: Some patients with a fever may experience milder symptoms in the morning and worse in the afternoon, while some patients with depression often experience worse symptoms in the morning and milder at night. When they wake up in the morning, they feel tired both physically and mentally. As the sun sets in the evening, their physical and mental conditions gradually improve. In fact, our respiratory, blood pressure, heart rate, endocrine activity and digestive function all have circadian rhythms.

《素问·八正神明论》："月始生，则血气始精，卫气始行；月郭满，则血气实，肌肉坚；月郭空，则肌肉减，经络虚，卫气去，形独居。"当满月时，人体气血充盛，肌肤致密，腠理闭合。这时，人体即使遇到贼风邪气的侵袭，也较表浅而患病轻微。如在月亏之时，人体气血虚弱，肌肤松弛，腠理开泄，此时遇贼风邪气的侵袭，多急陷入里，发病急骤。《灵枢·岁露论》认为："故月满……虽遇贼风，其入浅不深。至其月郭空……遇贼风则其入深，其病人也卒暴。"

Su Wen Ba Zheng Shen Ming Lun (Chapter 26 of the Basic Questions) states: "At the beginning of a lunar month, blood and qi become refined, and the Wei-defensive qi begins to circulate; at the full moon, blood and qi are abundant, and the muscles are firm; at the end of a lunar month, the muscles are weakened, the meridians are empty, the Wei-defensive qi disappears, and the body is vulnerable." According to Ling Shu, during the full moon, the human body has abundant qi and blood, with compact skin and closed pores. At this time, even if the body is invaded by pathogenic wind, the disease is relatively mild and superficial. However, during the waning moon, the body's qi and blood are deficient, with loose skin and open pores. If the body is invaded by pathogenic wind, it is likely to rapidly penetrate deeply and cause a sudden onset of illness.

朔望月变化对人身心的影响：月亮绕地球一周约需28天，这是月亮盈亏变化的周期，叫作"朔望月"。每一个农历月份中，一个月相周期分为朔日（新月）、上弦月、下弦月、望日（圆月）。因为新月和满月的时候，月象对地面上江河湖海的影响是不一样的。上弦月是初七，下弦月是阴历二十三，因此，一个月里江河湖海的涨潮，就出现大小消涨的进退四个周期，这样就把一个月二十八天多一点点分成了四份，一份正好是七天。根据月亮盈亏的改变，不同时段的养生重点也各有不同。

The effects of the synodic month on human physical and mental health: The moon takes about 28 days to orbit around the earth, which is the cycle of the moon's phases, known as the synodic month. In each lunar month, a lunar phase cycle consists of the new moon, the first quarter moon, the last quarter moon, and the full moon. The lunar influence on rivers, lakes, and seas on the ground is different during the new moon and full moon phases. The first quarter moon occurs on the seventh day of a lunar month, while the last quarter moon occurs on the twenty-third day of a lunar month. Within a month, tides are divided into four stages: spring tide, neap tide, ebb tide, and flood tide. This effectively divides the slightly over 28-day lunar month into four parts, with each part spanning exactly 7 days. Based on the changing phases of the moon, different periods have distinct focuses on health preservation.

朝日（新月）：农历的每月初一。此时月缺无光，白天阳气渐弱，夜间阴气渐虚，此时人体特点是阳气弱，气血也处在比较亏虚的状态，抵抗力相对较弱。

The new moon falls on the first day of a lunar month. At this time, there is no moon light. During the day, yang qi gradually weakens, and at night, yin qi gradually becomes weaker. At this time, the human body is characterized by weakened yang qi and relatively deficient qi and blood, resulting in poor immunity.

上弦月：当月球转到与太阳呈90°角时，出现的月相叫"上弦月"，即农历初七前后，从上弦月到圆月，月亮由缺到圆、月光由暗到亮，人体之气也逐渐旺盛、充盈，人们精神良好、体力充沛，抗病能力较强。

The first quarter moon occurs when the moon is at a 90-degree angle to the sun. It usually falls around the seventh day of a lunar month. From the first quarter moon to the full moon, the moon's light increases from darkness to brightness, and the body's energy gradually becomes stronger and fuller. Thus, we tend to have good spirits, strong physical energy, and a relatively strong ability to resist diseases.

望日（圆月）：望日即圆月，是在农历十五前后，此时月圆光亮，精气充足。人体白天阳气旺盛，夜间阴气充盈，人的精神亢奋、体力较强，机体抗病能力增强；但是由于血气上浮，一方面头痛、头昏、失眠、多梦等病症高发，另一方面高血压病、上消化道出血、脑出血、肺结核、支气管扩张咯血等病症也容易在此时发作和加重。

The full moon occurs around the fifteenth day of a lunar month when the moon is round and bright. During this time, the body is filled with vitality, both physically and mentally. During the day, yang qi is strong, while at night, yin qi is abundant. People are energetic and have a strong ability to resist diseases. However, due to the upward flow of blood and qi, such diseases as headache, dizziness, insomnia, and disturbed sleep are more likely to occur. Moreover, such diseases as hypertension, upper gastrointestinal bleeding, cerebral hemorrhage, pulmonary tuberculosis, and bronchiectasis are also prone to occur or worsen during this time.

下弦月：农历二十三前后，从圆月到下弦月，月亮由圆到缺，月光由亮到暗，接着月亮渐渐亏缺，到二十三左右为下弦月，三十的时候月亮全亏，即为"晦"。人体之气亦逐渐虚弱、衰减，人们精神、体力较差，机体抵抗力较弱。

The last quarter moon occurs around the twenty-third day of a lunar month. During this phase, the moon gradually transitions from the full moon to the last quarter moon, with moonlight fading from bright to dark. As a result, the body's qi and vitality weaken and decline, and people may experience poorer mental and physical states, and a weaker immune system.

四季变化对人身心的影响：《素问·四气调神大论》："春三月……夜卧早起，广步于庭，被发缓形""夏三月……夜卧早起，无厌于日""秋三月……早卧早起，与鸡俱兴""冬三月……早卧晚起，必待日光。"顺应天时节气变化规律，随阴消而息，随阳长而起，除"春夏养阳，秋冬养阴"。中医讲脉象，春天的脉以弦为主，夏天的脉以洪为主，秋天的脉是毛浮的，冬天的脉是沉实的。从脉象上看，它有四季的变化。地球上生物体的生理活动，与地球以及和地球相关的日月星辰的运动周期有关。

The influence of seasonal changes on the human body

and mind: *Su Wen Si Qi Tiao Shen Da Lun* (Chapter 5 of the Basic Questions) states, "In spring...one should sleep early at night and get up early in the morning, take a leisurely walk in the courtyard, do not tie up the hair, and relax the body." "In summer ... one should sleep early at night and get up early in the morning to follow the day-night change." "In autumn...one should go to bed early at night and get up early in the morning." "In winter...one should go to bed early and get up late, waiting for the daylight." To conform to the laws of seasonal changes in accordance with the Heavenly Stems and Earthly Branches, one should rest during yin periods and get up during yang periods, in order to "nourish yang in spring and summer and nourish yin in autumn and winter." In TCM, the pulse varies with the change of seasons. In spring, the pulse is mostly string-like; in summer, it is mostly surging; in autumn, it is mostly floating and superficial; in winter, it is mostly deep and forceful. The physiological activities of living organisms are related to celestial cycles and movements.

当我们看到第一缕阳光，透出地平线，心胸徒然开阔；当我们在沉浸在月光里，清晖如水，思绪渐渐宁静，而仰望星空，竟然会生起归家般的亲切。天地变化，人相应就会产生感受，人皆有之。唯有将这些变化感受提升到理论，形成规律与模式，才能付诸实践应用，如中医理论经络、穴位。

As we catch the first glimpse of sunlight piercing through the horizon, the heart suddenly expands with a sense of liberation. As we immerse ourselves in the moonlight, the clear brightness of it gradually calms the mind. Looking up at the starry sky, we may suddenly feel a warm sense. The changes in nature affect people and evoke certain feelings, which is a common human experience. However, it is only by elevating these experiential changes to theoretical insights and establishing regularities and patterns that they can be applied practically, such as in TCM.

（4）万物运化的规律

(4) The Laws of Transformation and Movement of all Things

事物之间的内在的必然联系，决定着事物发展的必然趋向。世界上的万事万物虽然千变万化，但都有它的规律可循。如，"人之道，损不足而奉有余"。"天之道，损有余而补不足"。

The inherent connections between things determine the trends of their development. Although everything in the world may seem diverse, there are underlying patterns to follow. For example, the way of humans is to diminish the insufficient and supplement the excessive, while the way of the heavens is to diminish the excessive and supplement the insufficient.

中医亦如此，"泻有余而补不足"，注重阴阳矛盾而统一。没有最好的药，最标准的动作，只有最合适的。"大黄救人无功，人参杀人无过"。大黄是苦寒泻下的药，应用得当能救人性命，但一般人避之唯恐不及，即使救人性命，大家也不认为是大黄的功劳，所以说大黄救人无功。人参是贵重的滋补之品，应用不当能取人性命，但一般人只知其利不知其弊，即使应用不当杀人了，大家也不认为是人参的过错。所以说人参杀人无过。砒霜，人皆知为毒药，古用之于哮喘，今用之于白血病。杀人剂而成活人术，皆为知物性、人性，行阴阳和合之理。

TCM also follows the principle of balancing excess and deficiency, and emphasizes the unity of yin and yang. There is no single "best" medicine or standard treatment method, but only the most appropriate one that can meet the needs of each individual patient. "The efficacy of rhubarb is unrecognized even when it saves lives, and the harm of ginseng is excused even when it kills." Rhubarb is a bitter and cold purgative herb that can save lives when used appropriately, but people generally avoid it and do not give it credit for saving lives. Therefore, the efficacy of rhubarb goes unrecognized. Ginseng is a valuable tonic that can cause harm when used inappropriately and even lead to death, but people only know its benefits and do not realize the risks. Even if it causes harm, people do not blame ginseng. Therefore, ginseng is excused for its harm. Arsenic, known to all as a poisonous substance, was used in ancient times to treat asthma and is now used to treat leukemia. The ability to use a deadly substance to save lives requires understanding its properties, as well as knowledge of human nature and the principles of yin and yang.

《易经·说卦》曰:"穷理、尽性,以至于命。" 穷究天下万物的根本原理,彻底洞明万物的体性,掌握万物运行的规律,才能把握生命的本源,改变生命的方向与形式。

Yi Jing (Book of Changes) says: "To thoroughly investigate the fundamental principles of all things in the world, to thoroughly understand the nature of all things, and to grasp the laws of their operation, is the only way to grasp the essence of life, and to change the direction and form of life."

(5) 万化本源
(5) The Origin of all Transformations

如果说思路决定出路,那么高度格局决定思路。站在山巅,山河尽收眼底,不再有怀疑,不再需要揣度,是什么就是什么,该怎么做就怎么做,故谓之自然。

If we say that mindset determines the way forward, then a high level of perspective will determine the mindset. Standing at the summit of a mountain, with the rivers and mountains all in view, there is no longer any doubt or need for speculation. What is, is what it is, and what needs to be done is done naturally.

本源,是有规律的,但又超越规律;本源是有名相的,又超越名相的。故夫子曰:从心所欲,不逾规矩。老子云:道可道,非常道。名可名,非常名。回到本源,什么都是平等的,什么又都是美的,故庄子说:天地有大美而不言。

The origin has its own rules, but it transcends these rules. The origin has its own names and forms, but it transcends these names and forms. Therefore, Confucius said, "One should pursue the heart's desires within the bounds of propriety." Laozi said, "The *Dao* that can be spoken of is not the eternal *Dao*. The name that can be named is not the eternal name." Returning to the origin, everything is equal and everything is beautiful. Hence, Zhuangzi said, "The heaven and the earth have great beauty but do not speak of it."

天人感应的内在本质是天、地、人一体,《素问·宝命全形论》:"夫人生于地,悬命于天,天地合气,命之曰人。"站在"一体"的角度上看,故能彼此感应,自然而然。《老子》:"道生一,一生二,二生三,三生万物矣。"——道(无极)之中自然而然地转化,产生真灵一气;一气自然含有阴阳二气,阴阳和合变化则万物生长老死。

The internal essence of man-nature correspondence is that man and nature are a unified whole. As stated in *Su Wen*,

"Man is born of the earth, sustained by the heaven, and the combination of heaven qi and earth qi is called human destiny." From the perspective of this "unity", the ability to interact with one another arises naturally. *Lao Zi* said: "*Dao* gives birth to one, one gives birth to two, two gives birth to three, and three gives birth to all things." Within *Dao* (the infinite and eternal), a natural transformation occurs, producing the true spirit and the unity of qi. This qi naturally contains the dual qi of yin and yang. The merging and the transformation of yin and yang lead to the birth, growth, aging, and death of all things.

天人感应是人的天赋、本能。天人感应的本质就是一气。故《老子》:"天得一以清,地得一以宁,神得一以灵,谷得一以盈,万物得一以生。"

Man-nature correspondence is an inherent and instinctive aspect of human nature, and its essence is the unity of qi. Therefore, *Lao Zi* said: "The heaven attains oneness and becomes pure; the earth attains oneness and becomes peaceful; spirits attain oneness and become divine; millet attains oneness and becomes full; all things attain oneness and come to life."

2. "天人感应"理论在导引术教学中的运用
2. Man-Nature Correspondence in Teaching Daoyin

导引之术,是研究生命本质和生命在不同的时空下种种变化的。其核心是天人感应。《素问·天元纪大论》曰:"太虚寥廓,肇基化元,万物资始。五运终天,布气真灵,捴统坤元。九星悬朗,七曜周旋,曰阴曰阳,曰柔曰刚,幽显既位,寒暑弛张,生生化化,品物咸章。"意为无边无际的太虚(道),是宇宙造化的原始基础，是万物化生的根本。其间五运往复循行，真灵之气遍布，主宰着一切生命生长的根源。由此九星明朗地悬耀于虚空，七曜循着天道有规律地运行，于是天运有了阴阳的迁移变化，大地有了刚柔的生杀现象，昼夜有了幽暗和明亮的变化，四时有了寒暑的更迭，如此不断生长变化，才有了丰富多样的万物生长。

Daoyin explores the essence of life and the various transformations of life across different times and spaces, with man-nature correspondence as its core. *Su Wen* states, "The boundless and infinite *Dao* is the primordial foundation of the universe and the fundamental source of all things' transformation and growth. Within it, the five elements revolve and cycle, and the true spirit's qi permeates, governing the root of birth and growth. As a result, the stars shine brightly in the void, and the celestial bodies follow the orderly path of the heavens. This gives rise to the migration and transformation of yin and yang in celestial movements, as well as the phenomenon of hardness and softness in the earth. The cycle of day and night brings about changes in brightness and darkness, and the alternation of the four seasons brings about changes in temperature. It is through these constant transformations and growth that the rich and diverse growth of all things is made possible."

外在的现象，呈现各种各类，多姿多彩，万千变化，而其内在，不过是天地气机之间的相互转化而已。其精微本质是浑然一体的，是不二的。导引术的教学，是通过知识、技术等方法，来认识自然——自然而然，本来如此。天地人一体，不是后天造作的，而是本就具备的，就像是岩石里的清泉，需要的只是挖掘；就像是高山的冰川，需要的只是融化，融化成一滴水，汇成小溪，并成江河，终成大海。导引术的教学不同于一般学问，是超越表象的, 是内趋性的, 是自然的。导引术教学实践, 灵机感应大致概括, 若作细致探讨, 可从三个方面加以阐述: 一曰变化, 二曰阴阳, 三曰整体。

The external phenomena demonstrate themselves in varying forms, colorful and ever-changing, while their internal essence is nothing but the mutual transformation between the qi and mechanisms of the heavens and earth. At the subtlest level, they are integrated as one. The teaching of daoyin involves the use of knowledge, skills, and other methods to gain an understanding of nature, which is natural and inherent. The unity of the heavens, earth, and humans is not something artificially constructed but rather something inherent and innate, much like a clear spring hidden within a rock, waiting to be discovered through excavation, or like a glacier atop a mountain that needs only to melt into a single drop of water, which then gathers into a stream, a river, and eventually an ocean. The teaching of daoyin is different from ordinary knowledge. It goes beyond surface appearances and is focused on intrinsic qualities, naturalness, and spontaneity. It can be broadly summarized as a process of intuitive resonance. However, if we examine it more closely, there are three key aspects that deserve further exploration: change, yin and yang, and holism.

（1）变化
(1) Change

生命, 近至个人, 远至浩瀚宇宙, 都是在不断地变化的。生命的内核——精、气、神, 或无形有相, 或无形无相, 难以言状, 是在不断地自我净化、否定、升华、归元的过程获得的认识与经验; 是从万物回到三, 三回到二, 二回到一, 一则归元的过程的感应体悟。这决定了导引术教学是注重变化与多层次的。

Life is constantly changing, from the microcosmic level of individuals to the vastness of the universe. Essence, qi, and spirit are essential for life. They may manifest in tangible or intangible forms. We acquire the understanding and experience of them through a continuous process of self-purification, negation and refinement, and then we return to the original state. They are the intuitive realization of returning to one's origin from a myriad of things. This determines that the teaching of daoyin emphasizes change and multi-level perspectives.

以功法论，一套功法动作完成，不同学生间动作各有差异，甚或一个老师，不同阶段，同一动作，也会有差别。这是由于每个人在不同的时空下，内外气机交感，对天地道感悟深度不同，以至内在精神变化，而表象必有差异。故而没有一个"绝对到位，固定不变"的动作，外在的形式，如导引、吐纳、存思，只是手段、方法，它是服从于内核——天、地、人、精、气、神的变化规律的。

Different students practicing the same set of qigong exercise display distinct movements. Moreover, even a teacher, when practicing the same set of qigong exercise at different stages, will exhibit differences in the movements. This is due to the fact that each individual, in different temporal and spatial contexts, interacts with the internal and external qi movements, has different levels of insight into the *Dao* of the heaven and the earth, and therefore undergoes different internal spiritual changes, resulting in differences in external manifestations. Therefore, there is no "absolutely precise and fixed" movement. The external forms, such as daoyin, breathing, and meditation, are the only methods that are subject to the internal core of the changing laws of the heavens, earth, humans, essence, qi, and spirit.

以练功目的论，导引术教学的目的内在本质是为了让学生认识自己、天地，掌握精气神；外化为有的为了治疗疾病，有的为养生保健，有的为内心宁静，有的为了解传统文化而来等，自然不能一概而论。故当因机而发，因机而教。

From the perspective of the purpose of practicing, the internal essence of teaching daoyin is to help students understand themselves and the universe, and master their own essence, qi, and spirit. The external manifestation varies, including treating illnesses, maintaining health, seeking inner peace, exploring traditional culture, etc., which cannot be generalized. Therefore, teaching should be based on the individual's needs and abilities.

以治疗为例，因辨证施功。

In the case of treatment, the approach should be tailored based on pattern identification.

辨证，就是根据四诊所收集的资料，通过分析、综合，辨清疾病的病因、性质、部位，以及邪正之间的关系，概括、判断为某种性质的证。这个过程当视作医生与病人之间的感应，从这个角度来看的话，证是医生以视觉、听觉、触觉、嗅觉了解病人外在基本情况，进而感受病人内在生命状态。

Pattern identification refers to the process of identifying a patient's illness by analyzing and synthesizing the information gathered from the four diagnostic methods (inspection, auscultation & olfaction, inquiry, and palpation). Based on the identified pathogenesis, nature, location, and the relationships between pathogenic factors and healthy qi, a specific pattern of syndrome is diagnosed, and corresponding treatment methods are then prescribed. From this perspective, the process can be seen as a resonance between the doctor and the patient. The doctor uses visual, auditory, tactile, and olfactory senses to understand the patient's external basic conditions, and then perceives the patient's internal life state.

以学生论，由于每一个学生的体质秉性、生活习惯等不同，即使是同一套功法，可以从不同角度入手，如由静入手，或由动入手；又有对"天人感应"体悟的深浅不同，天赋差异，可以直接从整体（道）入手，可以从局部入手，可以从无为入手，可以从有为入手，可以以神意为先，也可以从肢体开始。

From the perspective of individual students, their physical constitutions, temperaments, and lifestyles vary. Therefore, even the same set of daoyin exercise can be approached from different angles, such as starting from a static or dynamic approach. Different students have different understandings of man-nature correspondence, so they can approach the study of daoyin in various ways. They can start directly with the whole (*Dao*), focus on specific aspects, start with non-action (*Wu Wei*), begin with action (*You Wei*), prioritize spiritual intention, or even start with body movements.

导引术教学中变化的特质，决定了必须通过老师不断地引导来激发学生的自主性。导引术教学是一定是启发性的。老师善于使教学内容更为生动有趣。多做体验教学，比如让学生感受体验同样动作、同样的发音，老师身体的变化与学生的差异。老师善于学会巧设疑问，引导质疑，用疑问来激起学生的学习兴趣,这样学生就能更加积极主动地参与到学习中来。

The variability in teaching daoyin determines that teachers must continually guide students to stimulate their autonomy. The teaching must be inspirational. Teachers are adept at making the teaching content more vivid and interesting. More experiential teaching should be done, such as allowing students to experience the same movements and pronunciation, and observing the differences between the teacher and the students. Teachers should be good at asking thought-provoking questions, guiding students to question and doubt, and using questions to stimulate their interest in learning so that students can actively and proactively participate in their learning.

导引术从教与学两个方面而言都是有难度的。如何挖掘其内涵,拓展外在的形式;在不断地变化中,何时否定,何时肯定,既不能让学生困于表象,又不能伤害学生的求知欲,对老师和学生都是种历练。

Teaching and learning daoyin are both challenging. How to explore the essence of the practice and expand its external forms? How to discern when to reject and when to affirm amidst constant changes? It is a challenge for both teachers and students. Teachers must avoid letting students be trapped in superficialities while nurturing their thirst for knowledge, and students must learn to navigate this journey of self-discovery.

（2）阴阳

(2) Yin and Yang

"阴阳二气交感化生万物,万物生生而变化无穷焉。"万化宇宙无非阴阳二气之变幻。教与学就是阴阳,再如身与心、表象与内涵、道与术等。此处着重讨论老师与学生之间阴阳的关系。

"Yin and yang interact and give birth to all things, and all things are born and transformed endlessly." A myriad of changes in the universe are nothing but the transformation of yin and yang. Teaching and learning, body and mind, appearance and nature, as well as *Dao* and technique are like yin and yang. Here we focus on the yin-yang relationship between teachers and students.

老师与学生:老师和学生就是对阴阳关系。从普通的意义上来说,"师者,所以传道授业解惑也",师生从客观上存在上下级关系,导引术教学则不仅如此。导引术教学的目的是让学生认识、掌握精气神。要达到这一步,不仅仅需要外在的知识,更需要内化于心。外在的知识、技术只是桥梁,是为了通向内在本质真理。在教学中老师应与学生实现流畅的互动,创造自然、和谐的教学气氛。老师主观上应当确立平等地尊重每一位学生的观念,老师较学生之学问多寡与功夫深浅,仅仅是学有先后、术有专攻而已。在教学中,学生真诚地提出他的问题,老师应放下"师"之观念,以学生的"不知"为"师",返照自身之精气神,而自然流露出答案。而这样的答案,事先并未准备,无非灵机感应一动,却能更深得加强了对经典理论的理解,实践了教学互长——阴阳对立和互化、统一。

From a conventional perspective, "teachers are individuals who impart wisdom, teach academic subjects, and provide answers to challenging questions." In this sense, there is an objective hierarchical relationship between teachers and students. However, in the context of teaching daoyin, it is more than that. The purpose of teaching daoyin is to enable students to understand and master essence, qi and spirit. To achieve this, it is not only necessary to acquire external knowledge, but also to internalize it deeply. External knowledge and techniques are merely bridges that lead to the inner truth and essence. In teaching, teachers should establish smooth interactions with students and create a natural and harmonious learning atmosphere. Subjectively, teachers should establish respect for each student's ideas. The difference in knowledge and skill level between teachers and students is merely a matter of who have learned or practiced more, and what specific areas of expertise they have focused on. In teaching, when a student sincerely poses questions, the teacher should set aside the identity as a teacher, instead regard the student's questions as the teacher, and naturally give the answer. Such an answer, however, is not prepared in advance. It arises spontaneously and can deepen the understanding of classical theory, and promote mutual growth in teaching.

导引术教学过程应是师生积极互动、共同发展的过程。因此,在课堂教学中,师生之间、生生之间通过积极的对话、交流,可以分享彼此的思考、经验和知识,交流各自的情感、体验与观念,从而达成共识、共享。教学中的引导不应生拉硬拽,学生应在没有强迫、处于自由学习的状态中,自然地接纳老师给予的观念与方法。

The process of teaching daoyin should be an active interaction and collaborative development between teachers and students. Therefore, in classroom teaching, through active dialogue and communication between teachers and students, as well as among students, they can share their thoughts, experiences and knowledge, exchange emotions and ideas, and ultimately reach consensus and share together. Daoyin in teaching should not be forceful or coercive. Students should naturally accept the ideas and methods provided by the teacher in a state of free learning, without any pressure.

（3）整体

(3) Holism

《老子》:"人法地,地法天,天法道,道法自然。" 反映了局部统一于整体。天地万物,一以贯之。《素问·生气通天论》:"天地之间,六合之内,其气九州、九窍、五藏、十二节,皆通乎天气。其生五,其气三。数犯此者,则邪气伤人,此寿命之本也。"《素问·阴阳应象大论》:"其在天为玄,在人为道,在地为化。化生五味,道生智,玄生神。神在天为风,在地为木,在体为筋,在藏为肝。"

Dao De Jing states: "Man follows the earth, the earth follows the heaven, the heaven follows *Dao*, and *Dao* follows nature." This reflects the unity of the part and the whole. The myriad things in the world are unified by one principle. *Su Wen* states: "Between the heaven and the earth, from the vast expanse of China to the minute details of every organ in the human body, there exists a connection with natural rules and principles. If one frequently violates the rules and principles, pathogenic factors can harm the body. Therefore, adapting to these principles is fundamentally important for the continuation of one's lifespan." It also states, "In the heaven, it is mystery; in man, it is *Dao*; on earth, it is transformation. The transformation gives rise to the five tastes, *Dao* gives rise to wisdom, and the mystery gives rise to spirit. The spirit in the heaven is the wind, on earth it is wood, in the body it represents tendons, and in the organ it is the liver."

变化、阴阳以整体为基础；整体以阴阳、变化为表达。导引术是研究生命变化的，要注重细节，更要把握整体。导引术教学不仅仅需要接受知识，重复练习。更需要在这一过程中如何返本还元，又做到顺应万物——整体。导引术的教学是生命当下的体悟。体悟四时万物皆一气的变化——整体。

Changes and the concept of yin and yang are based on the whole; the whole is expressed through the concept of yin and yang and changes. Daoyin focuses on the study of changes in life, emphasizing attention to details while also grasping the overall picture. Learning daoyin not only requires acquiring knowledge and repeating exercises, but also involves understanding how to return to the original source and adapt to all things in the process. Teaching daoyin is a realization of life in the present moment, and a realization of changes in all things.

整体、自然、不妄作的思路，应贯穿于整个教学过程中，或隐或现。当学生困于观念，迷于表象，失之正气，应不断地予以棒喝，或轻或重，或缓或急；有时应故设迷局，有时亦可于化城中稍作停留。例如练功中身心先后与主次的问题。本质上讲导引术练的是内心的正气，精神的净化，升华；身心合一。对于初学，身心未得净化，身体的感觉反而是很大的迷惑。此时若依从身，表面上越有凭据可抓，往往却会离内心宁静合一越远。练功，即身心相应，从这个角度，又可鼓励初学多从身心两方面去体悟。不要怕错，对的经验、抉择的智慧恰恰是在错的基础上得来的。老师则应当依学生之机，在不同的角度，不断地予以纠正，使之身心合一。

The idea of holism and naturalness should be integrated throughout the entire teaching process, either implicitly or explicitly. When students are trapped in concepts, confused by appearances, or lose their sense of righteousness, they should be constantly scolded, lightly or heavily, slowly or quickly. Sometimes it may be necessary to set up a puzzle to mislead them, while at other times it may be appropriate to pause for a while in the midst of transforming their mindset. For example, in qigong practice, should body movements go first or mind exercises? Its essence lies in practicing inner righteousness, purifying the mind, elevating the spirit and thus achieving the integration of body and mind. For beginners, if their body and mind have not been purified, the physical sensations can be a great confusion. At this time, if one relies on the body, although there may be more tangible things to grasp, it often leads further away from inner peace and unity. The practice of daoyin is the harmonization of body and mind. From this perspective, beginners are encouraged to comprehend from both physical and mental aspects. Do not be afraid of making mistakes, as the experiences of being right and the wisdom of making choices often come after making mistakes. Teachers should rely on students' potential and provide continuous corrections from different angles to help students achieve the harmony between body and mind.

教学中,老师应当使学生的学习导引术方法符合太极文化的认识规律。教学的目的应该是让学生知道为什么学习、怎么学习,而不仅仅是停留在学习什么上。更重要的是让学生在获取知识的过程中掌握方法,探索规律,学习和掌握整体的思维方式和学习策略。在研究学法的基础上探索教法,从而使教师的教学方法和学生的学法皆合于太极基本规律。于课堂中培养学生整体、自然的习惯,于生活中历练,使生命契于太极,身体得以健康,内心得以宁静,道德得以升华。

In teaching, teachers should make sure that students' learning methods are in accordance with the cognitive laws of Taiji culture. The purpose of teaching should be to make students aware of why and how to learn, rather than just what to learn. It is crucial to help students acquire methods, explore rules, and learn and master the holistic thinking approach and learning strategies. Exploring teaching methods based on the study of learning methods can make both teachers' teaching methods and students' learning methods conform to the basic principles of Taiji. In the classroom, cultivate in students the habit of being whole and natural, and in life, let them experience and integrate their lives with Taiji, so that their bodies can be healthy, their hearts peaceful, and their morality elevated.

导引术，笔者以为：感天地万物一气尔；并于万物万化之中，直入此一气，不取不舍，逍遥自然，即应。

As for daoyin, in my opinion, it is to perceive the oneness of the heaven, the earth, and all things, and to directly enter this oneness amidst the infinite changes of all things, without attachment or rejection, and to be free and natural.

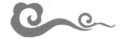

《诸病源候论》导引术 ● *Zhu Bing Yuan Hou Lun Dao Yin Shu* (Explanations for the Daoyin Exercises in *Zhu Bing Yuan Hou Lun*)

Characteristics and Essential Principles

特色与要领

操作性强

Daoyin with Practicability

《诸病源候论》全书共载导引术289条，导引记载丰富且较为全面，是隋朝以前导引术集大成者，导引动作主要来自《养生经要集》《真诰》《无生经》《太清导引养生经》等。《养生经要集》现已失传，有节本《养性延命录》可参。全书所载导引术动作可操作性强，85%以上动作基本没有难度，普通人士容易完成，适用于普通患者和中老年人群。同时，由于《诸病源候论》具有一定专业性，少量动作在操作过程具有一定难度，如"蹲式（下蹲），臀部离地一尺左右，两手从大腿外侧经膝内弯入，放于脚背，迅速握两脚脚趾，令脚趾背曲，尽力做到极势，1次。可以通利腰部和髋部，治疗淋症"。该条动作难度较大，不适合未接受过传统功法训练的普通患者。

Zhu Bing Yuan Hou Lun contains a total of 289 entries on daoyin exercises. The record is rich and comprehensive, and it is the culmination of daoyin exercises before the Sui Dynasty. The movements of daoyin mainly come from such works as *Yang Sheng Jing Yao Ji* (Essentials Collection on Health Preservation), *Zhen Hao* (Teachings by Immortals), *Wu Sheng Jing* (Sutra of Imperishable), and *Tai Qing Dao Yin Yang Sheng Jing* (Taiqing Daoyin of Health Preservation). *Yang Sheng Jing Yao Ji* is now lost, but there is a segmented version called *Yang Xing Yan Ming Lu* (The Record of Nurturing Nature for Prolonging Life) that can be consulted. The daoyin movements in *Zhu Bing Yuan Hou Lun* are highly practical, with over 85% of the movements having no difficulty, making them easy for ordinary people to do. They are suitable for ordinary patients and middle-aged and elderly people. A small number of movements may be somewhat difficult to finish. For example, a movement is finished in a squatting position. Squat down (The distance between the buttocks and the ground is about 30 centimeters), place the hands on the insteps, quickly and fully grasp the toes until the toes are bent, and hold for a few seconds. Do this exercise once. It can help unblock the lower back and hips, and treat strangury. This movement is relatively difficult and is not suitable for ordinary patients who did not practiced traditional qigong exercises.

辨证施功

Daoyin Based on Pattern Identification

《诸病源候论》对不同疾病的病因、病机、证候均有系统阐述,对阴阳、虚实、邪正关系等均有一定判断。全书所载289条导引术基本依据不同疾病证候选用,五脏六腑诸病候均有不同导引术。如"肝病候"所载导引术为"有肝病的人,容易忧愁不快乐,有悲伤、思虑、不满、恼怒的情绪,也会有头晕眼痛的症状。用'呵'字音出气,病就可以痊愈"。"心病候"所载导引术为"有心病的人,身体有发冷发热的症状。如果身体发冷,用'呼'字音吸气;如果发热,用'吹'字音出气"。"腹胀候"所载导引术为"腹中苦于发胀且有寒气,用'呼'字音出气,做30次"。"肺病候"所载导引术为"有肺病的人,躯体、胸背有疼痛胀满的症状,四肢感到烦闷不适,用'嘘'字音出气"。"肾病候"所载导引术为"有肾病的人,有咽喉阻塞、腹部胀满、耳聋不聪的症状,用'呬'字音出气"。

Zhu Bing Yuan Hou Lun systematically elaborates on the etiology, pathogenesis, and patterns of varying diseases, and makes certain judgments on the relationships between yin and yang, deficiency and excess, and pathogenic factors and healthy qi. The 289 daoyin exercises in the book are mainly selected according to corresponding disease conditions, with corresponding methods for the various diseases. For example, to treat liver diseases: People with a liver disease are prone to feeling unhappy and have emotional symptoms such as sadness, worry, dissatisfaction, and anger, as well as symptoms such as dizziness and eye pain. Exhale with the sound "he" to recover from the illness. To treat heart diseases: People with a heart disease may experience symptoms such as chills and fever. If the body feels cold, inhale with the sound "hu"; if the body feels hot, exhale with the sound "ci". To treat abdominal distension: For abdominal fullness with pathogenic cold, exhale with the sound "hu" 30 times. To treat lung diseases: People with a lung disease may experience pain and swelling in the body and chest, and discomfort in the limbs. To alleviate these symptoms, exhale with the sound "xu". To treat kidney diseases: For those with a kidney disease experiencing such symptoms as a foreign body sensation in the throat, abdominal fullness, and impaired hearing, exhale with the sound "hei".

以传统经典理论
"天人感应" 为指导

Daoyin Guided by Man-Nature Correspondence

　　传统经典理论认为,人生天地之间,宇宙之中,一切生命活动与大自然息息相关,故天、地、时空和人是互相感应、互为反应、互为映照。《素问·脉要精微论》:"从阴阳始,始之有经,从五行生,生之有度,四时为宜,补泻勿失,与天地如一。"《灵枢·邪客》:"此人与天地相应者也。"《老子》:"人法地,地法天,天法道,道法自然。"《诸病源候论》中记载的导引术以"天人感应"为指导。

Traditional theory holds that life activities are closely related to the heaven, the earth, and everything between them. Therefore, the heaven, the earth, time, space, and human beings are interdependent, responsive, and reflective of each other. *Su Wen Mai Yao Jing Wei Lun* (Chapter 17 of the Basic Questions) states that "The subtle changes of yin and yang are evident in the four seasons. It all begins with distinguishing between yin and yang. By analyzing and studying the twelve meridians in the human body, we can understand their connection to the five elements and their dynamic nature. The scale for observing this dynamic nature is based on the principles of yin and yang in the four seasons. By adhering to the laws of yin and yang in the four seasons, the human body can maintain a relative balance and achieve harmony between the yin and yang of the heaven and the earth." *Ling Shu Xie Ke* (Chapter 71 of the Spiritual Pivot) states, "Humans correspond with the heaven and the earth." *Lao Zi* says: "Man follows the earth, the earth follows the heaven, the heaven follows *Dao*, and *Dao* follows nature." The daoyin methods recorded in *Zhu Bing Yuan Hou Lun* are guided by man-nature correspondence.

(1)遵循时间与经络脏腑的规律。如"践行养生大道,常常根据日月星辰运行的规律。在凌晨1~3点间内心清净纯澈,身体安卧,漱液满口分3次咽下。可以调和五脏,杀蛊虫,令人长寿,也能治心腹痛"。

(1) Follow the rules between time and meridians & zang-fu organs. For instance, to practice health preservation, it is important to follow the rules of the movement of the sun,

moon, and stars. Between 1 am and 3 am, with a clear and calm mind and a relaxed body, produce some saliva in the mouth and swallow it in 3 times. This exercise can regulate the five zang organs, treat schistosomiasis, promote longevity, and also alleviate abdominal pain.

（2）遵循地理方位的规律。如"坐式（正坐）。向东而坐。鼻微微纳气，闭起嘴巴，迫气下行，留置脐下，然后以口微微出气，分12次吐出。适用于结聚。低头不呼不吸，12次。可助饮食消化、身轻体强。长期练习可使人冬天不怕冷。"

(2) Follow the rules of geographic orientation. For example, sit facing east. Inhale slightly through the nose, close the mouth, force the breath downward to the navel, and then exhale through the mouth in 12 parts (Figure 19–4). This exercise can help eliminate accumulation and obstruction in the body. Lower the head, and passively hold the breath 12 times (Figure 19–5). This exercise can help digest and strengthen the immune system. Long-term practice can make people less susceptible to cold in winter.

（3）遵循日月星辰与人体阴阳的规律。如"站式（立正）。吸收月亮的精华，在月亮初升，太阳将落尽时候，面向月亮站立，不呼不吸8次。仰头面向月亮吸收月光的精华，（因循着月光）咽下，8次。可以增长人的阴气，妇人吸收月亮精华，阴气更加旺盛，可使子道通畅。阴气增长可以益精补脑。"

(3) Follow the rules of the sun, moon, stars, and the yin-yang of the human body. For example, take an upright standing posture. Stand facing the moon when it rises at the beginning of the moon phase and the sun is about to set, and passively hold the breath 8 times. Look up and absorb the moonlight

essence by swallowing it, and do this 8 times. Legend goes that this can increase a person's yin qi, and for females, absorbing the essence of the moon can make their yin qi more vigorous, which can promote conception. Increasing yin energy can also nourish the essence and improve brain function.

特 色 与 要 领

Movements

功法操作

基础操作
Basic Postures

调身
Body Regulation

外形基本姿势主要分为站式、卧式、坐式。着重讲解坐式的几种基本姿势。

The basic postures mainly include standing postures, lying postures and sitting postures. This book focuses primarily on elucidating several fundamental sitting postures.

正坐：又称端坐，把两足跟竖起向上，（臀部）坐在足跟上，脚趾并拢，反方向朝外。

Sit upright: Upright lift the heels, sit on the heels and close the toes.

踞坐：又称"蹲踞"，两膝竖于胸前，臀部、两脚同时落于地面。

Sit with the knees raised and the feet on the ground.

蹲坐：蹲（犹虚坐也），屈膝下蹲，蹲身而坐，臀部离开地面。

Squat: Sit on the heels with the knees bent up close to the body.

箕坐：席地而坐，伸开两脚，并向两侧分开，其形如箕。
Sit by stretching out and separating the legs like a winnowing pan.

箕踞：交叉两脚成踞，两脚底和臀部着地。
Sit by crossing the legs with the feet on the ground.

平跪：双膝着地，大腿和躯干伸直，大腿与小腿成90°角。
Kneel: Place the knees on the ground, straighten the thighs and upper body, and form a 90° angle between the thighs and the lower legs.

胡跪：又称"互跪"，右膝着地，竖起左膝，臀部坐于右脚跟上。
Kneel by placing the right knee on the ground, erecting the left knee and sitting on the right heel, almost like getting down on one knee.

偏跏：即单盘，盘膝而坐，一足触地，另一足压于对侧大腿根上，又称偏跏趺坐。
Half-lotus posture: Place the sole of one foot up on the opposite thigh. Next, place the other foot beneath the other leg.

调息
Breath Regulation

吐纳：古代称亦称服气，主要分为自然呼吸、纳气、不呼不吸、闭气、发音呼吸。通过呼吸以沟通物我、内外、天地与脏腑气机。

In ancient times, breath exercises were also referred to as qi ingestion. Breath was mainly divided into natural breath, inhalation, passive breath-holding, breath-holding, and breath with pronunciation. Through breath, one can connect the physical and spiritual, the internal and external, the heaven and earth, and the internal organs' qi movements.

纳气：主要分为口纳气与鼻纳气。口纳气，指在内心安静后，放松口腔、胸腔、腹腔，而后通过口部引气入内。鼻纳气，指在内心安静后，放松鼻腔、口腔、胸腔、腹腔，而后通过鼻部引气入内。

Inhalation can be categorized into two forms based on the pathway of entry: oral inhalation and nasal inhalation. Oral inhalation refers to the process of inhaling air into the body through the mouth after relaxing the oral cavity, chest, and abdomen, once the mind is calm. Nasal inhalation refers to the process of inhaling air into the body through the nose after relaxing the nasal cavity, oral cavity, chest, and abdomen, once the mind is calm.

不呼不吸：入静之后，心息相依，自发地停止呼吸的一种状态。

Passive breath-holding refers to a state where, after

entering a state of meditation, the heart and breath become interdependent and the breath stops spontaneously.

闭气：主动吸气后，停止呼吸，尽可能地维持一段时间。

Breath-holding refers to the deliberate act of ceasing to breathe after inhaling, and attempting to maintain this state for a period of time.

发音呼吸：呼吸时，同时发音，以吐气发音为主。主要的字音包括嘘、呵、呼、呬、吹、嘻。发音呼吸方法有助于沟通气机。在练功中特殊的发音能调和脏腑，沟通人与人、天地与人之间的精神往来。中医素有五音与五行、五藏相配的理论。如《灵枢·脉度》曰："肾气通于耳，肾和则耳能闻五音矣。"五音，即宫、商、角、徵、羽，是我国古代五声音阶的名称。清代喻嘉言《医门法律》："《内经》本宫商角徵羽五音、呼笑歌哭呻五声，以参求五脏表里虚实之病。"又如《史记》所言："故音乐者，所以动荡血脉，通流精神，而和正心也。故宫动脾而和正圣，商动肺而和正义，角动肝而和正仁，徵动心而和正体，羽动肾而和正智。"其所言"五音内动五脏"之义，正与《内经》所论同。

Breath with pronunciation refers to the technique of making sounds while breathing, with the emphasis on exhaling to produce sounds. The main sound syllables include "xu", "he", "hu", "hei", "ci" and "xi". This technique can be helpful in promoting qi movements. Special pronunciations used in qigong practice can help harmonize the zang-fu organs and facilitate spiritual communication between individuals and between humans and the universe. Traditional Chinese medicine has a theory that matches the five tones and five elements with the five zang organs. For example, *Ling Shu Mai Du* (Chapter 17 of the Spiritual Pivot) states: "Since kidney qi flows to the ears, when kidney qi is

Zhu Bing Yuan Hou Lun Dao Yin Shu (Explanations for the Daoyin Exercises in Zhu Bing Yuan Hou Lun) • 《诸病源候论》导引术 • 功法操作 • Movements

54

in normal functions, the ears can hear the five tones." *Jué* (mi), *zhǐ* (sol), *gōng* (do), *shāng* (re), and *yǔ* (la) are the names of the five tones in ancient China. In the medical book *Yi Men Fa Lv* (Medical Laws), it is recorded that "In *Huang Di Nei Jing*, the five musical notes are associated with cheer, laughter, singing, crying, and groaning, respectively. These associations are used to diagnose the deficiency or excess of the five zang organs." As stated in *Shi Ji* (Records of the Grand Historian), "Music serves to promote the circulation of blood and qi, and calm down the mind. The note *gōng* corresponds to the spleen, *shāng* corresponds to the lung, *jué* corresponds to the liver, *zhǐ* corresponds to the heart, and *yǔ* corresponds to the kidney." The meaning of "the five tones corresponding to the five zang organs" mentioned in *Shi Ji* is consistent with that discussed in *Huang Di Nei Jing*.

调心
Mind Regulation

《诸病源候论》调心方法以存思为主。存思，一名"存想"，简称"存"，道教修炼方术之一。要求闭合双眼或微闭双眼，存想内观某一物体或神真的形貌、活动状态等，以期达到集中思想，去除杂念，进入心物合一境界。存思的对象很广泛，主要包括以下3类。

In *Zhu Bing Yuan Hou Lun*, the method of mind regulation focuses on inward contemplation. It is one of the Taoist cultivation practices. For mind regulation, close or partially close the eyes and visualize the form and activity of a certain object or deity in order to achieve focused thinking, eliminate distracting thoughts, and enter a state of unity between the mind and the body. The objects of inward contemplation can be wide-ranging, including celestial bodies (the sun, the moon, stars and clouds), natural scenery (qi and flames), human body parts (the five zang organs and *Dantian*), and divine beings (deities inside and outside the body).

（1）存思天象（日、月、五星，云雾）：如：卧式（仰卧）。舒展手脚，心中观想月亮犹如油囊裹着朱砂的颜色。适用于阴囊肿大、少腹重、便秘。腹中有热的情况，以口纳气，鼻出气，做几十次，不需要小咽气。腹中不热的情况，做7次呼吸，使气温暖后再咽下，做十几次。

(1) Celestial bodies (the sun, the moon, stars and clouds): For example, take a supine position. Stretch the limbs and visualize the moon in the mind, as if it were the color of cinnabar wrapped in an oil bag. This can help alleviate such conditions as swollen scrotum, lower abdomen heaviness, and constipation. To relieve a hot sensation in the abdomen, inhale through the mouth, exhale through the nose and repeat several tens of times. For those without a hot sensation in the abdomen, breathe 7 times, warm the air in the mouth, swallow the warm air, and repeat more than 10 times.

（2）存思景物（气、炎火）：如：卧式（俯卧）。脚自然舒展，肚腹贴于地面，内视气缓缓向下行，心中当觉察气有去处。此时两手掌撑地，尽力撑起使手臂伸直，脊背放松使气之缓缓下行，反复做14次。适用于脏腑内宿冷、筋脉拘急、腰背肩臂风冷。

(2) Natural scenery (qi and flames): For example, take a prone position. Extend the feet naturally and bring the belly close to the ground. Focus on the inward flow of qi, feeling it gradually descending. Place both hands flat on the ground and lift up to straighten the arms while relaxing the spine to

allow qi to flow downward. Repeat 14 times. This exercise can help treat cold retention in the zang-fu organs, muscle/tendon spasm, and cold wind in the lower back and shoulders.

（3）存思人体（五脏、丹田），如："《无生经》曰：治百病、邪鬼、蛊毒，当仰卧。闭眼闭气，内视丹田，鼻缓缓纳气，令腹部胀满至极点，以口缓缓吐气，不要听到气息声，吸气多吐气少，气息轻柔。内视五脏，看到五脏的形色，再内视胃中，令神光充盈，鲜活明晰洁白如丝绢。做到疲倦至极并且出汗就可以停止了，用粉轻扑于身上，按摩身体。汗未出但感到疲倦的，也可以停止。待第二天再做。

(3) Human body parts (the five zang organs and *Dantian*): For example, *Wu Sheng Jing* (Sutra of Imperishable) states that to treat varying diseases, evil spirits and schistosomiasis, take a supine position. Close the eyes, hold the breath, focus on the *Dantian*, and inhale slowly through the nose to make the abdomen full. Then exhale slowly through the mouth without making any sound. The inhalation should be longer than the exhalation, and the breathing should be gentle and soft. Look at the five zang organs, and observe their forms and colors. Then look at the stomach, and make it bright, lively, clear and white as silk. Continue until exhaustion and sweating are present, then stop, lightly apply powders to the body, and massage the body. If exhaustion is felt but sweating has not yet occurred, stop and repeat the practice the following day."

存思有助于寂然入静，感而遂通。

Inward contemplation helps to enter a state of meditation and clarity, leading to insight and enlightenment.

具体操作

Specific Daoyin Exercises for Dealing with Corresponding Disorders

一、风病诸候提要
Daoyin Exercises for Disorders Induced by Wind

本节论述风病诸候的导引术。风，是四季气候的一种自然现象。但风有时又可以成为一种病邪，能伤人致病。风邪留于人体腠理，则阻碍气血运行，导致脏腑之气不能宣通，外来邪气不得发泄。风侵入经络，危害脏腑则致病。

This chapter introduces the daoyin exercises for disorders induced by wind. Normally, wind is a natural phenomenon; however, it can sometimes become a pathogenic factor of some diseases. Retention of wind within interstices may block the circulation of blood and qi in the zang-fu organs. Under this condition, wind may invade the meridians and zang-fu organs, and subsequently lead to some disorders.

1. 风偏枯候提要
1. Hemiplegia induced by wind

风偏枯是由于正气衰弱，偏侧气血不足，又受风湿之邪侵袭，邪气独留所致。

Weakness of healthy qi, and deficiency of qi and blood on the side of the body, coupled with the invasion of wind-dampness, may cause hemiplegia.

（1）站式、坐式（立正或正坐）。靠墙，不呼不吸，行气，从头至脚（图1-1）。适用于疽、疝、大风、偏枯以及由风邪引起的各种痹证。立正或正坐。背靠墙，伸展两脚，舒展脚趾，把心安静下来，不呼不吸，行气，从头引气到十个脚趾和脚心，这样的引气做21次，等待脚心有得气的感觉就可以停止了。

（1）Take a standing or sitting position. Stand straight or sit upright. Lean against a wall, passively hold the breath, and circulate qi from the head to the feet (Figure 1-1). This exercise can help treat deep-rooted ulcer, hernia, blood deficiency stirring wind, hemiplegia and varying *Bi*-impediment patterns caused by pathogenic wind. Take a standing or sitting position. Stand straight or sit upright. Lean against a wall, stretch the legs and toes, calm the mind, passively hold the breath, and circulate qi from the head to the feet 21 times until the arrival of qi in the soles is present.

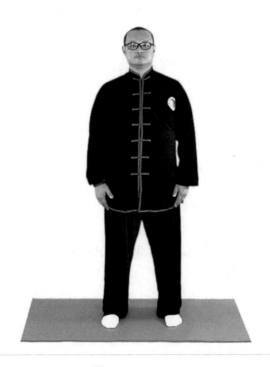

图1-1　Figure 1-1

［操作要领与注意事项］① 行气的原则：自然放松，气自然向下行。② 此动作站、坐皆可，靠墙完成，非常适用于体质虚弱的偏枯患者及平衡能力弱的人。

[Tips and notes] ① The principle of qi circulation: Relax the body and promote qi downward naturally. ② This movement can be done by leaning against a wall in a standing or sitting position. It is very suitable for hemiplegia patients with a weak constitution and for those with a weak balance ability.

（2）卧式（仰卧）。勾起十个脚趾，做5次自然呼吸（图1–2）。适用于腰背痹症、偏枯，可以让耳朵听得见声音。经常练习这样的导引，能使人眼耳清静，不易被外物干扰。

(2) Take a supine position. Fully stretch the toes, naturally inhale and exhale 5 times (Figure 1–2). This exercise can help treat *Bi*-impediment involving the lower back, hemiplegia, and deafness. Regular practice can keep the eyes and ears clear and reduce disturbance from the environment.

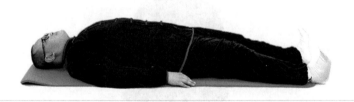

图1-2　Figure 1-2

［操作要领与注意事项］完成此动作时，脚趾要往上抬、往上勾，可助肾气强盛。

[Tips and notes] During the exercise, fully stretching the toes can strengthen kidney qi.

（3）站式、坐式（立正或正坐）。靠墙，不呼不吸，行气（图1-3），从口部把气引至头部（图1-4）。适用于痈疽、风痹、大风病、偏枯等。

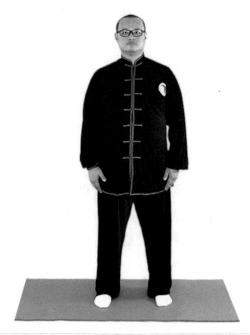

图1-3　Figure 1-3

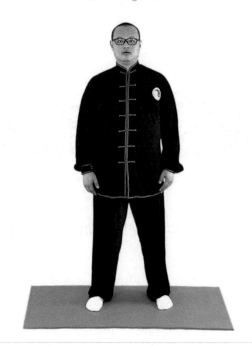

图1-4　Figure 1-4

(3) Take a standing or sitting position. Stand straight or sit upright. Lean against a wall, passively hold the breath, and circulate qi (Figure 1–3) from the mouth to the head (Figure 1–4). This exercise can help treat such disorders as abscesses, wind *Bi*-impediment, blood deficiency stirring wind, and hemiplegia.

［操作要领与注意事项］这个导引动作如同打哈欠一般，引清气上入脑窍。

[Tips and notes] This movement is like yawning. It ascends clear qi to the brain.

（4）站式。一脚踏地，另一脚向旁侧打开（成丁字步）（图1-5）。身体旋转侧身，一手从上往下，使两手并拢，尽力做到最大幅度（图1-6），然后两手快速收回，左右手脚互换做上述动

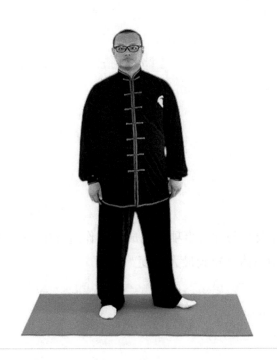

图1-5　Figure 1-5

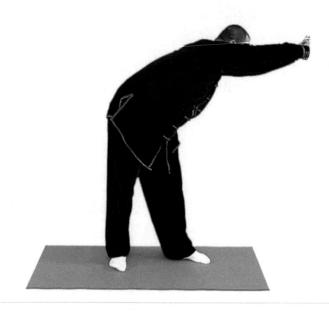

图1-6　　Figure 1-6

作,各14次。适用于脊柱中的风冷,以及半身偏枯导致的气血
不能畅通和濡养的病症。

(4) Take a standing position. Take a step to the side with
one foot (T-shape stance) (Figure 1–5). Turn the upper body
to the side, fully lift and put down the hands one by one, and
put them together (Figure 1–6). Quickly retract the hands and
repeat the movements on the other side, 14 times on each side.
This movement can help dispel wind and cold in the spine,
and deal with the obstruction and malnutrition of qi and blood
caused by hemiplegia.

[操作要领与注意事项] 完成此动作过程中,一手从上往下
运动,可使身体牵拉到最大幅度。

[Tips and notes] Lifting and putting down the hands can
fully stretch the body.

2. 风四肢拘挛不得屈伸候提要

2. Spasticity of the hands and feet with impaired flexion and extension

---

四肢拘挛不得屈伸是由于身体虚弱，腠理开泄，风邪乘虚而入，损伤于筋所致。

Insecurity of the skin pores due to a weak constitution may allow pathogenic wind to damage the tendons, and subsequently lead to this condition.

（1）站式、坐式。① 两手一前一后依次极力上托，做21次（图1-7）。两手掌心向下，低头向下，行气先到涌泉穴再到仓门，带动全身向后用力。维持这个状态一段时间（图1-8），然后放松身体，心平气和。② 头部运动带动两肩部做前后转动，14次（图1-9）。适用于肩部的风冷瘀血、筋脉拘急。

(1) Take a standing or sitting position. ① Lift the hands in turn with the palms facing upward 21 times (Figure 1-7). Put down the hands with the palms facing downward, lower the head, circulate qi from the point Yongquan (KI 1) to the left side of the sub-costal region, drive the whole body backward, keep this state for some time (Figure 1-8), then relax the body and keep a peaceful mind. Move the head to rotate the shoulders back and forth 14 times (Figure 1-9). This exercise can help eliminate wind, cold and blood stasis in the shoulders, and also relieve muscle/tendon spasm.

［操作要领与注意事项］① 动作一：手肘尽量往后拉，带动重心往后靠，才能做到全身向后发力。② 动作二：由头部带动整个脊柱的运动，动作须柔和、缓慢。

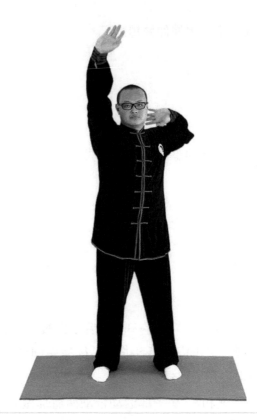

图1-7　Figure 1-7

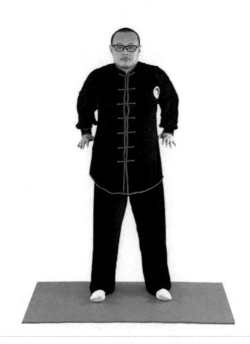

图1-8　Figure 1-8

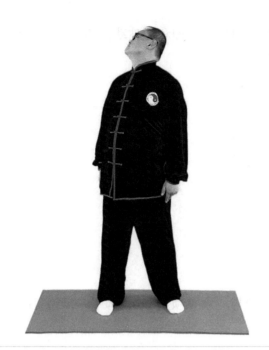

图1-9　Figure 1-9

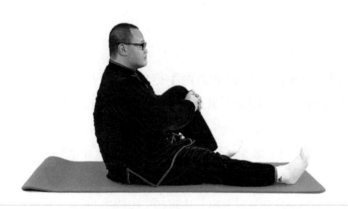

图1-10　Figure 1-10

[Tips and notes] ① Fully stretch the elbows backward to drive the center of body weight backward, so that the whole body can exert force backward. ② The head drives the movement of the whole spine, and the movement should be soft and slow.

（2）坐式（踞坐）。伸出右脚，两手抱住左膝，鼻纳气，腰部自然舒展，做7次这样的呼吸，同时向外侧舒展右脚（图1-10）。

Zhu Bing Yuan Hou Lun Dao Yin Shu (Explanations for the Daoyin Exercises in Zhu Bing Yuan Hou Lun) · 《诸病源候论》导引术 · 功法操作 · Movements

66

适用于腿脚难以完成屈伸和跪站动作的症状,以及小腿疼痛和痿软的病症。

(2) Take a sitting position. Sit with the knees raised and the feet on the ground. Stretch out the right foot, hold the left knee with both hands, extend the waist naturally, breathe through the nose 7 times, and stretch the right foot outward at the same time (Figure 1–10). This exercise can help treat the difficulty of the legs and feet in flexion, extension, kneeling and standing, and can also help treat pain and flaccidity in the lower legs.

操作要领与注意事项:呼吸与动作做到位后,腰部会自然舒展伸起。

[Tips and notes] Breathe and do the movement correctly to extend the waist naturally.

(3) 站式、坐式、卧式。两手抱住左膝,尽量把大腿贴紧胸口(图1–11)。适用于下肢困重和难以屈伸的症状。

(3) Take a standing, sitting or lying position. Hold the left knee with both hands, and fully bring the thigh close to the chest (Figure 1–11). This exercise can help treat lower limb heaviness and difficulty in flexion and extension.

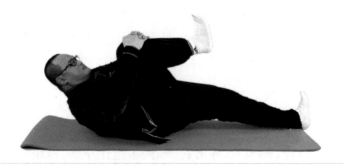

图1–11　Figure 1–11

［操作要领与注意事项］大腿紧贴胸口是关键。此动作站、坐皆可,靠墙完成,非常适用于体质虚弱的偏枯患者及平衡能力弱的人。

[Tips and notes] The key point lies in fully closing the thigh to the chest. This movement can be done by leaning against a wall in a standing or sitting position. It is very suitable for hemiplegia patients with a weak constitution and for those with a weak balance ability.

（4）坐式（踞坐）。伸出右脚,两手抱住左膝,鼻纳气,至满,腰部自然舒展,做7次这样的呼吸,同时向外侧舒展右脚(图1-10)。适用于腿脚难以完成屈伸和跪站动作的症状,以及小腿痛痹的病症。

(4) Take a sitting position. Sit with the knees raised and the feet on the ground. Extend the right foot, hold the left knee with both hands, inhale through the nose deeply, and naturally extend the waist. Repeat this breathing pattern 7 times while extending the right foot outward (Figure1-10). This exercise can help treat the difficulty of the legs and feet in flexion, extension, kneeling and standing, and can also help treat pain and flaccidity in the lower legs.

［操作要领与注意事项］此导引动作中做到鼻纳气至满,呼吸与动作做到位后,腰部会自然舒展伸起。

[Tips and notes] Inhale deeply through the nose. Once the breathing and movements are done correctly, the waist will be naturally stretched and extended.

（5）站式。立身中正，一手上托，一手下按，仰手如推，按手如压，尽量用力，左右手交换做上述上托下按的动作，共28次（图1-12）。适用于肩内的风邪、肩部的冷血，两腋下的筋脉挛急。

(5) Take a standing position. Stand upright, lift a hand with the imagination of pushing the sky and drop the other hand with the imagination of pressing the earth. Change the position of the hands to do the same movement and repeat 28 times (Figures 1–12). This exercise can help dispel pathogenic wind and blood stasis in the shoulders, and relieve contracture in the armpits.

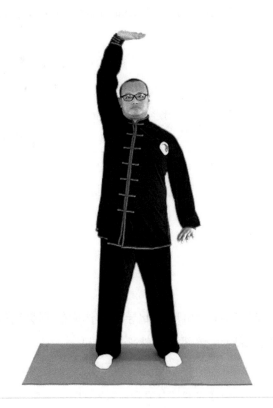

图1-12　Figure 1-12

［操作要领与注意事项］两手一上一下交叉动作，可将身体做斜向的撑拔。

[Tips and notes] This exercise can stretch the body obliquely.

（6）坐式（踞坐）。伸出左脚，两手抱住右膝，鼻纳气至满，腰部自然舒展，做7次这样的呼吸，同时向外舒展左脚（图1-13）。适用于腿脚难以完成屈伸和跪站动作的症状，以及小腿痛痹的病症。

(6) Take a sitting position. Sit with the knees raised and the feet on the ground. Extend the left foot, hold the right knee with both hands, inhale through the nose deeply, and naturally extend the waist. Repeat this breathing pattern 7 times while extending the left foot outward (Figure1-13). This movement can help treat the difficulty of the legs and feet in flexion, extension, kneeling and standing, and can also treat pain in the lower legs.

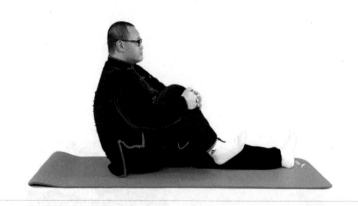

图1-13　Figure 1-13

［操作要领与注意事项］呼吸与动作做到位后，腰部会自然舒展伸起。

[Tips and notes] Once the breathing and movements are done correctly, the waist will be naturally stretched and extended.

3. 风身体手足不随候提要

3. Impaired movement of the body, hands, and feet due to wind

身体手足不随是由于身体虚弱，腠理开泄，风邪乘虚而入，损伤于脾胃经络所致。

Insecurity of the skin pores due to a weak constitution may allow pathogenic wind to damage the meridians of stomach and spleen, and subsequently lead to this condition.

（1）卧式（俯卧）。极力振动两臀，不呼不吸，连续做9次（图1-14）。适用于臀痛、劳累疲乏、风气不遂、久行麻木不觉痛痒而出现各种病症。

(1) Take a prone position. Fully shake both hips, passively hold the breath, and repeat the movement 9 times (Figure 1-14). This exercise can help treat pain in the buttocks, fatigue, lassitude, difficulty in movement due to pathogenic wind, as well as numbness and insensitivity upon prolonged walking.

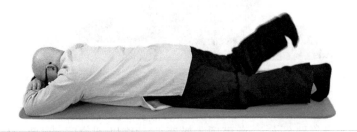

图1-14　Figure 1-14

［操作要领与注意事项］完成此动作，如同普通人入眠之前，两腿会突然抽动般自然地振动两臀。如果难以完成，可模仿动物㧓蹶子一样左右来回交替踢动两腿以振动两臀。

[Tips and notes] Shake the hips naturally, as if one is experiencing sudden muscle twitches before falling asleep. If it is difficult to do, try kicking your legs alternately back and forth, imitating the movement of an animal kicking its legs.

（2）卧式（仰卧）。两膝靠拢，两脚伸展，舒展腰部，口纳气，振腹至极，做7次这样的呼吸（图1–15）。适用于高热、疼痛、两腿动作不便。

(2) Take a prone position. Bring the knees together, stretch the feet outward, stretch the waist, inhale through the mouth and fully vibrate the abdomen. Repeat this breathing exercise 7 times (Figure 1–15). This exercise can help treat high fever, pain, and impaired leg movements.

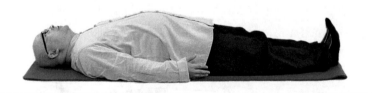

图1–15   Figure 1–15

［操作要领与注意事项］完成此动作时，通过口纳气做到振腹。

[Tips and notes] Vibrate the abdomen by inhaling through the mouth.

（3）卧式（仰卧）。治疗四肢疼闷、行动不便、腹中胀气。可以采用下面的方法：床席平稳，仰卧，松解衣带，枕高三寸，两手握固，伸展两手，各距离身体五寸（图1–16）。安心定意，调和气息，不想杂事，专注气息，慢慢地漱醴泉。所谓漱醴泉，即是用舌在口唇齿间转动（图1-17），使津液满口，而后缓缓咽下，然后徐徐以口吐气，再以鼻纳气。这些动作都须轻且慢，不要匆促硬做。调和呼吸，渐至自己听不到呼吸声后，以心行气，引气至脚趾端而出。每吸5或6次，呼1次，为一息。初学，由一息渐做到十息，以后慢慢增加到一百息、二百息。

(3) Take a supine position. To treat oppressive pain in the limbs, difficulty in movement, and abdominal distension, lie on a flat bed, wear loose clothes, use a pillow with 3 *cun* high, make fists with the hands, and stretch the arms outwards, with each hand being about 5 *cun* away from the body (Figure 1-16). Keep a peaceful mind, regulate and focus on the breath, close the mouth, and slowly rotate the tongue to make saliva fill the mouth, then slowly swallow, then slowly exhale through the mouth, and inhale through the nose (Figure 1-17). These movements should be done gently and slowly. Regulate the breath and gradually make it so quiet that you cannot hear it. Then focus the mind on guiding qi to the tips of the toes. Inhale 5 or 6 times and exhale once to complete a breath cycle. For

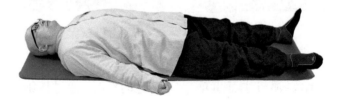

图1-16　Figure 1-16

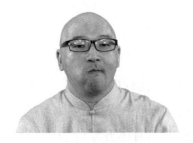

图1-17　Figure 1-17

beginners, start with 1 breath cycle and gradually increase to 10, and then slowly increase to 100 or 200 breath cycles.

［操作要领与注意事项］握固，将大拇指弯曲，其余四指向内握住大拇指。完成此动作过程中，可从无为法和有为法着手。无为法：清静自然，以心行气，浊气自然下行，引气至脚趾端而出；有为法：虚心自谦，亦可使浊气下行，至脚趾端而出。练功期勿食生的蔬菜、鱼、肥肉。过饱和喜怒忧忿时都不可行气。在凌晨清静时候行气最好，适用于各种疾病。

[Tips and notes] The method of making a fist is to bend the thumb and grasp it with the other four fingers. During the exercise, you can approach it using either the non-action (*Wu Wei*) method or the action (*You Wei*) method. For the *Wu Wei* method, stay calm and natural, circulate qi with the mind, descend the turbid qi naturally, and guide qi to exit from the toes. For the *You Wei* method, keep a humble and open mind, or descend the turbid qi naturally, and guide qi to exit from the toes. During the exercise period, avoid eating uncooked vegetables, fish, or fatty meat. Do not circulate qi when you are overly full or emotional. The best time to circulate qi is in the early morning, which can help treat various disorders.

4. 风痹手足不随候提要
4. Impaired movement of the hands and feet due to wind *Bi*-impediment

风邪偏多者为风痹。风邪侵袭肌肤，随其经气虚弱处停滞，内犯经脉关节，以致麻木不仁，手足不随。

Excessive pathogenic wind may cause wind *Bi*-impediment. Pathogenic wind may invade the skin and stagnate at the area with weak meridian qi, and thus further invade the meridians and joints, resulting in numbness and insensitivity of the limbs.

站式(立正)。两手合抱,拱起两臂,不呼不吸9次(图1-18)。适用于臂足疼痛、劳倦、风痹不遂。

Take an upright standing position. Hold both hands together, raise both arms, and passively hold the breath 9 times (Figure 1–18). This exercise can help treat pain in the arms and feet, fatigue, lassitude, as well as impaired movement due to wind *Bi*-impediment.

［操作要领与注意事项］完成此动作时,两手合抱拱起两臂,类似于"作揖"。

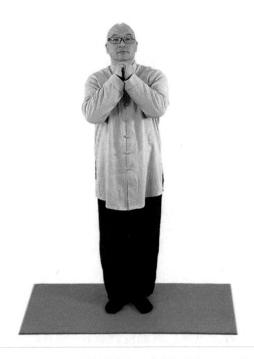

图1-18　Figure 1-18

[Tips and notes] During the exercise, clasp the hands together and raise both arms, similar to the gesture of making a bow.

5. 偏风候提要
5. Hemiplegia

身体虚弱,腠理开泄,风邪乘虚而入,伤其一侧,而成偏风。

Insecurity of the skin pores due to physical weakness may allow pathogenic wind to damage one side of the body, and subsequently lead to this condition.

（1）站式。一手舒展打开,手掌向上;另一手握住下颌向外侧推拉。每次做到极势,左右手交换做上述动作14次。然后手不动,身体向两侧快速尽量转动,做14次(图1-19)。适用于颈

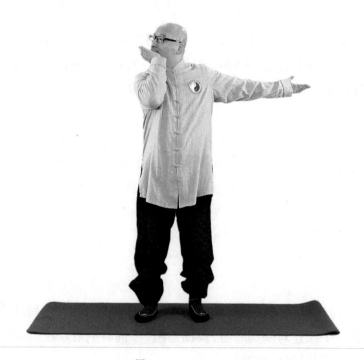

图1-19　Figure 1-19

椎活动障碍、头痛脑眩、喉痹、肩部冷痛、偏风的病症。

(1) Take a standing position. Fully extend and open one hand with the palm facing upward, grip the jaw and push and pull it outward with the other hand. Change the position of the hands and do the above movement 14 times. Then, keep the hands still, and quickly rotate the body to both sides 14 times (Figure 1–19). This exercise can help treat impaired cervical movement, headache, dizziness, throat *Bi*-impediment, pain and cold in the shoulders, and hemiplegia.

［操作要领与注意事项］完成此动作过程中，容易导致颈椎小关节错位，宜缓做。忌爆发力。

[Tips and notes] Since this movement is easy to cause dislocation of the small joints in the cervical vertebrae, do it slowly and avoid using brute force.

（2）站式。一脚踏地，一手向后用力伸展，另一手前抓住脚底涌泉穴快速上拉，手脚同时尽力做到极势（图1–20）。左右手脚互换做上述动作，14次。适用于上下偏风、阴气不和的病症。

(2) Take a standing position. Fully stretch one hand backward, grab the point Yongquan (KI 1) located in the sole and pull it up quickly with the other hand (Figure 1–20). Change the position of the hands and feet to repeat the above movements 14 times. This exercise can help treat hemiplegia, and disharmony between yin and qi.

［操作要领与注意事项］完成此动作过程中，首先需站稳，然后一手抓住对侧脚底时，脚向前蹬，手同时向后牵拉，形成一个对拉劲，以利气血循行。

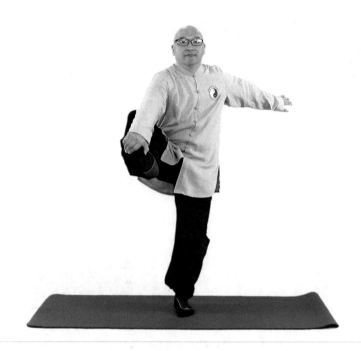

图1-20　Figure 1-20

[Tips and notes] To do this exercise, first stand firmly. When grasping the sole with one hand, push the foot forward while pulling the hand backward to stretch, in order to facilitate the circulation of qi and blood.

6. 风不仁候提要
6. Numbness and insensitivity

风邪侵袭肌肤,血气运行不畅,以致麻木不仁。

The invasion of pathogenic wind in the skin may obstruct the circulation of blood and qi, and subsequently result in numbness and insensitivity.

（1）卧式（仰卧）。伸展两腿两手,脚跟向外,脚趾相对,鼻纳气，至满，做7次这样的呼吸（图1-21）。适用于肌肤枯槁、麻木和足部寒冷的病症。

(1) Take a supine position. Extend both legs and arms with the heels facing outward and the toes touching each other, inhale through the nose deeply, and repeat this breathing pattern 7 times (Figure 1–21). This exercise can help treat skin dryness, numbness, and cold in the feet.

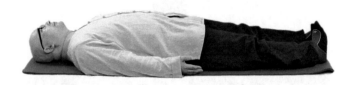

图1-21　Figure 1-21

［操作要领与注意事项］完成此动作过程中，通过鼻纳气至满来舒展腰膝。

[Tips and notes] During this exercise, deeply inhale through the nose to stretch the waist and knees.

(2) 卧式（仰卧）。伸展两脚向上（图1-22），适用于肌肤麻木不仁、小腿寒冷。

(2) Take a supine position. Stretch both legs upwards (Figure 1–22), which can help treat skin numbness and insensitivity, and cold in the lower legs.

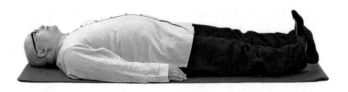

图1-22　Figure 1-22

［操作要领与注意事项］完成此动作过程中，要保持脚趾向上，以利气血行至腰膝部。

[Tips and notes] During this exercise, keep the toes upward to help the flow of qi and blood to the waist and knees.

7. 风湿痹候提要
7. Wind-dampness *Bi*-impediment

气血不足，外邪侵袭，风湿邪偏多、寒邪少者为风湿痹。

Deficiency of qi and blood, coupled with strong pathogenic wind-dampness and mild pathogenic cold may result in this condition.

（1）卧式（仰卧）。放松两臂，不呼不吸12次（图1-23）。适用于足湿痹不能行走、腰脊痹痛。又仰卧。两手叠放背下，伸展两脚，不呼不吸12次（图1-24）。适用于腿脚湿痹不能行走、腰脊痹痛。有一侧肢体患病，如病在左侧，左脚压右脚；如病在右侧，右脚压左脚（图1-25，图1-26）。要经常反复练习这样的导引动作。如果上肢有病，练习方法同下肢。练习这样的导引动作，做10次才能停止。

(1) Take a lying position. Relax both arms and passively hold the breath 12 times (Figure 1-23). This exercise can help treat the inability to walk due to dampness *Bi*-impediment involving the feet, and also treat pain in the lower back and spine. Take a supine position. Make both hands stacked beneath the lower back, extend both legs, and passively hold the breath 12 times (Figure 1-24). This exercise can help treat the inability to walk due to dampness *Bi*-impediment involving the feet and legs, and also treat pain in the lower back and spine. If

the left side is affected, place the left foot on the right leg; if the right side is affected, place the right foot on the left leg (Figure 1–25 and Figure 1–26). It is necessary to regularly practice these movements. If the upper limbs are affected, the same method as for the lower limbs should be used. Practice these movements 10 times.

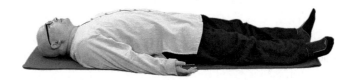

图1–23　Figure 1–23

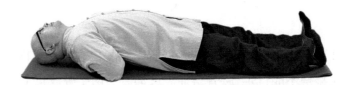

图1–24　Figure 1–24

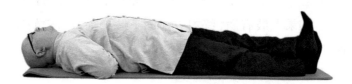

图1–25　Figure 1–25

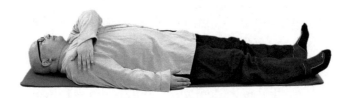

图1–26　Figure 1–26

[操作要领与注意事项] 完成此动作过程中, 不呼不吸松静自然, 气机通畅故可行气至患侧。

[Tips and notes] During the exercise, passively hold the breath, relax the body and keep a peaceful mind. Since qi flows smoothly, it is possible to guide it to the affected side.

（2）卧式（仰卧）。从脚向头的方向摩腹（图1-27）。屈伸两手臂导引, 屈膝, 以手攀脚底（图1-28）, 然后两臂放松, 两腿伸直, 闭气12次（图1-29）。适用于湿痹、行动不便、腰脊痛。

(2) Take a supine position. Massage the abdomen upward (Figure 1–27). Bend and stretch both arms, bend the knees, hold the soles with the hands (Figure 1–28), then relax both arms, extend both legs, and hold the breath 12 times (Figure 1–29). This exercise can help treat dampness *Bi*-impediment, impaired movement, and pain in the lower back and spine.

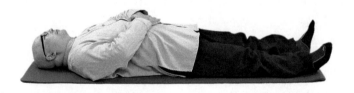

图1-27　Figure 1-27

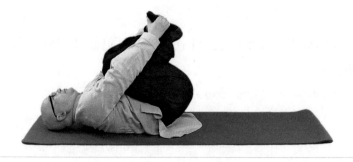

图1-28　Figure 1-28

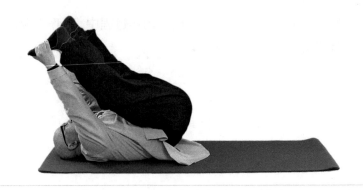

图1-29　Figure 1-29

[操作要领与注意事项] ① 用手做从脚至头方向的单向摩腹。② 屈膝以手攀脚,须大腿贴近腹部(手从外侧抱脚底效果更佳)。③ 此处闭气为刚猛有为法。初学若掌握不好,可以减少操作的次数与时间。

[Tips and notes] ① Massage the abdomen upward. ② When holding the soles with the hands, bend the knees and make sure the thighs are close to the abdomen. Better results can be achieved by holding the feet from the outside with the hands. ③ Holding the breath here should be done with force and purpose. Beginners can reduce the frequency and duration of the exercise.

8. 风痹候提要
8. Wind *Bi*-impediment

身体虚弱,风邪侵袭,外伤腠理,内犯血脉而致筋骨,为风痹。

Physical weakness coupled with the pathogenic wind may damage the interstices and further invade blood, meridians, tendons and bones, subsequently resulting in this condition.

（1）卧式。① 仰卧。以右脚跟勾住左脚拇指，鼻纳气，至满，做7次这样的呼吸。适用于风痹（图1–30）。② 仰卧。以左脚跟勾住右脚拇趾，鼻纳气，至满，做7次这样的呼吸。适用于厥痹（图1–31）。③ 两手交替拉两脚背放膝盖上，适用于体痹（图1–32）。

(1) Take a lying position. ① Take a supine position. Hook the right heel around the left big toe, inhale through the nose deeply, and repeat this breathing 7 times. This exercise can help treat wind *Bi*-impediment (Figure 1–30). ② Take a supine

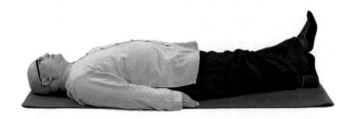

图1–30　Figure 1–30

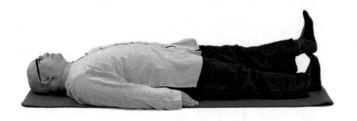

图1–31　Figure 1–31

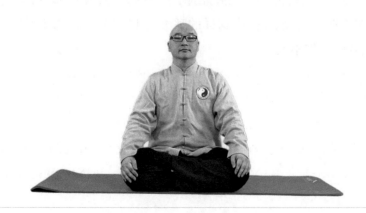

图1–32　Figure 1–32

position. Hook the left heel around the right big toe, inhale through the nose deeply, and repeat this breathing 7 times. This exercise can help treat *Bi*-impediment due to syncope (Figure 1–31). ③ Alternate pulling the back of both feet and placing them on the knees. This exercise can help treat *Bi*-impediment (Figure 1–32).

［操作要领与注意事项］完成此动作过程中，通过鼻纳气至满来舒展腰膝。勿用拙力。① 动作一：可养精血祛风。② 动作二：可补气行气，利气机下行。③ 动作三：可松解腰部、骶部和胯部，利于周身气机运行。

[Tips and notes] During the exercise, inhale deeply through the nose to stretch the waist and knees. Do not use brute force. ① The first movement can nourish essence and blood and dispel pathogenic wind. ② The second movement can tonify and circulate qi, and facilitate the downward movement of qi. ③ The third movement can relax the waist, sacrum, and hip area, which is beneficial for the circulation of qi throughout the body.

（2）卧式（仰卧）。两膝靠拢，翻起两脚，舒展腰部，口纳气，使腹部胀满至极，做7次这样的呼吸（图1–15）。适用于风痹热痛、两腿动作不便。

(2) Take a supine position. Close the knees, lift both feet up, stretch the waist, inhale through the mouth until the abdomen is completely full, and repeat this breathing 7 times (Figure 1–15). This exercise can help relieve fever and pain caused by wind *Bi*-impediment and treat impaired leg movements.

［操作要领与注意事项］完成此动作过程中，翻起两脚更利腰部舒展；口纳气，引气入腰腹，利于周身气血运行。

[Tips and notes] During the exercise, lift the legs to stretch the waist area; breathing in through the mouth allows qi to go into the waist and abdomen, facilitating the circulation of qi and blood throughout the body.

（3）坐式（踞坐）。两手攀两脚跟，鼻纳气，至满，做7次这样的呼吸；然后放松两手，置于膝部（图1-33）。用这样的方式舒展腰部，利于除痹止呕。

(3) Take a sitting position. Sit with the knees raised and the feet on the ground. Grasp the heels of both feet with both hands, inhale deeply through the nose, and repeat this breathing 7 times; then relax both hands and place them on the knees (Figure 1–33). This way of stretching the waist can help treat *Bi*-impediment and nausea.

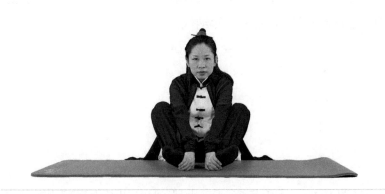

图1-33　Figure 1-33

［操作要领与注意事项］此动作以手从两膝内攀足，以助开胯后利于气血下行。

[Tips and notes] In this movement, grasp the heel of each foot from the inside of the corresponding knee to help open the hips and facilitate the downward flow of qi and blood.

（4）卧式（仰卧）。舒展手脚，鼻纳气，至满，做7次这样的呼吸；然后脚掌转动30次（图1-34）。适用于胸寒、脚寒、周身痹、厥逆。

(4) Take a supine position. Extend the arms and legs, inhale through the nose deeply, and repeat this breathing 7 times; then rotate the soles of the feet 30 times (Figure 1-34). This exercise can help alleviate cold in the chest and feet, *Bi*-impediment involving the general body, and syncope.

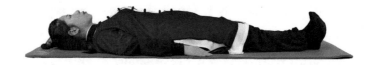

图1-34　Figure 1-34

［操作要领与注意事项］伸展两脚，膝关节可微微放松，以脚趾带动脚掌转动，使鼻自然纳气。

[Tips and notes] Extend both feet and slightly relax the knee joints. Use the toes to drive the rotation of the feet and inhale through the nose naturally.

（5）站式、坐式（立正或正坐）。靠墙，不呼不吸，行气，从头至脚（图1-1）。适用于疽、疝、大风、偏枯以及由风邪引起的各种痹证。

(5) Take a standing or sitting position. Stand straight or sit upright. Lean against a wall, passively hold the breath, and guide the qi from the head to the toes (Figure 1-1). This exercise can help treat deep-rooted ulcer, hernia, blood deficiency stirring

wind, hemiplegia, and varying *Bi*-impediment patterns caused by pathogenic wind.

［操作要领与注意事项］①行气的原则：自然放松，气自然向下行。②此动作站、坐皆可，靠墙完成，适用于体质虚弱的偏枯患者及平衡能力弱的人。

[Tips and notes] ① The principle of circulating qi is to relax naturally and let qi flow downward naturally. ② This exercise can be done by leaning against a wall in a standing or sitting position. It is very suitable for hemiplegia patients with a weak constitution and for those with a weak balance ability.

（6）坐式（踞坐）。两手撑地，仰头舒展腰部，做5次自然呼吸（图1-35）。适用于痿症、痹症，通利九窍。

(6) Take a sitting position. Sit with the knees raised and the feet on the ground. Push the ground with the hands, lift the head, stretch the waist, and breathe 5 times naturally (Figure 1-35). This exercise can help relieve *Wei*-flaccidity and *Bi*-impediment disorders, and promote the smooth flow of qi and blood in the nine orifices.

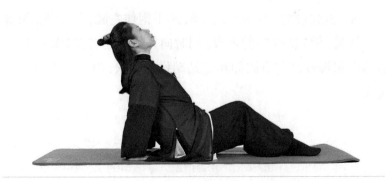

图1-35　Figure 1-35

［操作要领与注意事项］手撑地、仰头,鼻自然吸气,腰部自然舒展。完成此动作过程中,腰部不主动用力。

[Tips and notes] Support the upper body with both hands on the ground and lift the head to stretch the waist, and breathe naturally through the nose. During this movement, the waist should not exert force actively.

（7）卧式(仰卧)。勾起十个脚趾,做5次自然呼吸(图1-2)。适用于腰背痹症、偏枯,可以让耳朵听得见声音。经常练习这样的导引,有助于眼耳清静,不易被外物干扰。

(7) Take a supine position. Fully stretch the toes, naturally inhale and exhale 5 times (Figure 1–2). This exercise can help treat *Bi*-impediment involving the lower back, hemiplegia, and deafness. Regular practice can help keep the eyes and ears clear and reduce disturbance from the environment.

［操作要领与注意事项］完成此动作时,脚趾要往上抬、往上勾,可助肾气强盛。

[Tips and notes] During the exercise, fully stretching the toes can strengthen kidney qi.

（8）坐式(踞坐)。伸出右脚,两手抱住左膝,鼻纳气,腰部自然舒展,做7次这样的呼吸,同时向外侧舒展右脚(图1-10)。适用于腿脚难以完成屈伸和跪站动作的症状,以及小腿痛痹的病症。

(8) Take a sitting position. Sit with the knees raised and the feet on the ground. Extend the right foot, hold the left knee with both hands, inhale through the nose deeply, and naturally extend the waist. Repeat this breathing pattern 7 times while

extending the right foot outward (Figure1–10). This movement can help treat the difficulty of the legs and feet in flexion, extension, kneeling and standing, and can also treat pain in the lower legs.

[操作要领与注意事项] 呼吸与动作做到位后，腰部会自然舒展伸起。

[Tips and notes] Proper breathing and movements can lead to the natural stretching of the waist.

（9）站式。两手合抱，拱起两臂，不呼不吸9次（图1-18）。适用于臂足疼痛、劳倦、风痹不遂。

(9) Take a standing position. Hold both hands together and raise both arms, and passively hold the breath 9 times (Figure 1–18). This exercise can help treat pain in the arms and feet, fatigue, lassitude, as well as impaired movement due to wind *Bi*-impediment.

[操作要领与注意事项] 完成此动作时，两手合抱拱起两臂，类似于"作揖"。

[Tips and notes] Raise both arms and clasp the hands together, similar to making a bow.

（10）站式、坐式。有人觉得脊背僵紧不舒憋闷，无论什么时节，可以缩咽于肩（图1-36），仰面，肩胛骨上抬，头顺着左右两个方向移动，做21次（图1-37），然后稍停，待气血平复再做下一次。开始时要慢做再逐渐加快，不能先快后慢。如果是无病之人，可以在清晨3点至5点、中午11点至13点、下午17点至19点三个时间段操作，每个时段做14次。适用于寒热病、脊腰颈项痛、风痹、口内生疮、牙齿风、头眩。

(10) Take a standing or sitting position. For back rigidity, tuck in the throat (Figure 1–36), raise the head and scapula, and rotate the head to both sides 21 times (Figure 1–37). Then take a break to calm down qi and blood and do it again. Begin slowly and gradually increase the speed. Avoid starting fast and then slowing down. People in good health can do this exercise 14 times during each of the three time periods: 3–5 am, 11 am–1 pm, and 5–7 pm. This exercise can help treat chills, fever, and pain in the lower back, neck and shoulders, and can also help treat wind *Bi*-impediment, mouth ulcer, toothache, and dizziness.

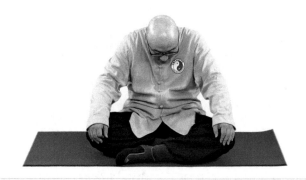

图1–36　Figure 1–36

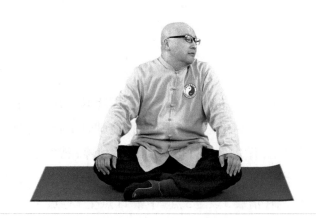

图1–37　Figure 1–37

［操作要领与注意事项］腰背脊柱放松，肩部自然打开。即，仰面带脊背肩胛向后固定，在此基础上再缩咽。

[Tips and notes] Relax the lower back and spine, and open the shoulders naturally. Raise the head to fix the spine and scapula, and then tuck in the throat.

9. 风冷候提要

9. Disorders induced by pathogenic cold and wind

身体虚弱，气血不足，感受风冷之邪所致。

Deficiency of qi and blood due to physical weakness, coupled with the contraction of pathogenic cold and wind, may result in these disorders.

（1）站式。一脚踏地，另一脚向旁侧打开，成丁字步（图1-5）。身体旋转侧身，一手从上往下，使两手并拢，尽力做到最大幅度，然后两手快速收回，左右手脚互换做上述动作，各14次（图1-6）。适用于脊柱中的风冷，以及半身偏枯导致的气血不能畅通和濡养的病症。

(1) Take a standing position. Place one foot firmly on the ground while opening the other to the side to form a T-shape stance (Figure 1-5). Turn the body sideways, and move one hand from top to bottom to bring the hands together with full range of motion. Then, retract both hands quickly, and perform the same procedure on the other side. Repeat 14 times on each side (Figure 1-6). This exercise can help dispel wind and cold in the spine, and deal with the obstruction and malnutrition of qi and blood caused by hemiplegia.

［操作要领与注意事项］完成此动作过程中，一手从上往下运动，可使身体牵拉到最大幅度。

[Tips and notes] Moving one hand from top to bottom can fully stretch the body.

（2）蹲式（蹲坐）。保持头部和上半身正直，两手交叉放于下颌，头不动，两肘上下摆动，做49次（图1-38）。也可松开两手做上述动作21次，放松身心（图1-39）。适用于乳房冷肿闷、鱼际寸口部位不适、日渐亏损之病。

(2) Take a squatting position. Keep the head and upper body upright, cross the hands under the chin, and swing the elbows up and down without moving the head. Repeat 49 times (Figure 1-38). Alternatively, release the hands and do the same movement 21 times to relax the body and mind (Figure 1-39). This exercise can help alleviate swelling, cold sensation and tightness in the breasts, and can also treat discomfort in the *Cunkou* area and thenar eminence, and chronic consumptive conditions.

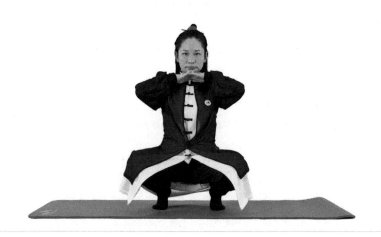

图1-38　Figure 1-38

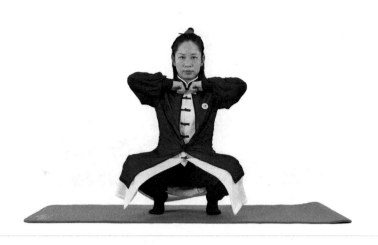

图1-39　Figure 1-39

［操作要领与注意事项］完成此动作过程中，两手托下颌，头颈轻轻拔起，有利于头、颈、肩放松。

[Tips and notes] Support the chin with both hands and gently lift the head and neck, which can help to relax the neck, shoulders, and head during the movement.

（3）坐式。两脚自然舒展，放松身心，纳气向下，内心柔和惬意（图1-40）。然后屈一脚，放于另一侧膝下；伸展的脚五趾尽力上翘，然后躺下仰卧，在头部还未接触地面时，两手臂立即尽力向前伸展，头部亦向上拉起，这一刻全身皆处于拉伸状态，这样做14次（图1-41）。左右脚互换再做上述动作。适用于脚疼、腰背肩臂冷、血冷、日渐亏损之病。

(3) Take a sitting position. Naturally extend the feet, relax the body, keep a peaceful mind, and inhale deeply (Figure 1-40). Then bend one leg and place it under the knee of the other leg. Raise the toes of the extended foot as high as possible and lie down on the back. Before the head touches the ground, immediately extend the arms forward and pull the head up to stretch the whole body. Repeat these movements 14 times (Figure 1-41). Change the position of the feet and repeat the

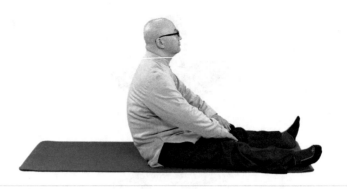

图1-40　Figure 1-40

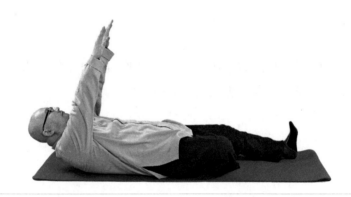

图1-41　Figure 1-41

above movements. This exercise can help relieve foot pain, cold sensation and blood stasis in the lower back and shoulders, and chronic consumptive conditions.

［操作要领与注意事项］动作外形与仰卧起坐相似，但此动作更注重身体内在气血运行，身体更为轻便。

[Tips and notes]　The movement is similar to sit-ups, but focuses more on the internal circulation of qi and blood in the body, making the body more relaxed.

（4）卧式（俯卧）。脚自然舒展，肚腹贴于地面，内视气缓缓向下行，心中当觉察气有去处（图1-42）。此时两手掌撑地，尽力撑起使手臂伸直，脊背放松使气之缓缓下行，反复做14次（图1-43）。适用于脏腑内宿冷、筋脉拘急、腰背肩臂风冷。

(4) Take a prone position. Extend the feet naturally and bring the belly close to the ground. Focus on the inward flow of qi, feeling it gradually descending (Figure 1-42). Place both hands flat on the ground and lift up to straighten the arms while relaxing the spine to descend qi. Repeat 14 times (Figure 1-43). This exercise can help alleviate cold retention in the zang-fu organs, muscle/tendon spasm, and wind cold in the lower back and shoulders.

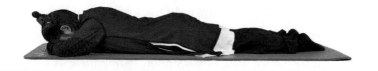

图1-42　Figure 1-42

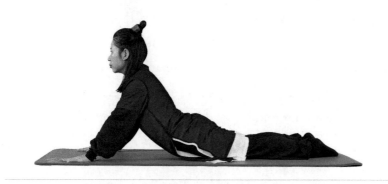

图1-43　Figure 1-43

［操作要领与注意事项］松静状态下内视气往脚趾方向下行。两手掌撑地时手不主动用力，而是通过脊柱向后放松使手臂自然伸直。

[Tips and notes] In a relaxed state, focus the internal vision on the direction of the toes and allow qi to flow downward. When supporting the ground with the palms, do not use force in the hands but naturally stretch the arms by relaxing the spine.

（5）卧式（侧卧）。手脚踡曲，闭气至极限，通过行气的方法使汗出；放松，待呼吸平稳，再次闭气，这样做反复至汗出为止（图1-44）。然后转身朝另一向侧卧，重复刚才的动作，汗大出即止。此法适用于身体内有风寒。有利于四肢疼痛的方法是：侧卧，踡曲健侧手脚，患侧手脚自然伸直，鼻纳气，而后闭气，以意推至腹部令腹部鼓起，观想气达患病处，感到有温热感即可。闭气至极限，建议医护人员在旁看护。

（5）Take a side-lying position. Bend the arms and legs, fully hold the breath, and promote sweating by circulating qi; relax to calm down the breath, hold the breath again, and repeat until sweating is present (Figure 1–44). Then repeat the same exercise on the other side. This exercise can help treat wind and cold retention in the body. To deal with pain in the limbs, take a side-lying position, curl the healthy limbs, extend the affected limbs naturally, inhale through the nose, then hold the breath and use the mind to push qi to the abdomen, causing it to bulge. Imagine the breath reaching the affected area until experience a warm sensation. Fully hold the breath, and it is recommended to do this exercise under the watchful eye of a person.

［操作要领与注意事项］手脚踡曲是人感受寒冷时的自然收紧状态，易聚气于背。踡曲侧卧更易形成腹式呼吸，帮助身体

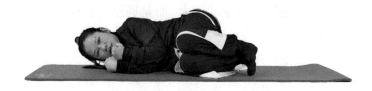

图1-44　Figure 1-44

Zhu Bing Yuan Hou Lun Dao Yin Shu (Explanations for the Daoyin Exercises in *Zhu Bing Yuan Hou Lun*) · 《诸 病 源 候 论》 导 引 术

97

功 法 操 作 · Movements

发热发汗。此法适用于初中风寒、虚弱之人，适用于外感风寒急证。操作时微微汗出即可，不宜大汗。此导引动作中的闭气为刚猛有为法。

[Tips and notes] The natural curled-up position of the hands and feet is a natural response to cold, and it is easier to gather qi at the back in this position. Taking a side-lying position with curled-up legs can facilitate abdominal breathing, helping the body generate heat and sweat. This method is suitable for people who have a common cold or have a weak constitution. It can help treat acute symptoms caused by external wind and cold. During the exercise, sweating slightly is sufficient, and sweating excessively should be avoided.

（6）卧式（俯卧）。肚腹贴于地面，一脚自然伸展，脚趾尽力后伸，对侧手臂尽力向前伸展，同侧手臂后伸，以手握住同侧脚踝，头部上仰，脊背拔伸：整个脊背斜向拉伸，向相反方向用劲，然后手脚和头皆尽力拔伸到最大幅度，做14次（图1-45）。左右手脚互换再重复刚才的动作。适用于颈、背、腰、膝、肩部的风冷疼闷、脊柱紧张强直。

(6) Take a prone position. Lie on the stomach, extend a leg naturally, fully extend the toes backward, fully extend forward the opposite arm, extend backward the arm on the same side, grasp the ankle of the same-side foot with the hand, and raise the head to stretch the spine. Stretch the entire spine diagonally in one direction, exert force in the opposite direction, then fully

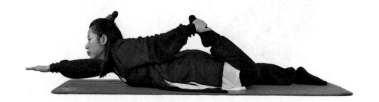

图1-45　Figure 1-45

stretch the hands, feet and head, and repeat 14 times (Figure 1–45). Change the position of the hands and feet to do the same movements. This exercise can help relieve pain in the neck, back, waist, knees, and shoulders caused by cold and wind, as well as rigidity and tension in the spine.

［操作要领与注意事项］完成此动作过程中，手臂后伸牵拉同侧脚踝，与对侧伸展的手臂呈反弓姿势，更利于整体拉伸。

[Tips and notes] During the exercise, extending the arm posteriorly to grasp the ankle on the same side can facilitate a more effective overall stretch.

（7）坐式（正坐）。两手于身后，一侧手握另一侧手腕，（被握住手腕一侧的）手掌反向撑地，身体尽力后仰，使腹部绷紧，上下反复做7次（图1-46）。两手姿势互换重复刚才的动作。可以减轻肚腹冷风、久宿气积、胃口冷、饮食反胃、呕吐不下。

(7) Take an upright sitting position. Place both hands behind the body, grasp the wrist of one hand with the other, and invert the palm of the grasped wrist to support the body weight on the ground. Lean the body backward, tighten the abdominal muscles, and repeat the movements 7 times in an up-and-down motion (Figure 1–46). Change the position of the hands

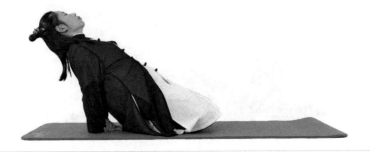

图1-46　Figure 1-46

and repeat the movements. This exercise can alleviate cold and wind in the abdomen, qi stagnation due to food retention, poor appetite, and stomach reflux.

［操作要领与注意事项］身体尽力后仰时，头部保持前视、不后仰；初学动作过程注重腹部绷紧，腰部放松，利于减轻肚腹疾患。

[Tips and notes] When leaning the body backward, avoid bending the head backward. For beginners, it is important to focus on tightening the abdominal muscles while relaxing the lower back, as this can help alleviate abdominal disorders.

（8）坐式。凡是学习调息的人，首先须正坐，并拢膝盖和脚。初学时，先将脚趾相对，脚跟向外扒开，（臀部）坐于脚跟上，坐得安稳（图1-47），再将两脚跟向内相对，（臀部）坐于脚跟上，脚趾向外扒开（图1-48）；感觉闷痛后逐渐起身，然后再坐回脚跟上。（练习）直至上述两种坐姿都不觉得闷痛，才开始把两脚跟向上竖起，（臀部）坐于脚跟上，脚趾并拢，反方向朝外（图1-49）。以上三种坐姿就是正坐的一般练习方式。适用于膀胱内冷气、膝冷、双脚冷痛，喘息上气、腰疼等病症。

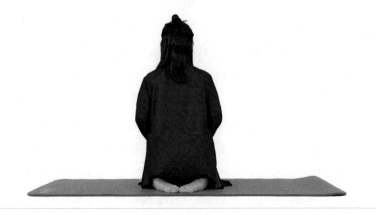

图1-47　Figure 1-47

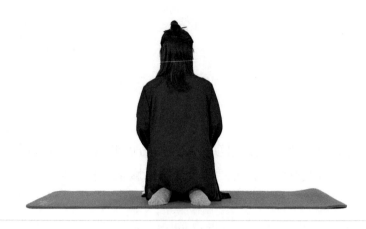

图1-48　Figure 1-48

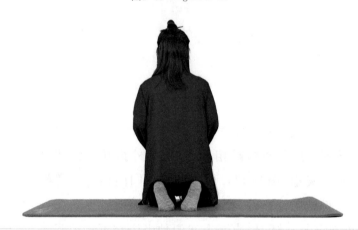

图1-49　Figure 1-49

(8) Take a sitting position. For those learning to regulate their breathing, it is important to sit upright and bring the knees and feet together. For beginners, start by positioning the toes facing each other and the heels turned outward, and sit on the heels for stability (Figure 1–47). Then, position the heels facing each other and the toes turned outward while sitting on the heels (Figure 1–48). Gradually stand up when experiencing oppressive pain, and then sit back on the heels. When there is no oppressive pain in the above-mentioned sitting positions, raise up the heels and sit on them with the toes together and facing outward (Figure 1–49). The above three postures are the typical practice methods of upright sitting. They can help

eliminate cold in the bladder, knees and feet, and alleviate such symptoms as shortness of breath and lower back pain.

[操作要领与注意事项] 学习此动作时，需循序渐进，按由易到难的顺序进行练习。

[Tips and notes] When learning this exercise, it is necessary to progress gradually and practice in order from easy to difficult.

（9）坐式（踞坐）。一脚舒展，一脚弯曲，两手牵拉足三里处，膝盖用力向前，身体后仰牵拉，这一刻全身皆处于拉伸状态，病气在内消散，就好像骨头完全松解散开一般。左右手脚互换做上述动作，各21次（图1-50）。有助于逐渐去除肩部脊背的风寒、血寒、筋脉拘急。

(9) Take a sitting position. Sit with the knees raised and the feet on the ground. Extend one leg and bend the other, put the hands on the point Zusanli (ST 36) to pull the leg, push the knee forward, and lean backward. At this moment, the whole body is in a stretching state, and illnesses are dissipated, just like the bones are completely relaxed and separated. Change the position of the hands and feet to do the exercise, and repeat 21 times on each side (Figure 1-50). This exercise can help

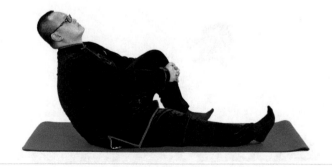

图1-50　Figure 1-50

gradually eliminate wind and cold in the shoulders and spine, cold in blood, and muscle/tendon spasm.

[操作要领与注意事项] 完成此动作过程中, 膝盖向前顶, 身体向后仰, 两向用力, 形成对拉劲, 利于周身气机运行。

[Tips and notes] During the exercise, push the knee forward and lean the body backward, exerting force in both directions to create a stretching sensation, which facilitates the circulation of qi throughout the body.

(10) 卧式(俯卧)。两手向后反方向尽量用力牵拉两脚, 仰头, 脚趾向外用力。拔伸时先缓慢, 做到极势后迅速放松(图 1-51)。上述动作反复做7次。两手向前伸直舒展, 脚自然摇动, 膝盖不动, 手和脚各做14次。适用于脊柱和腰部的闷痛、风冷病症。

(10) Take a prone position. Use both hands to fully pull the feet. Raise the head and extend the toes outward. When stretching, do it slowly and then quickly relax when reaching the maximum range of motion (Figure 1–51). Repeat the above movements 7 times. Extend both hands forward and stretch them out, sway the feet naturally, and keep the knees still. Repeat the movement 14 times. This exercise can help alleviate

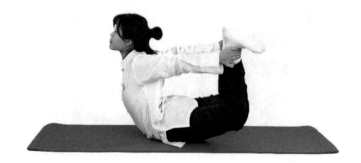

图1-51　Figure 1-51

oppressive pain and pathogenic cold and wind in the spine and lower back.

[操作要领与注意事项] 此动作利于全身气血流畅疏布。完成动作二时，体质虚弱的人，肘膝可不离开地面；体质较好的人，肘膝抬起离开地面，效果更佳。

[Tips and notes] This exercise facilitates the smooth flow and distribution of qi and blood throughout the body. For the second movement, people with a weak constitution can keep their elbows and knees on the ground, while those with a better constitution can lift them off the ground for better results.

（11）站式（立正）。① 两手尽力向后舒展，然后曲肘向后，手掌空按28次（图1-52）。② 转腰，两手自然下垂，手掌向四个方位做转动（图1-53）。适用于手臂的筋脉拘急。

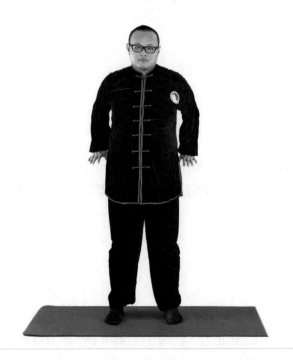

图1-52　Figure 1-52

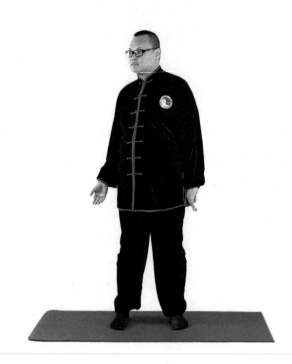

图1-53　Figure 1-53

(11) Take an upright standing position. ① Fully extend both hands backward, then bend the elbows backward and press the palms outward 28 times (Figure 1–52). ② Rotate the waist, hang both hands naturally, and then rotate the palms (Figure 1–53). This exercise can help alleviate muscle/tendon spasm in the arms.

［操作要领与注意事项］① 动作一：立身中正，注意腰臀部的放松。② 动作二：转腰与手部运动须彼此协调联动。

[Tips and notes] ① For the first movement, stand upright and relax the waist and hips. ② For the second movement, the waist and hand movements should be coordinated with each other.

（12）站式（立正）。① 两手与肩齐高，尽力舒展；合掌，手指指尖向下，当肩膀产生闷痛时，合掌上下摇摆，做14次（图1-

54）。② 手自然放下至髋部水平（图1-55），然后缓慢上举，再快速下落，手轻轻地做前后震颤放松，7次（图1-56）。有助于逐

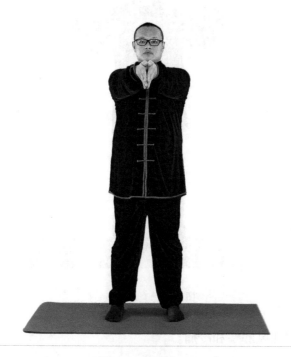

图1-54　Figure 1-54

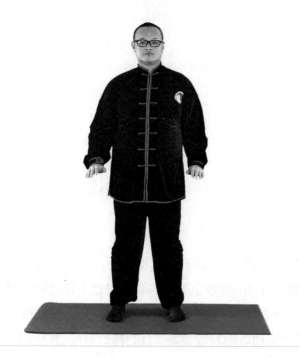

图1-55　Figure 1-55

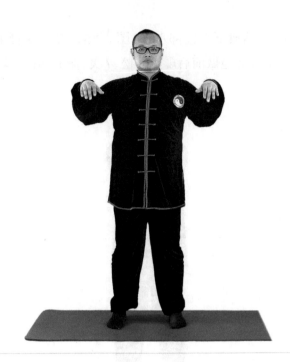

图1-56　Figure 1-56

渐去除肩部风邪寒和冷痛。

(12) Take an upright standing position. ① Raise the hands to shoulder level and fully stretch them out. Then clasp the hands together with the fingertips pointing downward. Swing the clasped hands up and down 14 times when experiencing an oppressive pain sensation (Figure 1–54). ② Drop the hands naturally to hip level (Figure 1–55), then slowly raise them up and quickly drop them down. Lightly shake them back and forth to relax 7 times (Figure 1–56). This exercise can help gradually relieve shoulder pain caused by pathogenic wind and cold.

［操作要领与注意事项］① 动作一：手指指尖向下才可以拔伸到肩胛与背部；合掌上下摇摆时要注意手和肩胛、脊柱的整体联动。② 动作二：手上举，须超过头顶，并尽力做到极势；手下落时，自然产生前后的轻轻震颤，放松脊柱、肩部、肘部、手腕、手指。

[Tips and notes] ① For the first movement, to stretch the

scapula and back, the fingertips must point downwards. When swaying the clasped hands up and down, pay attention to coordinating the movement of the hands with the scapula and spine as a whole. ② For the second movement, fully raise the hands above the head. Vibrate the hands slightly and naturally when dropping them to relax the spine, shoulders, elbows, wrists and fingers.

（13）站式。① 两手掌反方向托于两肩前，贴住两腋尽力做上下快速振摇，反复做21次（图1-57）。完成后，手不移动位，两肘部用力向上举，尽力做到极势，上下振摇14次（图1-58）。两手握拳做7次（图1-59），握拳后合拢做21次（图1-60）。适用于颈、肩部的筋脉拘急和劳损。② 一手握拳向左，另一手抓住对侧手肘，向内牵拉，尽力拔伸到极势（图1-61）；握拳的手放松，舒展手指3次；然后换手做28次，尽力做到极势（图1-62）。可调理肘部和肩部的筋脉痉挛。③ 两手向上托起，尽力做到极势，上下做21次（图1-63）。手不动，肘部尽力向上做到极

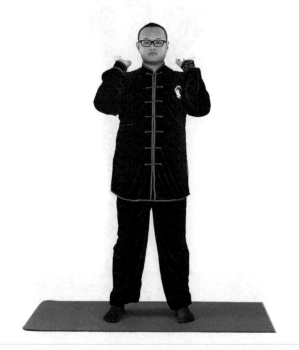

图1-57　Figure 1-57

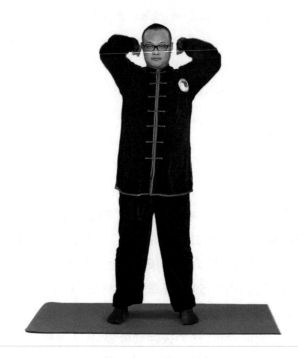

图1-58　Figure 1-58

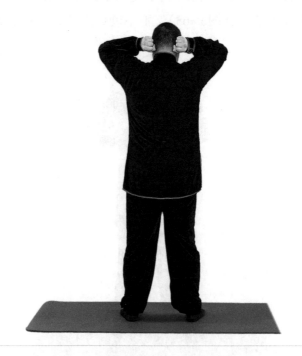

图1-59　Figure 1-59

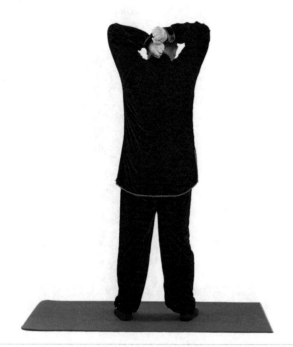

图1-60　Figure 1-60

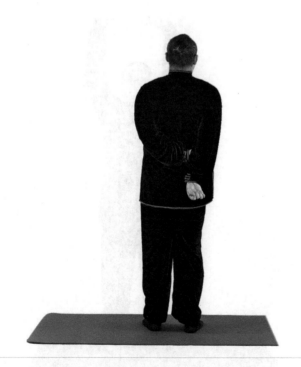

图1-61　Figure 1-61

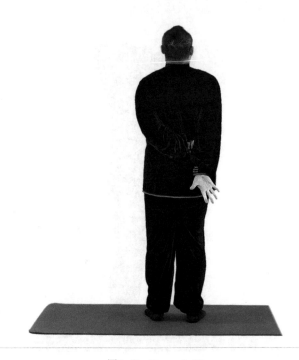

图1-62　Figure 1-62

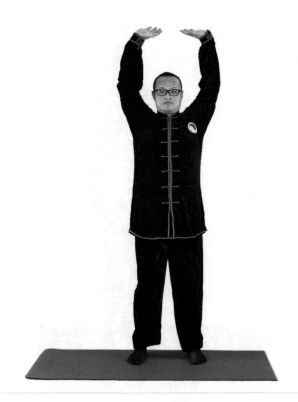

图1-63　Figure 1-63

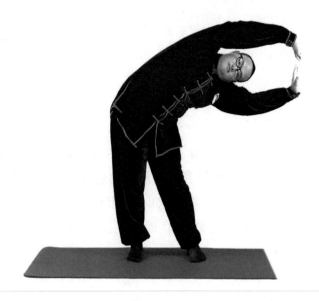

图1-64　Figure 1-64

势,做7次。手、肘、臂都不动,尽力侧身,左右来回做21次(图1-64)。适用于颈椎的风寒、拘急不舒。

(13) Take a standing position. ① Place the palms of both hands in front of both shoulders in opposite directions, press against both armpits, and shake up and down 21 times (Figure 1–57). Keep the position of the hands, fully lift both elbows upward, and shake up and down 14 times (Figure 1–58). Clench the fists with both hands 7 times (Figure 1–59), and then close the hands 21 times (Figure 1–60). This exercise can help alleviate muscle/tendon spasm and strain in the neck and shoulders. ② Make a fist with one hand and stretch towards the left, while grabbing the elbow with the other hand and fully pulling inward (Figure 1–61); relax the hand making a fist and stretch the fingers 3 times. Then change the position of the hands and repeat the exercise 28 times (Figure 1–62). This exercise can relieve muscle/tendon spasm in the elbows and shoulders. ③ Fully lift both hands up and stretch 21 times (Figure 1–63). Keep the hands still, and fully lift the elbows 7 times. Keep the hands, elbows and arms still, fully

lean sideways and repeat 21 times on each side (Figure 1–64). This exercise can help alleviate wind, cold and muscle/tendon spasm in the cervical vertebrae.

［操作要领与注意事项］① 动作一：手须贴住两腋做上下运动。② 动作二：肩胛与背脊在放松的前提下，以脊柱为中心做上下延展、左右延展。在极势时不用浊力，拔伸时肘部向后向内卷。忌将肩胛骨夹紧。③ 动作三：上臂尽量向脑后方向靠拢。

[Tips and notes] ① For the first movement, keep the hands close to the armpits and move them up and down. ② For the second movement, relax the shoulder blades and spine to extend up and down and left and right around the spine without using too much force. When extending, roll the elbows backward and inward. Avoid squeezing the shoulder blades too tightly. ③ For the third movement, try to bring the forearms as close as possible to the back of the head.

10. 风气候提要
10. Disorders induced by qi and wind

气虚感受风邪所致。

Qi deficiency coupled with pathogenic wind may result in these disorders.

站式。一手尽力前托，做到极势；一手放于乳房处，向后牵拉使胸部舒展。不能用僵力令胸口打开，（气）向下松沉，两手互换再做上述动作21次（图1–65）。将两手攀住膝盖，身体向后仰,尽力做到极势做21次(图1-66)。有助于去除风热导致的烦闷疼痛,使风府和云门的邪气散去。

Take a standing position. Fully stretch forward one hand, while placing the other hand on the breast to pull backward to stretch the chest. Do not use rigid force to open the chest.

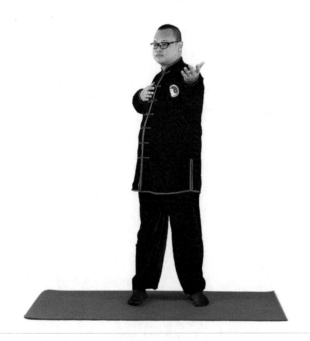

图1-65　Figure 1-65

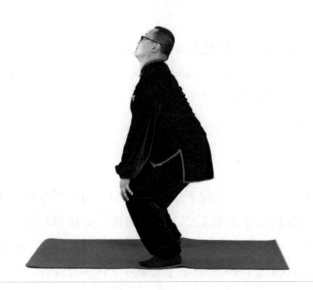

图1-66　Figure 1-66

Sink qi and then change the position of the hands to repeat the movements 21 times (Figure 1–65). Hold the knees with the hands and fully lean backward 21 times (Figure 1–66). This exercise can help relieve vexation and pain caused by wind and heat, and disperse pathogenic factors in the points Fengfu (GV 16) and Yunmen (LU 2).

［操作要领与注意事项］两手固定皆不可用力，肩膀也尽可能不动，以胸部运动带动肩、肘和手部的运动，不可单纯做扩胸运动。

[Tips and notes] Fix both hands without exerting force, and keep the shoulders still. Guide the movement of the shoulders, elbows and hands with the movement of the chest, and do not simply do chest expansion exercises.

11. 头面风候提要
11. Disorders in the head and face due to wind

身体虚弱，风邪侵犯头面诸阳经脉所致。

Pathogenic wind may invade the yang meridians in the face and head when the body is weak, and subsequently result in disorders.

（1）站式。一手托住下颌，极力向上，另一手尽量用力向后舒展，手掌向四个方位转动，这一刻皆尽力做到极势，做28次（图1–67）。两手互换做上述动作。两手托住下颌，使身体侧身旋转14次（图1–68），有助于去除手、肩、头部的风邪，适用于昏睡。

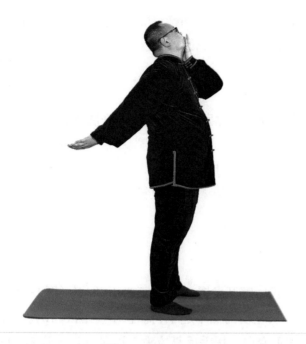

图1-67　Figure 1-67

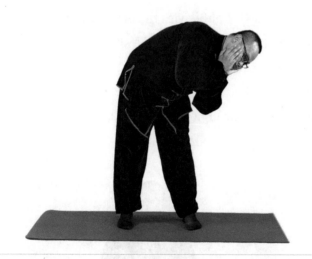

图1-68　Figure 1-68

(1) Take a standing position. Hold the chin with one hand and fully lift it. Fully extend the other hand backward and rotate the palm 28 times (Figure 1–67). Then change the position of the hands and repeat the above movements. Hold the chin with both hands and rotate the body sideways 14 times (Figure

1-68). This exercise can help dispel pathogenic wind in the hands, shoulders and head, and also treat lethargy.

[操作要领与注意事项] 此动作可舒展颈肩部的筋膜，利于气血运行。

[Tips and notes] This exercise can stretch the fascia of the neck and shoulders, and promote the circulation of qi and blood.

（2）坐式。解开发髻，握固，不吸不呼1次（图1-69）。然后向东而坐，从左右两侧举起手，掩住两耳（图1-70）。适用于头风，令头发不变白。用手反复梳头5次，使血脉流通（图1-71）。

(2) Take a sitting position. Untie the hair bun, bend the thumb, and grasp it tightly with the other four fingers. Passively hold the breath (Figure 1-69). Then sit facing east and raise the hands to cover the ears (Figure 1-70). This exercise can help treat head wind and prevent gray hair. Use the hands to comb the hair 5 times to promote blood circulation (Figure 1-71).

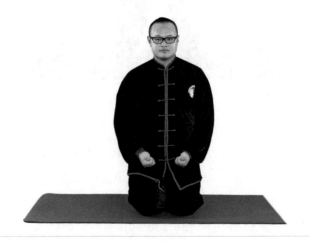

图1-69　Figure 1-69

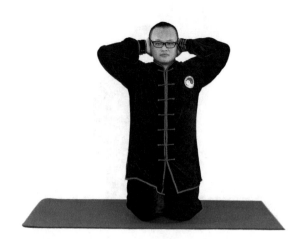

图1-70　Figure 1-70

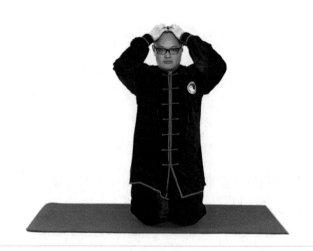

图1-71　Figure 1-71

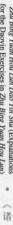
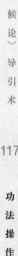
　　［操作要领与注意事项］向东而坐，以利气机生发。握固，将大拇指弯曲，其余四指向内握住大拇指。完成此动作过程中，两手上举起时，心中不能缺少向下内敛之意。

　　[Tips and notes] Sit facing east to facilitate the generation of qi. For each hand, bend the thumb and grasp it with the other four fingers. When raising the hands, sink the intention.

　　（3）坐式（端坐）。舒展腰部，头左右舒展（图1-72），闭眼，鼻纳气，至满，做7次这样的呼吸。适用于头风症。

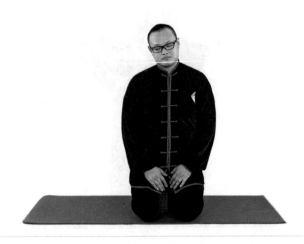

图1-72 Figure 1-72

(3) Take an upright sitting position. Stretch the lower back, stretch the head left and right (Figure 1–72), close the eyes, and inhale deeply through the nose 7 times. This exercise can help relieve head wind.

［操作要领与注意事项］此动作中,腰部舒展有强壮肾府之效,故有助于除头风。

[Tips and notes] Stretching the lower back can strengthen the kidney and help alleviate head wind.

(4) 站式、坐式、卧式。头痛,鼻纳气,以口缓缓吐气(图1- 73),这样的呼吸做30次才停止。

(4) Take a standing, sitting or lying position. To treat headache, inhale through the nose and exhale slowly through the mouth 30 times (Figure 1–73).

［操作要领与注意事项］鼻纳气之关键在于打开咽腔和鼻窍,有利于醒脑开窍,故适用于头痛。

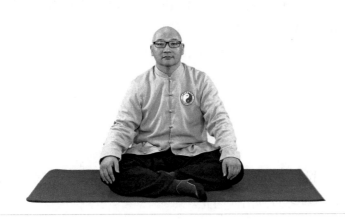

图1-73　Figure 1-73

[Tips and notes]　The key to breathing in through the nose lies in opening the throat and nose, which is beneficial for awakening the mind and treating headache.

（5）卧式。抱着两膝卧在地上，不吸不呼8次（图1-74）。适用于从胸到头的疾病，包括耳、目、鼻、喉的疼痛。

(5) Take a lying position. Lie on the ground, hold the knees with the hands, and passively hold the breath 8 times (Figure 1-74). This exercise can help treat such disorders located between the chest and the head as pain in the ears, eyes, nose and throat.

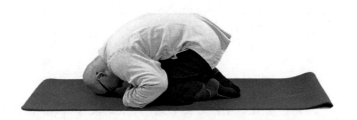

图1-74　Figure 1-74

［操作要领与注意事项］俯卧，内心宁静，不呼不吸，有利于醒脑开窍，故适用于诸上窍疼痛。

[Tips and notes] Taking a prone position, keeping a peaceful mind and passively holding the breath can help awaken the brain and treat pain in the upper orifices.

（6）卧式。治头痛，可仰卧（图1–75）。闭气至极限，而后鼻吸鼻呼。练习直到出汗为止。

(6) Take a lying position. To treat headache, take a supine position (Figure 1–75). Fully hold the breath, and then breathe through the nose. Practice until sweating is present.

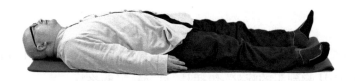

图1–75　Figure 1–75

［操作要领与注意事项］完成此动作过程中，闭气至极限，建议医护人员在旁看护。鼻吸鼻呼，有利于醒脑开窍，故适用于头痛。

[Tips and notes] Since this exercise needs to fully hold the breath, it is recommended to do this exercise under the watchful eye of a person. Nasal breathing can help awaken the brain and relieve headache.

（7）站式。立正，两手交叉于脑后，做到极势，振摇14次（图1–76）；手掌反复按头14次；然后两手拉头向后仰，并维持这个状态一段时间（图1–77），然后向四个角的方向，快速牵拉21

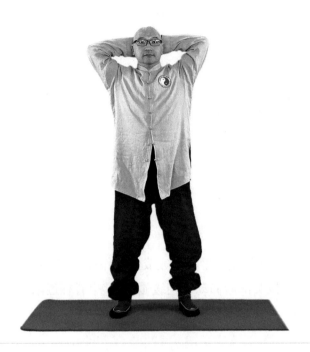

图1-76　Figure 1-76

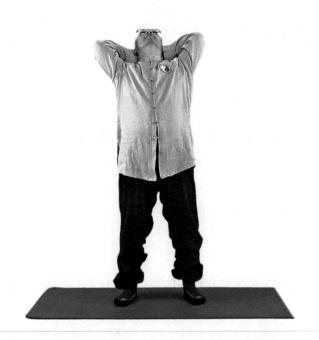

图1-77　Figure 1-77

次。有助于去除头、腋、臂、肘部的邪风。

(7) Take a standing position. Stand upright, fully cross the hands behind the head, and shake 14 times (Figure 1–76). Then use the palms to press the head 14 times. Next, use both hands to pull the head backward and maintain this position for a period of time (Figure 1–77), and then quickly pull it in the direction of the four corners 21 times. This exercise can help eliminate pathogenic wind in the head, armpits, arms and elbows.

［操作要领与注意事项］完成此动作过程中，两手振摇动作需快；两手拉头部后仰动作当缓慢，使整个脊柱逐渐拔起。

[Tips and notes] Shake the hands swiftly, and lean backward slowly to stretch the whole spine.

12. 风头眩候提要
12. Wind-induced dizziness

气血不足，风邪侵袭入脑，牵引目系所致。

Deficiency of qi and blood coupled with the invasion of pathogenic wind in the brain may influence the eyes and subsequently cause this disorder.

（1）卧式。两手抱右膝贴住胸口（图1–78），有助于去除风眩。

(1) Take a lying position. Hold the right knee with both hands and bring it close to the chest (Figure 1–78). This exercise can help treat wind-induced dizziness.

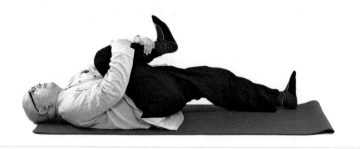

图1-78　Figure 1-78

［操作要领与注意事项］完成此动作时，仰卧为佳。抱右膝有利于壮精血。

[Tips and notes] Taking a supine position can better the efficacy of this exercise. Holding the right knee can strengthen the essence and blood.

（2）卧式（仰卧）。两手握住辘轳，身体倒悬，使脚比头高。适用于头晕风癫。坐在地上，伸展两脚，用绳扎住，再用粗绳扎好后并绑在辘轳上，转动辘轳使脚超过头而后放下，整个过程脚要离开地面。上述动作尽力做12次。适用于头晕风癫。经常这样练习，逐渐可使身体也能离开地面而不坠落。

(2) Take a supine position. Hold onto a windlass with both hands, and let the body hang down with the feet higher than the head. This exercise can help treat dizziness and epilepsy. Sit on the ground, stretch out the feet, tie them up with a rope, and then tie the rope securely to a windlass. Turn the windlass to make the feet go over the head and then back down again, making sure that the feet do not touch the ground throughout the process. Repeat 12 times. This exercise can help treat dizziness and epilepsy. Over time, practice to lift the entire body off the ground without falling.

［操作要领与注意事项］完成此动作需要外固定装置，在医护人员辅助下完成。

[Tips and notes] This exercise requires an external apparatus for fixation and should be done under the watchful eye of a person.

（3）站式。一手舒展打开，手掌向上；另一手握住下颌向外侧推拉。每次做到极势，左右手交换做上述动作14次。然后手不动，身体向两侧快速尽量转动，做14次（图1-19）。适用于颈椎活动障碍、头痛脑眩、喉痹、肩部冷痛、偏风的病症。

(3) Take a standing position. Fully extend and open one hand with the palm facing upward, grip the jaw and push and pull it outward with the other hand. Change the position of the hands and do the above movement 14 times. Then, keep the hands still, and quickly rotate the body to both sides 14 times (Figure 1-19). This exercise can help treat impaired cervical movement, headache, dizziness, throat *Bi*-impediment, pain and cold in the shoulders, and hemiplegia.

［操作要领与注意事项］完成此动作过程中，容易导致颈椎小关节错位，宜缓做。忌爆发力。

[Tips and notes] Since this movement is easy to cause dislocation of the small joints in the cervical vertebrae, do it slowly and avoid using brute force.

（4）站式、坐式。有人觉得脊背僵紧不舒憋闷，无论什么时节，可以缩咽于肩（图1-36），仰面，肩胛骨上抬，头顺着左右两个方向移动，做21次（图1-37），然后稍停，待气血平复再做下一次。开始时要慢做再逐渐加快，不能先快后慢。如果是无病之人，可以在清晨3点至5点、中午11点至13点、下午17点至19点三个时间段操作，每个时段做14次。适用于寒热病、脊腰颈项痛、风痹、口内生疮、牙齿风、头眩。

(4) Take a standing or sitting position. For back rigidity, tuck in the throat (Figure 1–36), raise the head and scapula, and swing the head to both sides 21 times (Figure 1–37). Then take a break to calm down qi and blood and do it again. Begin slowly and gradually increase the speed. Avoid starting fast and then slowing down. People in good health can do this exercise 14 times during each of the three time periods: 3–5 am, 11 am– 1 pm, and 5–7 pm. This exercise can help treat chills, fever, and pain in the lower back, neck and shoulders, and can also treat wind *Bi*-impediment, mouth ulcer, toothache, and dizziness.

[操作要领与注意事项] 腰背脊柱放松，肩部自然打开，即仰面带脊背肩胛向后固定，在此基础上再缩咽。

[Tips and notes] Relax the waist, back and spine, and open the shoulders naturally. Raise the head to fix the spine and scapula, and then tuck in the throat.

(5) 坐式。坐在地上，交叉两脚，两手从脚弯处伸入，低头，再把手交叉于项后（图1-79）。适用于久寒自身无力变暖、耳朵听不到声音。

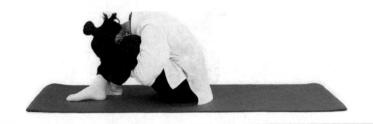

图1-79　Figure 1-79

Zhu Bing Yuan Hou Lun Dao Yin Shu (Explanations
for the Daoyin Exercises in Zhu Bing Yuan Hou Lun)

·

《诸病源候论》导引术

126

功法操作

·

Movements

(5) Take a sitting position. Sit on the ground with the feet crossed, then lower the head and cross the hands behind the neck (Figure 1–79). This exercise can help treat chronic cold sensations in the body and deafness.

［操作要领与注意事项］松解打开脊骨、胯骨，有利于督脉气血运行。此动作难度大，易受伤。初学者练习此动作时忌幅度大、速度快，宜循序渐进。

[Tips and notes] Relax and open the spine and hips to circulate qi and blood within the Governor Vessel. This exercise is difficult and can easily cause injury. Beginners should start slowly and gradually increase the range of motion.

（6）坐式。脚放于头上，不呼不吸12次（图1–80）。适用于身体大寒感觉不到暖热，顽固性冷疾、耳聋目眩。长期练此动作就能有效，每次做30次，不能改变。

(6) Take a sitting position. Place the feet on the top of the head and passively hold the breath 12 times (Figure 1–80). Persistent exercise can help treat extreme cold sensations in the body, intractable cold-related disorders, deafness and blurred

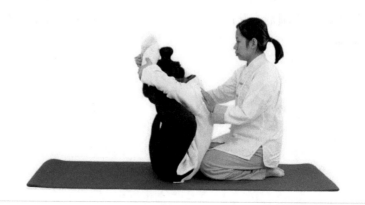

图1–80　Figure 1–80

vision. Do this exercise 30 times per session.

［操作要领与注意事项］松解打开脊骨、胯骨，有利于督脉气血运行。此动作难度大，易受伤。初学者完成此动作时忌幅度大、速度快，宜循序渐进，在医护人员辅助下完成。

[Tips and notes] Relax and open the spine and hips to circulate qi and blood within the Governor Vessel. This exercise is difficult and can easily cause injury. Beginners should start slowly and gradually increase the range of motion, and do this exercise under the watchful eye of a person.

（7）坐式。低头，不呼不吸6次（图1–81）。适用于耳聋、目癫眩、咽喉不利。

(7) Take a sitting position. Lower the head and passively hold the breath 6 times (Figure 1–81). This exercise can help treat deafness, blurred vision, and throat discomfort.

［操作要领与注意事项］内心宁静，不呼不吸，气机萌新。低头，放松颈椎，醒脑开窍。

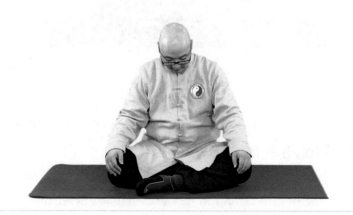

图1–81　Figure 1–81

[Tips and notes] Keeping a tranquil mind and passively holding the breath can promote the qi activity. Lowering the head and relaxing the neck can awaken the mind.

（8）卧式（跪伏）。侧身以耳贴地，不呼不吸6次（图1-82）。适用于耳聋目眩。以耳聋侧伏卧，两膝并拢，耳紧贴地，专心用力贴住至极限。长期练此动作可改善听力，耳闻十方；也可使头倒转向下时不觉眩晕，也适用于一些难治的疾病。

(8) Take a lying position. Lie on the side with the ear touching the ground, and passively hold the breath 6 times (Figure 1-82). This exercise can help treat deafness and blurred vision. Lie on the side with the deaf ear, bring both knees together, and press the ear firmly against the ground. Regular practice can improve hearing and also help relieve blurred vision when the head is inverted. In addition, this exercise can be used to help treat certain intractable disorders.

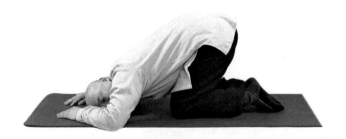

图1-82　Figure 1-82

［操作要领与注意事项］内心宁静，不呼不吸，气机萌新。耳聋侧贴地，有利于放松脊椎，开耳窍。

[Tips and notes] Keeping a tranquil mind and passively holding the breath can promote the qi activity. Lying on the side with the deaf ear touching the ground can help relax the spine and benefit the ears.

（9）站式。立正，转身向后看，然后不呼不吸7次（图1–83）。适用于咳逆、胸中病、寒热癫疾、喉不利、咽干咽塞。

(9) Take a standing position. Stand upright, turn the head to look back, and passively hold the breath 7 times (Figure 1–83). This exercise can help treat cough, chest disorders, chills and fever, convulsions, dry throat and other throat disorders.

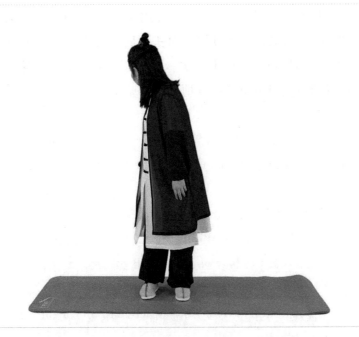

图1–83   Figure 1–83

［操作要领与注意事项］完成此动作过程中，以眼神带动整个脊柱运动，低头向后看，做连续动作。动作似狼顾，眼光内敛不外露，从下往上做下弦线弧度运动。

[Tips and notes] During this exercise, use the movement of the eyes to drive the movement of the spine. Keep the movements continuous and smooth.

13. 风癫候提要

13. Depressive psychosis

气血不足，风邪侵袭入阴经所致。

Deficiency of qi and blood coupled with the invasion of pathogenic wind in the yin meridians may induce this condition.

卧式（仰卧）。两手握住辘轳，身体倒悬，使脚比头高。适用于头晕风癫。坐在地上，伸展两脚，用绳扎住，再用粗绳扎好后并绑在辘轳上，转动辘轳使脚超过头而后放下，整个过程脚要离开地面。上述动作尽力做12次。适用于头晕风癫。经常这样练习，逐渐可使身体也能离开地面而不坠落。

Take a supine position. Hold onto a windlass with both hands, and let the body hang down with the feet higher than the head. This exercise can help treat dizziness and epilepsy. Sit on the ground, stretch out the feet, tie them up with a rope, and then tie the rope securely to a windlass. Turn the windlass to make the feet go over the head and then back down again, making sure that the feet do not touch the ground throughout the process. Repeat 12 times. This exercise can help treat dizziness and epilepsy. Over time, practice to lift the entire body off the ground without falling.

［操作要领与注意事项］完成此动作需要外固定装置，在医护人员辅助下完成。

[Tips and notes] This exercise requires an external apparatus for fixation and should be done under the watchful eye of a person.

14. 风邪候提要

14. Disorders induced by pathogenic wind

风邪是风气伤人致病的统称。起居失常、饮食不节、脏腑虚损、气血不足,都易感受风邪。

Contributing factors may include an improper diet, irregular lifestyle, deficiency of zang-fu organs, and insufficiency of qi and blood.

(1) 站式、坐式。脾主土,主肌肉,人身暖和则可以发汗,有助于去除风冷邪气。如果腹部胀气,必须先使脚暖和,肚脐与气海穴上下按摩,不限次数,以多为好,左回右转21次(图1-84)。中和之气发挥作用的原则是,用身内一百一十三法,回转三百六十骨节,经脉畅行筋骨活动,气血布散润泽,二十四脉气和润,脏腑协调。中和之气具体运用的方法是,活动、旋转、摇摆、振动头部,手气上行,心气下行,清楚察觉气的去和来。无论是平手、侧腰、转身、摩气、屈转、回缩、转动各种动作结束后,心气向下散,送至涌泉穴,每一步骤和动作都遵循气的运行规律,运用得好则有益身心。不懂运用气的原则和方法,反而导致气紊乱。

(1) Take a standing or sitting position. The spleen governs muscles. When the body is warm, sweating can help dispel pathogenic wind and cold. For abdominal distension, warm up the feet first and massage the area around the navel and the point Qihai (CV 6) up and down. There is no limit to the number of massage but more is better (Figure 1–84). To facilitate the functions of harmonious qi, adopt the 113 internal methods within the body to unblock the meridians, promote the circulation of qi and blood, and harmonize the zang-fu organs. The specific methods for utilizing the harmonious qi include

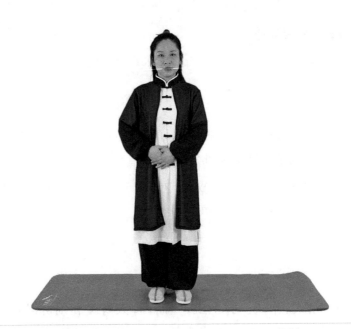

图1-84　Figure 1-84

moving, rotating, shaking and vibrating the head, ascending hand qi, descending heart qi, and keeping a clear mind on the coming and going of qi. At the end, descend heart qi to the point Yongquan (KI 1). Each step and movement should follow the rules of qi circulation, and using it properly can benefit the body and mind. Not understanding the principles or methods of using qi can lead to qi disorders.

［操作要领与注意事项］用身内一百一十三法（三十六天罡，七十二地煞，统以五行），意在以天人相应的规律引导气机运行。

[Tips and notes] Adopting the 113 internal methods within the body is to guide the flow of qi according to man-nature correspondence.

（2）站式、坐式、卧式。闭眼闭气，内视丹田，鼻缓缓纳气，令腹部胀满至极点，以口缓缓吐气，不要听到气息声，吸气多吐气少，气息轻柔（图1-85）。内视五脏，看到五脏的形色，再内视胃中，令神光充盈，鲜活明晰洁白如丝绢。做到疲倦至极并且出汗就可以停止了，用粉轻扑于身上，按摩身体。汗未出但感到疲倦的，也可以停止。待第二天再做。

(2) Take a standing, sitting or lying position. Close the eyes, hold the breath, focus on the *Dantian*, and inhale slowly through the nose to make the abdomen full. Then exhale slowly through the mouth without making any sound. The inhalation should be longer than the exhalation, and the breathing should be gentle and soft (Figure 1–85). Look at the five zang organs, and observe their forms and colors. Then look at the stomach, and make it bright, lively, clear and white as silk. Continue until exhaustion and sweating are present, then stop, lightly apply powders to the body, and massage the body. If exhaustion is felt but sweating has not yet occurred, stop and repeat the practice the following day.

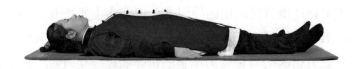

图1-85　Figure 1–85

［操作要领与注意事项］此导引动作中，闭气属有为法，然后纳气、吐气，气息须轻柔，再做观想。观想以丝绢形容白色的鲜活、流动、飘荡，不宜观想成实物。

[Tips and notes] In this exercise, holding the breath is considered an active method. After that, one should inhale and exhale gently, and the visualization should be done afterward. The visualization should describe the vividness, fluidity, and fluttering of white silk instead of a real object.

（3）站式、坐式、卧式。存想巨雷闪电，雷鸣电闪，进入腹中。能这样坚持存想，有助于疾病自然消除。

(3) Take a standing, sitting or lying position. Visualize great thunder and lightning, with thunderbolts and flashes entering into the abdomen. Persistent visualization can help treat disorders.

［操作要领与注意事项］完成此动作时，实地观察巨雷闪电，更利于感同身受，帮助观想自然流出。

[Tips and notes] During this exercise, observing real thunder and lightning can better help visualization.

二、虚劳病诸候提要
Daoyin Exercises for Consumptive Conditions

本节论述虚劳病诸候的导引术。虚劳病主要指五劳、六极、七伤。五劳，按五脏分证，包括肺劳、肝劳、心劳、脾劳、肾劳。六极指由疲劳引起的六种较为严重的机体病理变化，包括气极、血极、筋极、骨极、肌极、精极。七伤指七种对身心伤害的因素，按五脏分证，包括大饱伤脾、大怒伤肝、强力受湿伤肾、形寒寒饮伤肺、忧思伤心、风雨寒暑伤形、大恐伤志。

This chapter introduces the daoyin exercises for such consumptive conditions as the five exhaustions, six excesses, and seven damages. The five exhaustions are classified according to the five zang organs and include lung exhaustion, liver exhaustion, heart exhaustion, spleen exhaustion, and kidney exhaustion. The six excesses refer to six more severe pathological changes in the body caused by fatigue, including qi excess, blood excess, tendon excess, bone excess, muscle excess, and essence excess. The seven damages refer to seven pathogenic factors that lead to deficiency and consumption, including improper diet, anxiety, drink, sex, hunger, over-exertion, and damage to meridians, collaterals, *Ying*-nutrients, *Wei*-defense and qi.

1. 虚劳候提要
1. Consumptive conditions

虚劳病包括五劳、六极、七伤。

Consumptive conditions include the five exhaustions, six excesses, and seven damages.

（1）站式、坐式、卧式。两手托两颊，手不动，两肘向内使筋绷紧，腰内随之绷紧，维持这个状态一段时间（图2-1）。两肘头向外放松，使肘、肩、腰内气缓缓散去，放松到极势，当身体感到憋闷时再重新开始做，反复做7次。适用于肘臂劳损。

(1) Take a standing, sitting or lying position. Hold both cheeks with both hands, keep the hands still, pull the elbows inward to tighten the tendons, and tighten the waist accordingly. Maintain

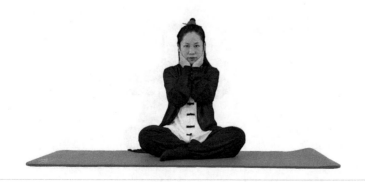

图2-1　Figure 2-1

this posture for a period of time (Figure 2-1). Relax the elbows to dissipate qi within the elbows, shoulders and waist, totally relax the body until an oppressive feeling is present, and repeat 7 times. This exercise can help treat strain in the elbows and arms.

［操作要领与注意事项］完成此动作过程中，阴（内）侧筋经延长产生紧促感，筋经鼓动肾气，故能治疗肘臂劳损。

[Tips and notes] During the exercise, the stretching of the yin (inner) meridians produces a tight sensation, and the stimulation of the meridians activates kidney qi, thus helping to treat strain in the elbows and arms.

（2）站式、坐式。两手抱两乳，快速用力前后振摇，尽力做14次。手不动摇，两肘头上下振摇21次。适用于两肘内的劳损，使心气向下行，血脉流畅布散全身，没有壅滞（图2-2）。

(2) Take a standing or sitting position. Hold both breasts with both hands, and quickly shake the body back and forth 14 times. Without moving the hands, shake the elbows up and down 21 times. This exercise can help treat strain in the elbows, promote the downward flow of heart qi, and circulate blood (Figure 2-2).

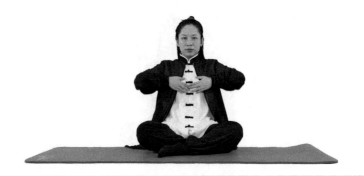

图2-2　Figure 2-2

［操作要领与注意事项］完成此动作过程中，手固定，肘部不主动用力，脊柱放松，肾气鼓动，以身体带动肘部运动则可带动全身气血流畅疏布。阴（内）侧筋经的运动带动外部肢体动作，才能使心气向下行。若为外部动作主动牵引，易使心气向上行。

[Tips and notes] During the exercise, fix the hands, the elbows do not actively use force, relax the spine, and use the body to drive the movement of the elbows, which can help promote the circulation of qi and blood. The movement of the yin (inner) meridians drives the movement of the body, allowing heart qi to flow downward. Actively moving the body is prone to cause heart qi to flow upward.

（3）坐式。两脚跟相对，臀部坐于脚跟上，两脚脚趾向外扒开，两膝跪地，尽力向外扒，然后两手自然舒展，做前后拉伸，足膝手皆尽力达到极限，做21次（图2-3）。适用于虚劳、腰脊膝疼痛、伤冷脾痹。

(3) Take a sitting position. Place the heels together, sit on them, extend the toes outward, kneel down with both knees, then fully stretch the arms forward and backward, and repeat 21 times (Figure 2–3). This exercise can help treat consumptive

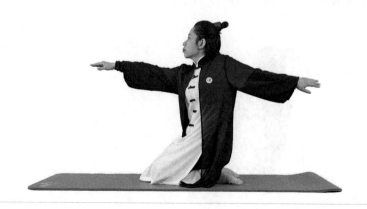

图2-3　Figure 2-3

conditions, pain in the lower back, spine and knees, and spleen *Bi*-impediment due to cold.

［操作要领与注意事项］此动作通过姿势外部拉伸完成，是动态舒展的过程。

[Tips and notes] This movement is a dynamic stretching.

（4）跪式。跪一脚，臀部坐于上，两手从大腿内侧扳脚上翻，脚跟向下用力。身体向外后侧，尽力做到极势，这一刻全身皆处于对拔拉伸状态，向心来去做14次（图2-4）。左右手脚互换再做上述动作。适用于五劳、足臂疼闷、膝冷阴冷。

(4) Take a kneeling position. Sit on one foot, use both hands to pull the other foot, exert downward pressure on the heel, fully lean the upper body outward and backward, and repeat 14 times (Figure 2–4). Change the position of the feet and repeat the above exercise. This exercise can help treat the five exhaustions, oppressive pain in the feet and arms, and cold in the knees.

［操作要领与注意事项］完成此动作时，扳脚上翻，内合于腰；对拔拉伸时，肘、脊柱、上肢放松打开。

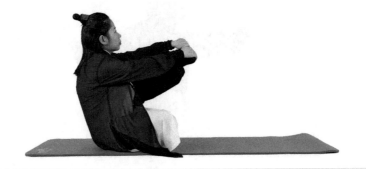

图2-4　Figure 2-4

[Tips and notes] During the exercise, when pulling the foot upward, relax and open the elbows, spine and upper limbs.

（5）坐式（踞坐）。两手抱膝下足三里穴下2寸，迅速抱膝贴身，尽量用力，脚朝两个方向悬起，就像折叠的胡床（图2-5）。保持这样的姿势一会，恢复踞坐姿势，再做抱膝动作上下反复14次。适用于腰足臂内虚劳、膀胱冷。

(5) Take a sitting position. Sit with the knees raised and the feet on the ground. Place both hands 2 *cun* below the point Zusanli (ST 36), and then quickly and fully bring the knees close to the body (Figure 2–5). Maintain this posture for a while, and then repeat 14 times. This exercise can help treat deficiency in the lower back, feet and arms, and can also treat cold in the bladder.

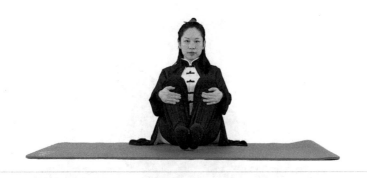

图2-5　Figure 2–5

［操作要领与注意事项］大腿与小腿折叠抱膝如胡床。由于横向抱膝之力，由折叠形成上下争力，利于上身拔起。

[Tips and notes] Fully bring the knees close to the body to lift the upper body.

（6）坐式。两脚对踏，脚掌合拢，向会阴侧做快速的轻微收缩，两手捧膝头，朝两个方向用力到极致，按捺14次（图2-6）。

然后身体尽力向两侧活动14次（图2-7），腰部前后活动7次（图2-8）。适用于心劳、痔病、膝冷。调理虚劳未完全恢复时，须谨言慎语、不怒不喜。

(6) Take a sitting position. Bring the soles together, quickly and slightly contract the pelvic muscles, hold both knees with both hands and pull the knees 14 times (Figure 2-6). Then fully bend the body to both sides 14 times (Figure 2-7), and move the waist forward and backward 7 times (Figure 2-8).

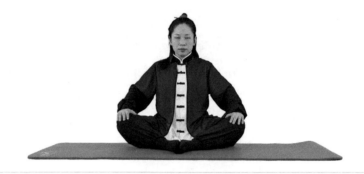

图2-6　Figure 2-6

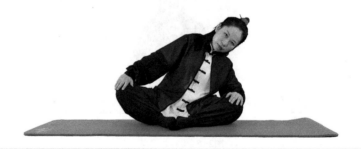

图2-7　Figure 2-7

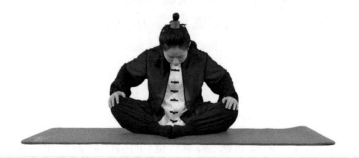

图2-8　Figure 2-8

This exercise can help treat heart deficiency, hemorrhoids, and cold in the knees. To treat consumptive conditions, talk less and keep a peaceful mind.

[操作要领与注意事项] 完成此动作过程中，膝关节向下，背部向上，两向极势，提中气故能治心劳；腰腹打开，阳气升促进气血旺盛，腰腹强，肾气充足，故能治膝冷。

[Tips and notes] During this exercise, fully drop the knee joints and lift the back to regulate middle qi and thus treat heart deficiency. Open the waist and abdomen to promote the ascending of yang qi, tonify qi and blood, and strengthen the kidney, lower back and abdomen, thereby treating cold in the knees.

（7）坐式（单盘）。两手抱住一侧膝头，膝用力向外，身体、手和膝部向相反的方向尽量用力，尽力牵拉到极势，头需仰起，做21次，左右脚互换再做上述动作（图2-9）。有助于去除背脊拘急和手臂劳损。

(7) Take a half-lotus position. Hold one knee with both hands and pull it outward while exerting force in the opposite direction with fully stretched hands and body, raise the head,

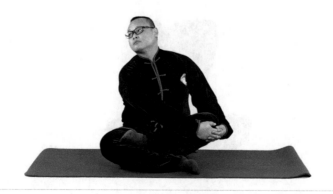

图2-9　Figure 2-9

and repeat 21 times. Change the position of the legs and repeat the movements (Figure 2-9). This exercise can help treat contracture in the back, and strain in the arms.

［操作要领与注意事项］两手抱一侧膝,膝向下向外做放松,与背形成对拔之势,肩背打开,气血运行,故可除背脊和手臂疾患。

[Tips and notes] Grasp one knee with both hands, and relax the knee downward and outward to form an opposing force with the back, which opens the shoulders and back and promotes the circulation of qi and blood. This exercise can help treat disorders in the back and arms.

(8) 坐式。① 两脚对踏,脚掌合拢,两脚尽量向内收,两手尽力舒展,从两侧打开,然后两手交叉于脑后,触碰于肩(图2-10);手牵拉头部,(身体向下低俯)使手和肩都朝向地,做7次(图2-11)。② 两手仰掌,做上述动作7次(图2-12,图2-13);两手合掌,做上述动作7次(图2-14,图2-15)。两手再从头部两侧向斜上方举起,尽力做到极势,腰正,脚不动(图2-16)。适用于五劳七伤、脐下冷暖不和,经常练此动作,可使身体调和舒适。

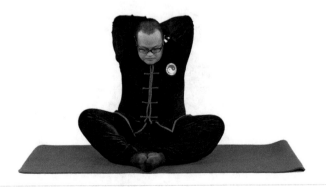

图2-10　Figure 2-10

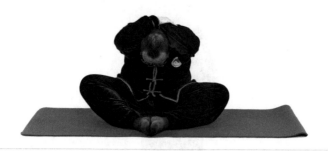

图2-11　Figure 2-11

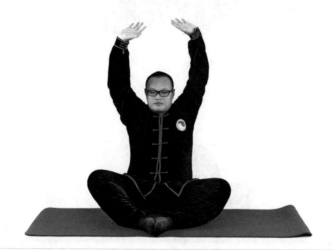

图2-12　Figure 2-12

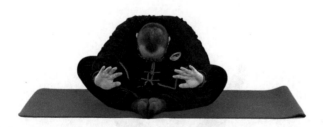

图2-13　Figure 2-13

(8) Take a sitting position. ① Bring the soles together, fully bring the feet close to the body, fully extend the hands along the sides of the body, and then cross both hands behind the head, touching the shoulders (Figure 2–10); pull the head with the hands (bend the body down) to make the hands and

Zhu Bing Yuan Hou Lun Dao Yin Shu (Explanations for the Daoyin Exercises in *Zhu Bing Yuan Hou Lun*) · 《诸 病 源 候 论》 导 引 术

144

功 法 操 作 · Movements

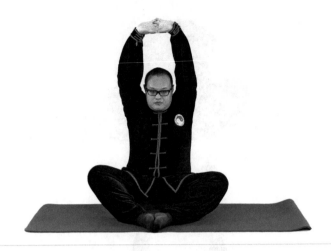

图2-14　Figure 2-14

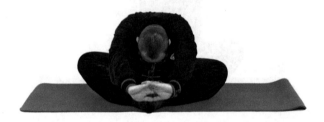

图2-15　Figure 2-15

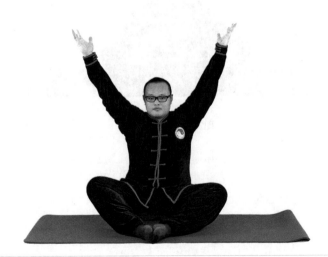

图2-16　Figure 2-16

shoulders face down towards the ground, and repeat 7 times (Figure 2–11). ② Lift the palms with them facing upward, and do the above movements 7 times (Figure 2–12 and Figure 2–13); cross the fingers, and do the above movements 7 times (Figure 2–14 and Figure 2–15). Fully raise both hands diagonally from the sides of the head, and keep the waist upright and the feet still (Figure 2–16). This exercise can help treat the five exhaustions, seven damages, and disharmony between cold and heat in the lower abdomen.

［操作要领与注意事项］① 动作一：两脚对踏，脚掌合拢，利于腹部气血运行；两手交叉于脑后，有助于脊柱打开。② 动作二：合掌是在仰掌的基础上将手指交叉。

[Tips and notes] ① The first movement: Bringing the soles together helps promote the circulation of qi and blood in the abdomen. Crossing the hands behind the head helps open the spine. ② The second movement: Cross the fingers on the basis of lifting the palms with them facing upward.

（9）站式、坐式。一脚踏地，另一腿屈膝，两手合抱在膝眼下，迅速用力向身体牵拉，尽力做到极势（图2–17）。左右脚交换做上述动作28次，适用于五劳所伤、足三里的气机不得下行。

(9) Take a standing or sitting position. Place one foot on the ground, lift the other leg, with both hands clasped under the lifted knee, and quickly and fully pull the knee towards the body (Figure 2–17). Change the position of the legs and repeat the movements 28 times on each side. This exercise can help treat the five exhaustions, and qi stagnation in the point Zusanli (ST 36).

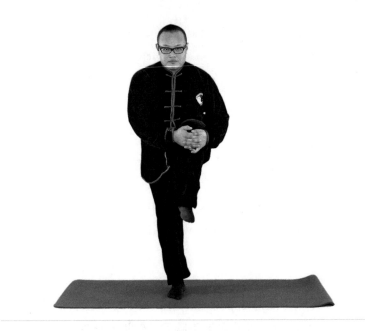

图2-17　Figure 2-17

[操作要领与注意事项] 完成此动作过程中, 自然纳气, 以利归元。

[Tips and notes] During the exercise, breathe naturally to guide qi into the *Dantian*.

（10）卧式、坐式。蛇行气。先曲身侧卧（图2-18），然后翻身仰卧，再起身踞坐（图2-19）。闭眼，身体随着内在气机缓缓自然流动运行，不吸不呼12次。少食，肠胃才可以畅通。服气为食，舌抵上腭，津液自生，如琼浆般饮下。适时养生，春天适合活动升发，冬天适宜收敛封藏。适用于五劳七伤。

(10) Take a lying or sitting position. Assume the posture of a snake to circulate qi. First, lie down on the side with the body bent (Figure 2-18), then lie on the back, and sit with the knees raised and the feet on the ground (Figure 2-19). Close the eyes, perceive qi movements within the body and passively hold the breath 12 times. Eat less food and ingest qi. Press the tongue against the palate to produce saliva and swallow it.

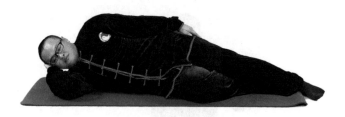

图2-18　　Figure 2-18

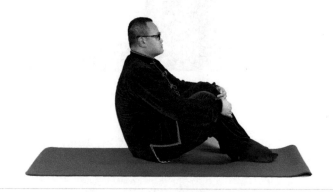

图2-19　　Figure 2-19

Health preservation should follow the rules of nature. Spring is suitable for promoting the upward flow of qi, while winter is best for consolidating and preserving. This exercise can help treat the five exhaustions and seven damages.

［操作要领与注意事项］侧卧，腰胯自然放松，利于呼吸。

[Tips and notes] Lying on the side with the waist and hips relaxed is conducive to breathing.

（11）坐式。虾蟆行气。正坐。摇动两手臂，不吸不呼12次（图2-20）。适用于五劳七伤和水肿病。

(11) Take an upright sitting position. Assume the posture of a toad to circulate qi. Shake the arms and passively hold the breath 12 times (Figure 2-20). This exercise can help treat the five exhaustions (Long-time observation damages blood; long-

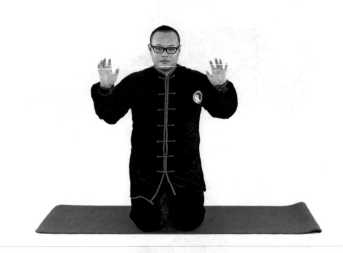

图2-20 Figure 2-20

time lying damages qi; long-time sitting damages muscles; long-time standing damages bones; long-time walking damages sinews) and seven damages (Refers to seven pathogenic factors that lead to deficiency and consumption, including improper diet, anxiety, drink, sex, hunger, over-exertion, and damage to meridians, collaterals, *Ying*-nutrients, *Wei*-defense and qi) as well as oedema.

[操作要领与注意事项] 完成此动作时，通过摇动双臂带动腰背部的运动。忌憋气。

[Tips and notes] During the exercise, use the movement of the arms to drive the movement of the waist and back. Avoid holding the breath.

（12）坐式。向外转动两脚，做10次（图2-21）。有助于去除心腹劳疾。向内转动两脚，做10次（图2-22）。有助于去除全身的劳损疾病、疹病。向外转动两个脚，两脚平踏而坐，用意鼓动膝关节，令骨关节中间（筋）鼓起。向外牵拉10次，不要旋转两脚（图2-23）。

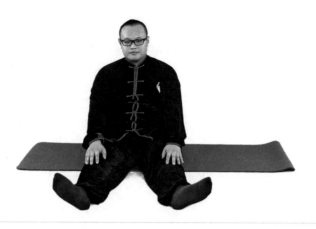

图2-21 Figure 2-21

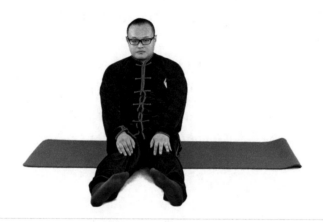

图2-22 Figure 2-22

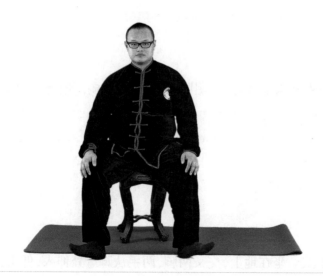

图2-23 Figure 2-23

(12) Take a sitting position. Rotate both feet outward 10 times (Figure 2–21). This exercise can help treat disorders in the heart and abdomen caused by overexertion. Rotate both feet inward 10 times (Figure 2–22). This exercise can help treat strain and skin rashes. Sit with both feet flat on the ground, rotate the two feet outward, and use the mind to stretch the knee joints (tendons) 10 times without rotating the feet (Figure 2–23).

［操作要领与注意事项］完成此动作过程中，从外打开向内转动两脚，有利于胸腹部气血运行；从内打开向外转动两脚，有利于腰背部气血运行。

[Tips and notes] During the exercise, rotating both feet inward from the outside facilitates the circulation of qi and blood in the chest and abdomen. Rotating both feet outward from the inside facilitates the circulation of qi and blood in the waist and back.

2. 虚劳寒冷候提要
2. Consumptive conditions with cold

虚劳病人血气虚衰，阴阳失衡，脏腑衰弱。阳虚则内寒。

Patients with consumptive conditions may experience exhaustion of qi and blood, along with an imbalance between yin and yang and weakness in the zang-fu organs. Yang deficiency often leads to internal cold.

坐式。坐在地上，交叉两脚，两手从脚弯处伸入，低头，再把手交叉于项后（图1-79）。适用于久寒自身无力变暖、耳朵听不到声音。

Take a sitting position. Sit on the ground with the feet crossed, then lower the head and cross the hands behind the neck (Figure 1–79). This exercise can help treat chronic cold sensations in the body and deafness.

[操作要领与注意事项] 松解打开脊骨、胯骨，有利于督脉气血运行。此动作难度大，易受伤。初学者练习此动作时忌幅度大、速度快，宜循序渐进。

[Tips and notes] Relax and open the spine and hips to circulate qi and blood within the Governor Vessel. This exercise is difficult and can easily cause injury. Beginners should start slowly and gradually increase the range of motion.

3. 虚劳少气候提要
3. Consumptive conditions with shortness of breath

虚劳病人肺气虚损，肺主气，气属阳，阳气不足故引起少气。

Patients with consumptive conditions may experience deficiency of lung qi. The lung governs qi, and qi belongs to yang. The deficiency of yang qi leads to shortness of breath.

站式、坐式、卧式。不宜随意吐津液，应当随有随咽，如同经常含着一颗枣核一般，口内产生津液，而后咽下（图2–24）。要爱惜精气、津液，这是养生的关键。

Take a standing, sitting or lying position. Swallow the saliva, imagine holding a jujube pit in the mouth to produce saliva and then swallow it (Figure 2–24).

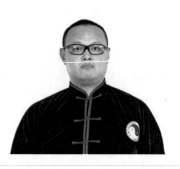

图2-24　Figure 2-24

[操作要领与注意事项] 完成此导引动作过程中，"恒含枣核"使口腔维持张开的感觉，促进口内津液生成。

[Tips and notes] During the exercise, "constantly hold a jujube pit in the mouth" to open the oral cavity and promote the generation of saliva.

4. 虚劳里急候提要
4. Consumptive conditions with tenesmus

虚劳病人肾气虚损，冲脉失于濡养，故腹内拘挛紧缩不舒。

Patients with consumptive conditions may experience deficiency of kidney qi. This condition may result in malnutrition of the *Chong* meridian, leading to abdominal spasm.

卧式（仰卧）。口缓缓纳气，鼻出气（图2-25，图2-26）。有助于去除腹内拘急疼痛、饱食不消化。然后小咽气几十口，起到温中的效果。如果受寒邪，使人干呕腹痛，以口纳气70次，腹部充盈则可扶正祛邪。再小咽气几十口，两手掌摩擦，温热后摩腹，令气下行（图2-27）。

Take a supine position. Inhale slowly through the mouth and exhale through the nose (Figure 2-25 and Figure 2-26).

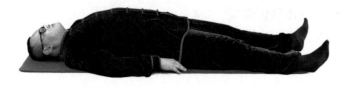

图2-25　Figure 2-25

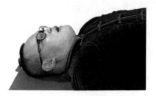

图2-26　Figure 2-26

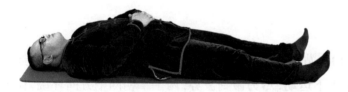

图2-27　Figure 2-27

This exercise can help treat abdominal cramps and pain, as well as indigestion. Then, swallow the air dozens of times to warm the stomach. For retching and abdominal pain caused by contraction of pathogenic cold, inhaling through the mouth 70 times to make the abdomen full can reinforce healthy qi to eliminate pathogenic factors. Then, swallow the air dozens of times, rub the hands to generate warmth and knead the abdomen in order to promote the downward movement of qi (Figure 2–27).

[操作要领与注意事项] 完成此导引动作时，空气要优良，气温不能过低。

[Tips and notes]　During the exercise, the air quality should be excellent, and the temperature should not be too low.

5. 虚劳体痛候提要

5. Consumptive conditions with body pain

虚劳病人阴阳皆虚，气血运行不畅。假使感受风邪，正气与其相争，遇寒则身体疼痛，遇热则皮肤发痒。

Patients with consumptive conditions may experience deficiency of both yin and yang as well as unsmooth circulation of qi and blood. Healthy qi may fight against the invading pathogenic wind. As a result, they may experience body pain when exposed to cold and itchiness when exposed to heat.

（1）站式、坐式。① 两手向上舒展手指，手掌、脸面朝南，曲肘做上下运动，尽力做到极势，两手掌朝四个方向环绕，做28次（图2-28）。② 然后双臂放松，自然向下垂落，两手向后振动，使气舒缓放松，做14次（图2-29）。两肩做上下运动，14次。适用

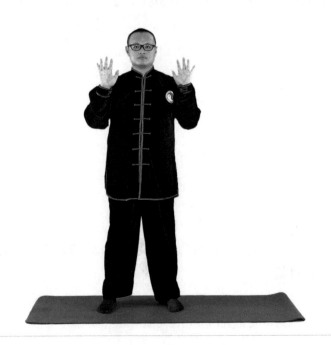

图2-28　Figure 2-28

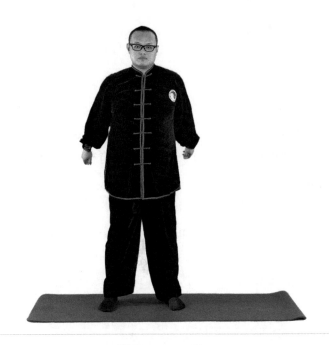

图2-29　Figure 2-29

于身体、手臂和肋区的疼闷不适。日积月累练习,有助于消除这些病痛。

(1) Take a standing or sitting position. ① Stand facing south, extend the fingers upward, bend the elbows and move them up and down, and rotate the palms 28 times (Figure 2-28). ② Then relax both arms and hang them down naturally, vibrate both hands backward to relax, and repeat 14 times (Figure 2-29). Move both shoulders up and down 14 times. Long-term exercise can help treat oppressive pain in the body, arms and sub-costal region.

[操作要领与注意事项] ① 动作一:上半身的动作要靠腰胯来完成。② 动作二:两手振动要靠腰腹脚的振颤来完成,是全身的振颤,是整体的运动。

[Tips and notes] ① The first movement: Use the movement of the hips and waist to drive the movement of the upper body. ② The second movement: Use the vibration of the waist, abdomen, and feet to drive the vibration of the hands. Vibrate the whole body.

（2）坐式（跽坐）。两手抓住两脚脚趾，尽力做到极势，低头，不吸不呼9次（图2-30）。适用于颈、脊柱、腰和脚的疼痛及虚劳病症。

(2) Take a sitting position. Sit by stretching out and separating the legs like a winnowing pan. Fully grab the toes of both feet with both hands, lower the head and passively hold the breath 9 times (Figure 2–30). This exercise can help treat pain in the neck, spine, lower back and feet, and can also help treat consumptive conditions.

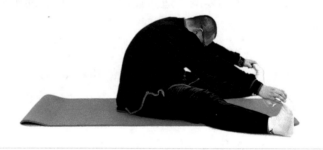

图2-30　Figure 2-30

［操作要领与注意事项］跽坐，坐姿的一种。席地而坐，伸开两脚，并向两侧分开，其形如箕。完成此动作过程中，低头时弯腰后坐，自然能产生不呼不吸的状态。

[Tips and notes] During the exercise, lowering the head while bending forward can help passively hold the breath.

（3）卧式（仰卧）。伸展两腿，两脚脚趾向右，两手伸直放于身旁，鼻纳气7次（图2-31）。适用于骨痛病症。

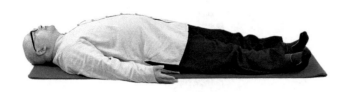

图2-31　Figure 2-31

(3) Take a supine position. Extend the legs and toes, stretch and put the arms by the sides, and breathe in through the nose 7 times (Figure 2–31). This exercise can help treat bone pain.

［操作要领与注意事项］仰卧，有利于放松全身；脚趾右旋，有利于壮精血；鼻纳气，有利于督脉气血运行。

[Tips and notes] Taking a supine position can relax the whole body. Rotating the toes to the right can strengthen the essence and blood. Inhaling through the nose can promote the circulation of qi and blood in the Governor Vessel.

（4）坐式（端坐）。舒展腰部，举右手，仰掌向上，左臂从后面覆盖住右手。鼻纳气，至满，7次，呼吸中稍稍振劲左手（图2-32）。有助于去除手臂及背的疼痛。

(4) Take an upright sitting position. Stretch the waist, lift the right hand with the palm facing upward, and put the left hand on the right arm along the back of the head, inhale deeply through the nose 7 times, and slightly vibrate the left hand during the breathing (Figure 2–32). This exercise can help treat pain in the arms and back.

［操作要领与注意事项］完成此动作过程中，仰掌有利于放松腰部，利于腰内气血行；左手覆右手，利于气血向右腰集中。

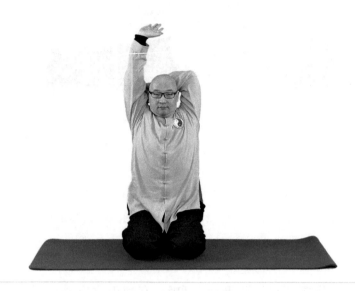

图2-32　Figure 2-32

[Tips and notes] During the exercise, turning the palm upward is conducive to relaxing the waist and promoting the flow of qi and blood within it. Placing the left hand on the right arm is conducive to directing the flow of qi and blood towards the right waist.

（5）跪式（互跪）。身体向下低俯,当头离地面5寸时,抬头仰面,两手同时抽出,先左手向身前舒展,右手向身后舒展,尽力做到极势（图2-33）。左右手脚互换做上述动作。有助于去除臂骨、脊柱和筋的气血不和、疼痛闷胀不适。

(5) Take a kneeling position. Kneel by placing the right knee on the ground, erecting the left knee and sitting on the right heel, almost like getting down on one knee. Bend the upper body forward until the head is 5 *cun* off the ground, lift the head, and fully extend the left hand forward and the right hand backward (Figure 2–33). Change the position of the hands and feet and repeat the movement. This exercise can help treat the disharmony between qi and blood as well as oppressive

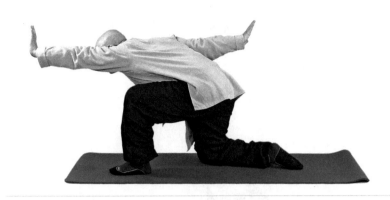

图2-33　Figure 2-33

pain in the arms, spine and tendons.

[操作要领与注意事项] 互跪后，缓缓抬头，有利于脊柱放松拔伸；一手向前，一手向后舒展，有利于打开骶胯关节，舒张腰背部。

[Tips and notes] Slowly lifting the head is beneficial for relaxing and stretching the spine. Stretching one hand forward and one hand backward is beneficial for opening the sacroiliac joints and extending the waist and back.

（6）坐式、跪式。臀部坐于一脚上，另一脚横放下压于另一脚的膝部。一手用力向下按上边的膝使腿掤紧，另一手向相反方向舒展；仰头向前，两手同时用力，这一刻尽力做到极势，按摇14次（图2-34）。左右手脚互换做上述动作。适用于大腿、胸、颈、腋的血脉迟涩和挛痛闷疼。互跪安稳后，抽出一脚尽力向前，头面尽力向前过两脚脚趾，上下来回做21次（图2-35）。左右脚互换做上述动作。有助于去除臂、腰、背、股、膝内的疼闷不适，使五脏六腑之气血津液调和。一脚屈向前，使小腹紧贴腿上；另一脚尽力后伸，用力伸脚趾。两手向后，形似飞仙，凌空昂头，这一刻尽力做到极势，做14次（图2-36）。左右脚互换做上述动作。有助于去除全身不适。

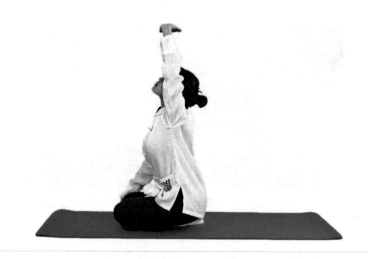

图2-34　Figure 2-34

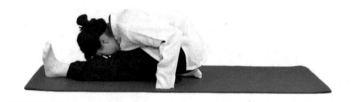

图2-35　Figure 2-35

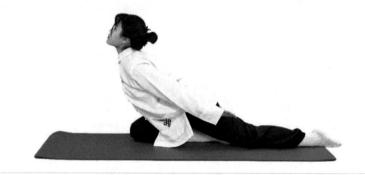

图2-36　Figure 2-36

(6) Take a sitting or kneeling position. Sit on one foot with the other foot beneath the knee, use one hand to press the upper knee to tighten the leg, stretch the other hand in the opposite direction, fully exert force with both hands, and press and shake 14 times (Figure 2–34). Change the position of the legs and hands, and repeat the above movements. This exercise

can circulate blood and qi and help treat oppressive pain in the thighs, chest, neck and armpits. Take a kneeling position, fully extend one leg forward, bend the upper body forward over the toes of both feet, and repeat 21 times (Figure 2–35). Change the position of the legs and hands, and repeat the above movements. This exercise can help treat oppressive pain in the arms, waist, back, thighs and knees, and also harmonize qi, blood and body fluids of the five zang organs and six fu organs. Bend one leg forward and bring the lower abdomen close to the thigh, stretch the other leg backward and stretch the toes. Fully extend both hands backward like a flying immortal, raise the head, and repeat 14 times (Figure 2–36). Change the position of the legs and hands, and repeat the above movements. This exercise can help treat general body discomfort.

［操作要领与注意事项］松解打开脊骨、胯骨，有利于全身气血运行。此动作难度颇大，易受伤。初学者练习此动作时忌幅度大、速度快，宜循序渐进。

[Tips and notes] Relax and open the spine and hips to circulate qi and blood. This exercise is difficult and can easily cause injury. Beginners should start slowly and gradually increase the range of motion.

（7）坐式。① 舒展两脚，两脚脚趾用力向上；舒展两手，掌心相对，手指伸直，仰头挺脊，尽力做到极势，3次（图2-37）。② 然后移动两脚相距一尺，手不移动位，手掌外翻，做7次（图2-38）。③ 过一会，再移动两脚相距两尺，手向下按地，尽力做到极势，3次（图2-39）。有助于去除全身的筋与关节的虚劳、骨髓痛闷。伸展两手，贴身向上，然后两手握住两脚脚趾，用力捏按脚趾，但此时心意不可用力，才能使心气走向脚下。手脚一起用力再放松,尽力做到极势,反复21次(图2-40)。有助于去除脚跟、臀部及腰部疼痛,以及解溪穴处的拘紧不适、日见消损之病症。

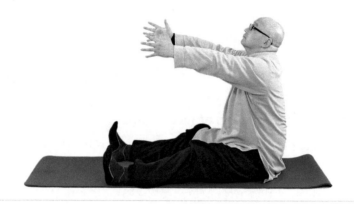

图2-37　Figure 2-37

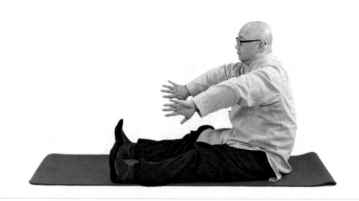

图2-38　Figure 2-38

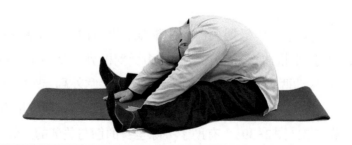

图2-39　Figure 2-39

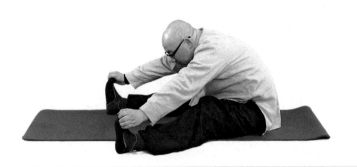

图2-40　Figure 2-40

(7) Take a sitting position. ① Stretch out both legs, fully extend the toes upward, stretch out both hands with the palms facing each other, extend the fingers, raise the head, keep the spine straight, and repeat 3 times (Figure 2-37). ② Then move the feet apart (The distance between the feet is about 33 cm.), keep the position of the hands, turn the palms outward, and repeat 7 times (Figure 2-38). ③ After a while, move the feet apart (The distance between the feet is about 66 cm.), fully bend the upper body to press the ground with the hands, and repeat 3 times (Figure 2-39). This exercise can help treat deficiency of the tendons and joints, as well as oppressive pain in the bones. Stretch and lift the hands to grasp the toes of both feet and pinch them. At this time, do not exert any force, in order to allow heart qi to flow towards the feet. Use both hands and feet together to exert force and then relax, and repeat 21 times (Figure 2-40). This exercise can help treat pain in the heels, hips and lower back, as well as tightness or discomfort in the point Jiexi (ST 41), and prevent gradual decrease in body weight.

　[操作要领与注意事项] ① 动作一：完成此动作过程中，舒展全身，如同伸懒腰。② 动作二：手掌外翻，有利于放松腰背部。③ 动作三：手向下按地，有利于放松肩膀与上肢；手指用力捏按脚趾时，须延展肌腱，忌收缩肌肉发力。

[Tips and notes] ① The first movement: During this movement, stretch the whole body. ② The second movement: Turning the palms outward helps to relax the whole back. ③ The third movement: Pressing the ground with the hands helps to relax the shoulders and upper limbs; when pinching the toes with the fingers, stretch the tendons and avoid contracting the muscles.

6. 虚劳口干燥候提要
6. Consumptive conditions with dry mouth

虚劳病人血气虚损,阴阳气机阻隔,冷热不能交通,故上焦生热,灼伤津液导致口干燥。

Deficiency of blood and qi may block the flow of and the interaction between yin qi and yang qi, and thus the upper jiao may generate heat to consume body fluids, leading to dry mouth.

坐式。向东而坐。仰头,不呼不息5次(图2-41),舌在口中转动(引发津液),漱口满14次,而后咽下。适用于口干。如同引动肾水上发为甘泉而至咽喉。津液甘美,能除口苦,使口腔香洁、吃东西甘美味正。经常练习这样的导引,能使津液味如甘露,人不会感觉饥渴。

Take a sitting position. Sit facing east, raise the head, passively hold the breath 5 times (Figure 2–41), rotate the tongue to produce saliva, rinse the mouth with saliva 14 times, and then swallow it. This exercise can help treat dry mouth. It is as if drawing up the kidney water to the throat. Saliva can help treat bitter taste in the mouth, making the mouth clean and feel

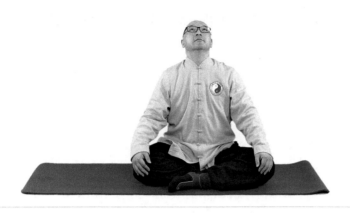

图2-41　Figure 2-41

the food delicious. Regular practice can relieve thirst.

[操作要领与注意事项] 向东而坐，以利气机生发。此导引动作中，舌头搅动，助肾气蒸腾，气机向上引发甘泉。

[Tips and notes] Sit facing east to ascend qi. During this exercise, stirring the tongue helps to steam kidney qi and guide the upward flow of qi.

7. 虚劳膝冷候提要

7. Consumptive conditions with cold in the knees

虚劳病人肾弱髓虚，又受风寒邪气侵袭，故引起膝冷。

Weakened kidney and marrow coupled with the invasion of pathogenic wind and cold may lead to cold in the knees.

（1）跪式。两手向后，手掌撑地，跪一脚，臀部坐于上，屈另一脚，脚掌上翻如仰面。内视气在各处流通自在，振动，尽力做到极势，做28次（图2-42）。左右脚互换做上述动作。然后两脚向前双踏，尽力做到极势，做14次（图2–43）。有助于去除胸腹病、膝冷脐闷。

(1) Take a kneeling position. Place both hands behind to support the body, kneel with one leg and sit on the foot, bend the other leg and turn the sole upward. Perceive the free flow of qi throughout the body, fully vibrate the body, and repeat 28 times (Figure 2–42). Change the position of the feet and do the above movements again. Then, fully stretch the feet, and repeat 14 times (Figure 2–43). This exercise can help treat disorders involving the chest and abdomen, cold in the knees, and stuffiness around the navel.

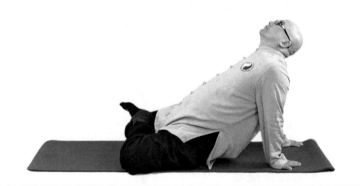

图2–42　Figure 2–42

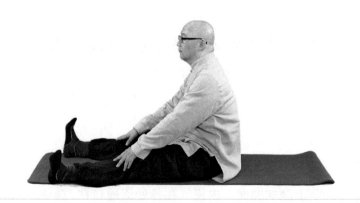

图2–43　Figure 2–43

［操作要领与注意事项］完成此动作过程中，松静自然，浊阴下沉，清阳上腾。两脚向前双踏，有利于松解全身。

[Tips and notes] During this exercise, keep a peaceful mind and relax the body to descend turbid yin qi and ascend clear yang qi. Stretching the feet can help relax the body.

（2）跪式（互跪）。调和心气，气向下到脚。观想气一索一索地流布到身体各处，然后慢慢平展身体，匍匐至地；手舒展地放于两肋旁，手掌好像会不停地吸气呼气；当脸上觉得有点紧与闷时，就挺起背脊，（过一会）再向下至地，如此上下起伏做21次（图2-44）。有助于去除膝关节冷、膀胱宿病、腰脊僵硬、脐下冷闷。

(2) Take a kneeling position. Kneel by placing the right knee on the ground, erecting the left knee and sitting on the right heel, almost like getting down on one knee. Harmonize heart qi and direct it downward to the feet. Visualize the flow of qi spreading smoothly throughout the body, and then slowly bend the body forward. Extend and place the hands on the sides of the ribcage, and imagine continuously inhaling and exhaling through the palms. When oppressive and tight sensations are present, return to the starting posture and hold the position for a moment. Repeat 21 times (Figure 2–44). This exercise can help

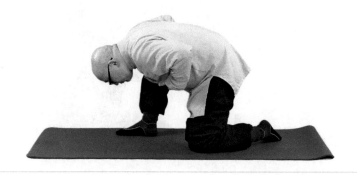

图2-44　Figure 2-44

treat cold in the knees, chronic bladder disorders, stiff waist and back, as well as oppression and cold in the lower abdomen.

［操作要领与注意事项］完成此动作过程中，松静自然，心气自然向下。气行各处，观之即可，勿忘勿助。

[Tips and notes] During this exercise, keep a peaceful mind to descend heart qi naturally.

（3）坐式。舒展两脚，散气到涌泉穴，3次。气彻底到了涌泉穴后，收屈右脚，两手握住涌泉穴向上拉，同时脚向下踏，这一刻手脚同时用力，尽力做到极势，送气至涌泉穴，做21次（图2-45）。完成上述动作的过程中，要有气的运行。有助于去除肾内冷气、膝冷、脚疼。

(3) Take a sitting position. Extend both legs and disperse qi to the point Yongquan (KI 1) 3 times. After qi has thoroughly reached the point, lift the right leg, and grip the point with both hands to fully pull upward while stepping down with the foot. Repeat 21 times (Figure 2–45). During the exercise, circulate qi. This exercise can help treat cold in the kidney and knees, and foot pain.

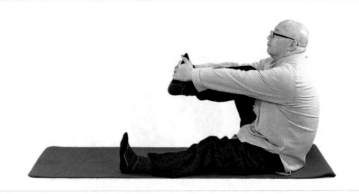

图2-45　Figure 2-45

［操作要领与注意事项］完成此动作过程中，自然放松地坐着，心气自然向下行至涌泉穴；两手抱脚向上牵拉时，须使大腿竖抱于腹前，不可横抱。

[Tips and notes] During this exercise, sit naturally and relax the body to make heart qi go downward naturally to the point Yongquan (KI 1). When pulling the foot upward with the hands, keep the thighs vertical and close to the abdomen.

（4）跪式。跪一脚，臀部坐于上，两手从大腿内侧扳脚上翻，脚跟向下用力。身体向外后侧，尽力做到极势，这一刻全身皆处于对拔拉伸状态，向心来去做14次（图2-4）。左右手脚互换再做上述动作。有助于去除痔疮、五劳、足臂疼闷、膝冷阴冷。

(4) Take a kneeling position. Sit on one foot, use both hands to pull the other foot, exert downward pressure on the heel, fully lean the upper body outward and backward, and repeat 14 times (Figure 2–4). Change the position of the feet and repeat the above exercise. This exercise can help treat hemorrhoids, the five exhaustions, oppressive pain in the feet and arms, and clod in the knees.

［操作要领与注意事项］完成此动作时，扳脚上翻，内合于腰；对拔拉伸时，肘、脊柱、上肢放松打开。

[Tips and notes] During this exercise, when pulling the foot upward, relax and open the elbows, spine and upper limbs.

（5）卧式（仰卧）。伸展两腿，两脚十趾相撑，两手伸展放于身旁，鼻纳气7次（图2-46）。可以去除两小腿冷、腿骨疼痛。

(5) Take a supine position, extend both legs with the toes of both feet supporting each other, extend both hands, place

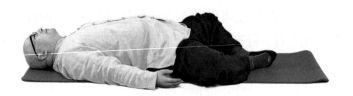

图2-46　　Figure 2-46

them on the sides of the body, and inhale through the nose 7 times (Figure 2–46). This exercise can help treat cold in the lower legs, and leg bone pain.

［操作要领与注意事项］十趾相撑利于打开胯骨，导引气血下行；鼻纳气，可开窍，通利脊骨。

[Tips and notes] The toes supporting each other are conducive to opening the hips and guiding qi and blood downward. Inhaling through the nose can open the orifices and unblock the spine.

（6）卧式（仰卧）。伸展两腿两手，脚跟向外，脚趾相对，鼻纳气，至满，做7次这样的呼吸（图1-21）。有助于去除两膝寒凉、胫骨疼痛、转筋。

(6) Take a supine position. Extend both legs and arms with the heels facing outward and the toes touching each other, inhale through the nose deeply, and repeat this breathing pattern 7 times (Figure 1–21). This exercise can help treat cold in the knees, shin bone pain, and leg cramps.

［操作要领与注意事项］完成此动作过程中，通过鼻纳气至满来舒展腰膝。

[Tips and notes] During this exercise, deeply inhale through

Zhu Bing Yuan Hou Lun Dao Yin Shu (Explanations for the Daoyin Exercises in Zhu Bing Yuan Hou Lun) ·〈诸病源候论〉导引术

170

功法操作 · Movements

the nose to stretch the waist and knees.

（7）坐式。两脚脚趾向下撑地，两脚底涌泉穴相踏，臀部坐于两脚跟上，两膝头向两侧外扒（图2-47），手与上身向前向下俯卧，尽力做到极限，做7次（图2-48）。有助于去除劳损、阴疼、膝冷、脾失运化、肾精枯槁。

(7) Take a sitting position. Use the toes to support the body weight, bring the points Yongquan (KI 1) on both feet together, sit on the heels, and extend the knees outward (Figure 2-47). Lift the hands, fully bend the upper body forward, and repeat 7 times (Figure 2-48). This exercise can help treat strain, pain, dysfunctions of the spleen, exhaustion of kidney essence, and cold in the knees.

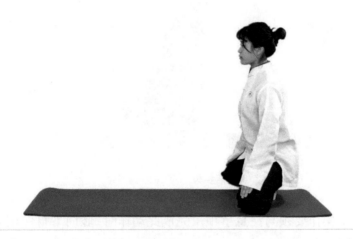

图2-47　Figure 2-47

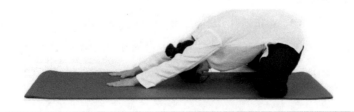

图2-48　Figure 2-48

［操作要领与注意事项］此动作利于开胯，导引气血下行，补肾填精。

[Tips and notes] This movement is beneficial for opening the hips, guiding the downward flow of qi and blood, and nourishing the kidney.

（8）蹲式（蹲坐）。两手抱两膝，仰头向后摇动尽力做到极限，摇动49次（图2-49）。有助于去除膝冷。

(8) Take a squatting position. Hold both knees with the hands, fully raise the head and shake the head backward 49 times (Figure 2-49). This exercise can help treat cold in the knees.

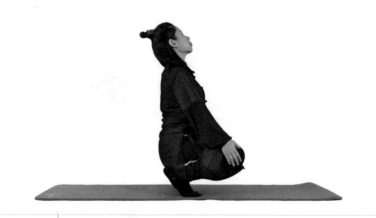

图2-49　Figure 2-49

［操作要领与注意事项］完成此动作时，膝向下自然用力，仰头通过头部（百会穴）向后牵引脊柱，膝与背形成对拔之势，助气血运行。

[Tips and notes] During this exercise, exert natural force downward with the knees. Raise the head to pull the spine backward. In this posture, stretch the knees and back to assist in the circulation of qi and blood.

（9）卧式（仰卧）。伸展两腿，两脚脚趾向左，两手伸直放于身旁，鼻纳气7次（图2-50）。有助于去除肌肉萎缩、小腿寒冷。

(9) Take a supine position. Extend both legs, turn the toes to the left, place both hands straight on the sides of the body, and inhale through the nose 7 times (Figure 2-50). This exercise can help treat muscle atrophy, and cold in the lower legs.

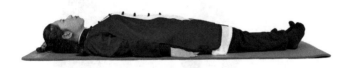

图2-50　Figure 2-50

［操作要领与注意事项］仰卧，有利于放松全身；脚趾左旋，有利于行气补气，利于阳明，故可治痿。

[Tips and notes] Taking a supine position is beneficial for relaxing the whole body. Turning the toes to the left can help circulate and tonify qi, especially in the Yangming meridians. Thus, this exercise can help treat atrophy.

（10）站式（立正）。两手托按整个腰部，使身体正直，骨节筋膜肌肉放松，气自然向下到达它该去的地方，脚前后振摇49次（图2-51）；双脚并拢，与头部朝两个方向振摇14次（图2-52）；头上下摇动，同时缩咽后仰，使两肩胛自然上抬，使脊背柔和，这样做7次（图2-53）。有助于冷气消散，脏腑之气向涌泉穴通彻。

(10) Take an upright standing position. Place both hands on the waist, hold and press the waist to straighten the body, relax the joints, tendons, fascia and muscles, sink down qi, and shake the feet back and forth 49 times (Figure 2-51). Bring

the feet together and shake the feet in the opposite direction of the head 14 times (Figure 2–52). Move the head up and down while tucking in the throat to lift the scapulae and soften the back, and repeat 7 times (Figure 2–53). This exercise can help disperse cold qi and facilitate the flow of qi in the zang-fu organs towards the point Yongquan (KI 1).

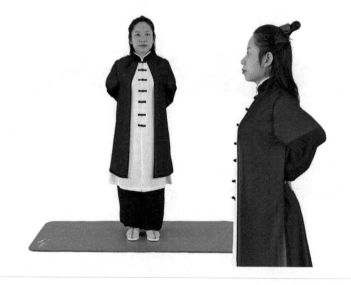

图2–51   Figure 2–51

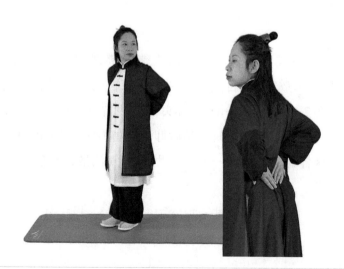

图2–52   Figure 2–52

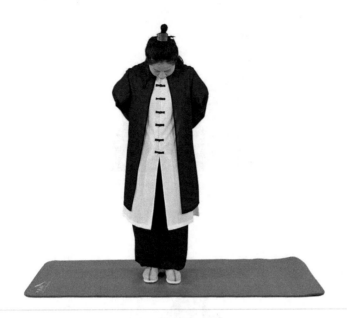

图2-53   Figure 2-53

［操作要领与注意事项］完成此动作过程中，脚正直，脊柱放松后带动身体其他部位运动。

[Tips and notes] During this exercise, keep the feet straight and relax the back to move other parts of the body.

（11）跪式（互跪）。两手向后，手掌撑地，鼻出气向下；然后腰腹逐渐向后下，觉得腰脊部气息滞胀时，再恢复向上，上下来回做14次（图2-54）。身体正直，左右散气，转腰21次（图2-55）。有助于去除脐下冷闷、膝头冷、解溪内疼痛。

(11) Take a kneeling position. Kneel by placing the right knee on the ground, erecting the left knee and sitting on the right heel, almost like getting down on one knee. Place both hands behind the body to support the body weight, exhale through the nose, gradually bend backward until a distending sensation is present in the waist, return to the starting position, and repeat 14 times (Figure 2–54). Stand upright, relax the body, and rotate the waist 21 times (Figure 2–55). This exercise

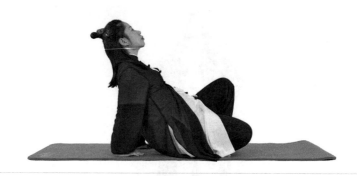

图2-54　Figure 2-54

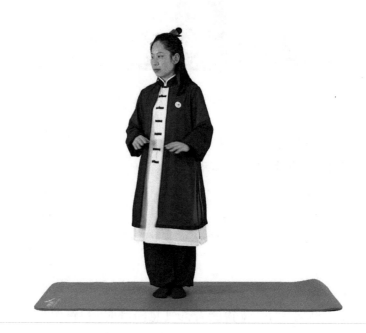

图2-55　Figure 2-55

can help treat oppression and cold in the lower abdomen, cold in the knees, and pain in the point Jiexi (ST 41).

［操作要领与注意事项］腰腹逐渐向后下，可松解腰背部，配合鼻出气，小腹微微向腰部收，可温化关元气海。

[Tips and notes] Gradually bend backward to relax the back. Exhale through the nose and slightly tuck in the lower abdomen to warm the points Guanyuan (CV 4) and Qihai (CV 6).

8. 虚劳阴痛候提要

8. Consumptive conditions with pain in the genitals

虚劳病人肾气虚损，又被风寒邪气侵袭，邪气侵入肾经与阴气相搏，正邪交争，故前阴疼痛。

Deficiency of kidney qi may allow pathogenic wind and cold to invade and fight against the yin qi within the kidney meridian, thus leading to this condition.

坐式。两脚脚趾向下撑地，两脚底涌泉穴相踏，臀部坐于两脚跟上，两膝头向两侧外扒（图2-47），手与上身向前向下俯卧，尽力做到极限，做7次（图2-48）。有助于去除劳损、阴疼、膝冷。

Take a sitting position. Use the toes to support the body weight, bring the points Yongquan (KI 1) on both feet together, sit on the heels, and extend the knees outward (Figure 2–47). Lift the hands, fully bend the upper body forward, and repeat 7 times (Figure 2–48). This exercise can help treat strain, pain, and cold in the knees.

［操作要领与注意事项］此动作利于开胯，导引气血下行，补肾填精。

[Tips and notes] This exercise is beneficial for opening the hips, guiding the downward flow of qi and blood, and nourishing the kidney.

9. 虚劳阴下痒湿候提要

9. Consumptive conditions with wet, itchy genitals

大虚劳损的病人肾气虚损，故前阴发冷，阴汗自出。假使再与风邪，风湿相搏，郁而生热，则致阴下发痒。

Deficiency of kidney qi may cause cold in the genitals and spontaneous sweating. With the invasion of pathogenic wind, the combined wind and dampness may produce heat and subsequently lead to itchy genitals.

卧式（仰卧）。屈膝，脚跟放于臀部下，两手轻放于两膝头，口纳气，使腹部快速舒张，至极，鼻出气，做7次（图2-56）。有助于去除阴下湿证、少腹里痛、膝冷不灵活。

Take a supine position. Bend the knees with the heels placed under the buttocks, place both hands on the knees, inhale quickly through the mouth to fully extend the abdomen, then exhale through the nose. Repeat 7 times (Figure 2-56). This exercise can help treat wet genitals, lower abdominal pain, cold in the knees and knee joint inflexibility.

［操作要领与注意事项］口纳气至腰腹，有利脾胃气血运化，土生金，又利于疏通肺部与大脑清窍。

[Tips and notes] Inhale through the mouth to guide qi to

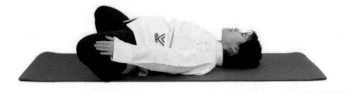

图2-56　Figure 2-56

the lower back and abdomen, which helps circulate qi and blood in the spleen and stomach, and also clear the lung and mind.

10. 风虚劳候提要
10. Consumptive conditions with wind

风为百病之长。虚劳病人血气虚弱，易被风邪侵袭。风邪入侵的部位不同，或浅表肌肤，或深入脏腑，可引发不同的病症。

Wind is the leading cause of diseases. Deficiency of blood and qi makes individuals susceptible to invasion by pathogenic wind that may affect superficial muscles and skin or penetrate deep into the zang-fu organs, leading to varying disorders.

（1）坐式。单脚跪坐，屈曲一脚，脚趾向地尽量用力，一手倒拉足部解溪穴，向心侧尽力拉，一手向后撑地，使腰部、足解溪穴部位、头部感觉骨解气散，这一刻全身皆处于拉伸状态，做21次（图2-57）。两手互换做上述动作。有助于去除手、脚、腰、肩部的风热急闷。

(1) Take a sitting position. Kneel with one leg, flex the other leg, place one hand on the point Jiexi (ST 41) to pull the

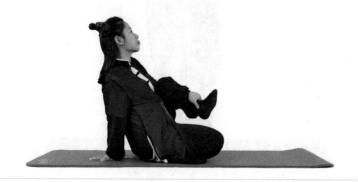

图2-57　Figure 2-57

Zhu Bing Yuan Hou Lun Dao Yin Shu (Explanations for the Daoyin Exercises in Zhu Bing Yuan Hou Lun) · 《诸病源候论》导引术 · 功法操作 · Movements

180

foot, push backward against the ground with the other hand to stretch the entire body, and repeat 21 times (Figure 2–57). Change the position of the hands and repeat the movements. This exercise helps alleviate the symptoms of wind, heat and oppression in the hands, feet, lower back and shoulders.

［操作要领与注意事项］完成此动作过程中，足部向下自然用力，手倒拉解溪穴，形成对拔之势。

[Tips and notes] During the exercise, apply natural downward force to the foot, and then use one hand to pull the point in order to stretch the whole body.

（2）站式。立正，弯腰低头（身体向下低俯），尽力做到极势，两手自然下垂达膝头的位置（图2–58），然后直起腰，使头身恢复正直，上下来回做21次。头身正直，两手自然放松向下，左右转动腰，做14次（图2–59）。脊背后仰，上下来回做7次（图2–60），有助于去除背脊、肩膀、腰冷不和。

（2）Take a standing position. Stand upright, bend forward, lower the head, and naturally hang down the arms to knee level

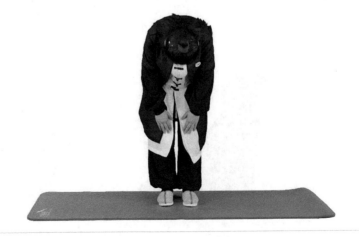

图2–58　Figure 2–58

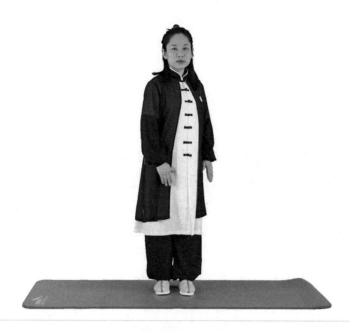

图2-59   Figure 2-59

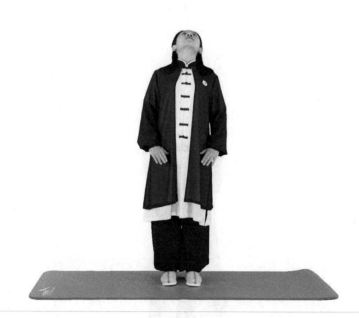

图2-60   Figure 2-60

(Figure 2–58). Then, stand up and repeat this up-and-down movement 21 times. Keep the head and body upright, relax the arms and naturally hang them downward, rotate the waist, and repeat the movement 14 times (Figure 2–59). Bend backward, and repeat 7 times (Figure 2–60). This exercise helps alleviate discomfort in the spine, shoulders, and lower back caused by pathogenic cold.

低头向下，两手自然舒展再向背后高举，渐渐向上距离头约5寸，尽力做到最大极限，然后两手向心前放下，再从背后高起。（这个过程）来去和谐，气力顺调，不使气强于力，也不使力强于气，做14次（图2-61）。适用于胸背前后筋脉不和、气血不调。

Lower the head, naturally extend the arms forward, raise the arms about 5 *cun* above the head, then drop them to the front of the chest, and repeat 14 times (Figure 2–61). Maintain natural and balanced movements. This exercise helps alleviate discomfort of the muscles and meridians in the chest and back, as well as disharmony between qi and blood.

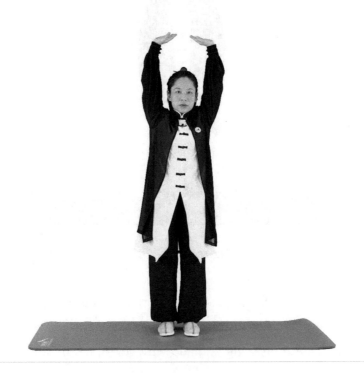

图2-61　Figure 2–61

［操作要领与注意事项］完成此动作过程中，做到肾纳气，脊柱放松带动身体从下向上运动。

[Tips and notes] During the exercise, relax the spine to drive the body movements.

（3）坐式。伸左腿，屈曲右膝内压在臀部下，做5次呼吸（图2-62）。引气入肺，头微微上仰，去风虚，令人目明。依据经络循行的规则练习，引肺中气，适用于风虚病，令人目明。

(3) Take a sitting position. Extend the left leg, flex the right leg, and breathe 5 times (Figure 2-62). By following the pathways of meridians, guide qi into the lung and raise the head slightly. This exercise can help treat deficiency due to wind and brighten the eyes.

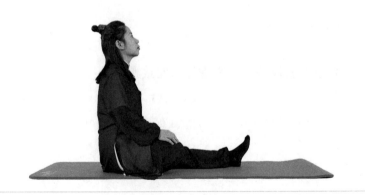

图2-62　Figure 2-62

［操作要领与注意事项］上额微微抬起（眼睛上翻），肺叶舒张，气向前走。

[Tips and notes] Raise the head slightly (roll the eyes upward), expand the lung lobes, and guide the breath forward.

三、腰背病诸候提要

Daoyin Exercises for Disorders Involving the Lower Back

本节论述腰背病诸候的导引术。腰痛的病因包括肾虚、风痹、劳损、受伤、卧湿。此外还论及胁痛。

This chapter introduces the daoyin exercises for disorders involving the lower back. Lower back pain can be induced by kidney deficiency, wind *Bi*-impediment, consumptive conditions, injury, and exposure to dampness. Additionally, this chapter also introduces pain in the sub-costal region.

1. 腰痛候提要

1. Lower back pain

肾经虚弱,风冷之邪乘虚侵入而致腰痛。

Weakness of the kidney meridian coupled with the invasion of pathogenic wind and cold may lead to lower back pain.

（1）站式。一手向上尽力伸展,手掌向四方回转,另一手向下用力（图3-1）,然后两手掌相合手指用力,侧身斜势,转身似乎向后看,手掌向上,心气向下放松布散（图3-2）,觉察气下行至极再上行时,身体拔伸到极致（图3-3）,这样左右做28次。有助于去除肩、肋、腰脊部的痛闷。

(1) Take a standing position. Fully raise one hand, rotate the palm, and press downward with the other hand (Figure 3-1). Then put both palms together, lean to one side, turn the

Zhu Bing Yuan Hou Lun Dao Yin Shu (Explanations for the Daoyin Exercises in *Zhu Bing Yuan Hou Lun*) · 《诸 病 源 候 论》 导 引 术

185

功 法 操 作 · Movements

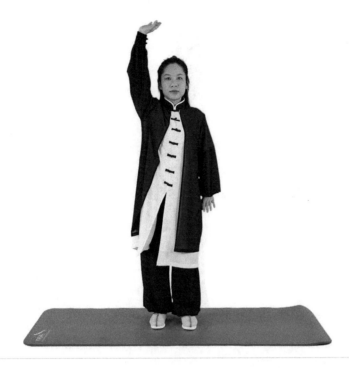

图3-1　Figure 3-1

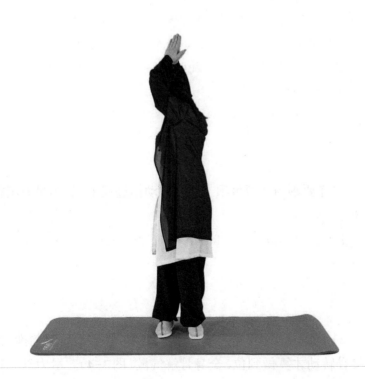

图3-2　Figure 3-2

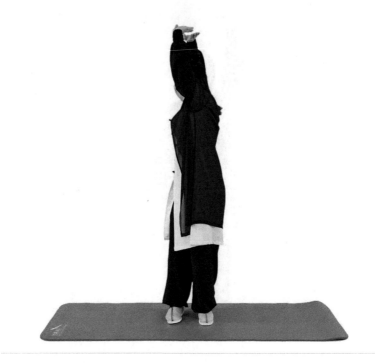

图3-3　Figure 3-3

body to look back, turn the palms upward, and disperse heart qi downward (Figure 3-2). Fully descend qi, then ascend it, and fully stretch the body (Figure 3-3). Repeat this exercise 28 times on each side to help alleviate oppressive pain in the shoulders, ribs and lower back.

［操作要领与注意事项］完成此动作过程中，身体呈螺旋状拔伸。

[Tips and notes] During the exercise, stretch the body in a spiral shape.

（2）坐式。平跪。两手向前伸直舒展，手着地后向前推，推至腰脊转动才算做到位，全身骨解气散（图3-4）。尽力舒展腰部，做到极势，然后才向后跪，就好像脊柱内的冷气向外散出。

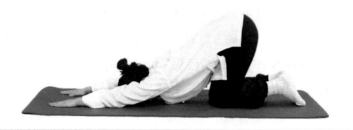

图3-4　Figure 3-4

当手臂有痛闷的感觉，再恢复平跪。上述动作反复做14次。适用于五脏不和，脊背闷痛。

(2) Take a sitting position. Place the knees on the ground, straighten the thighs and upper body, and form a 90° angle between the thighs and the lower legs. Extend and push both hands forward on the ground to drive the rotation of the spine. This can help release tension throughout the body and disperse qi (Figure 3–4). Fully stretch the lower back and then kneel backward to dissipate cold qi in the spine. When a sensation of oppressive pain is present in the arms, return to the kneeling position. Repeat these movements 14 times to help harmonize the five zang organs and alleviate oppressive pain in the back.

［操作要领与注意事项］完成此动作过程中，身体向前伸展是散气，向后跪坐是补气，故而能舒解全身关节，调和五脏。

[Tips and notes] During the exercise, stretching forward helps to disperse qi while kneeling backward helps to replenish qi. Therefore, it can relax the joints and harmonize the five zang organs.

(3) 站式、坐式。有人觉得脊背僵紧不舒憋闷，无论什么时节，可以缩咽于肩（图1-36），仰面，肩胛骨上抬，头顺着左右两个方向移动，做21次（图1-37），然后稍停，待气血平复再做下一次。开始时要慢做再逐渐加快，不能先快后慢。如果是无病之人，可以在清晨3点至5点、中午11点至13点、下午17点至19点三个时间段操作，每个时段做14次。适用于寒热病、脊腰颈项痛、风痹、口内生疮、牙齿风、头眩。

(3) Take a standing or sitting position. For back rigidity, tuck in the throat (Figure 1–36), raise the head and scapula, and rotate the head 21 times (Figure 1–37). Then take a break to calm down qi and blood and do it again. Begin slowly and gradually increase the speed. Avoid starting fast and then slowing down. People in good health can do this exercise 14 times during each of the three time periods: 3–5 am, 11 am–1 pm, and 5–7 pm. This exercise can help treat chills, fever, and pain in the lower back, neck and shoulders, and can also help treat wind *Bi*-impediment, mouth ulcer, toothache, and dizziness.

［操作要领与注意事项］腰背脊柱放松，肩部自然打开，即仰面带脊背肩胛向后固定，在此基础上再缩咽。

[Tips and notes] Relax the waist, back and spine, and open the shoulders naturally. Raise the head to fix the spine and scapula, and then tuck in the throat.

(4) 坐式。① 舒展两脚，两脚脚趾用力向上；舒展两手，掌心相对，手指伸直，仰头挺脊，尽力做到极势，3次（图2-37）。② 然后移动两脚相距一尺，手不移动位，手掌外翻，做7次（图2-38）。③ 过一会，再移动两脚相距两尺，手向下按地，尽力做到极势，3次（图2-39）。适用于全身的筋与关节的虚劳、骨髓痛闷。伸展两手，贴身向上，然后两手握住两脚脚趾，用力捏按脚趾，但此时心意不可用力，才能使心气走向脚下。手脚一起用力再放松，尽力做到极势，反复21次（图2-40）。有助于去除脚跟、臀部及腰部疼痛，以及解溪穴处的拘紧不适、日见消损之病症。

(4) Take a sitting position. ① Stretch out both legs, fully extend the toes upward, stretch out both hands with the palms facing each other, extend the fingers, raise the head, keep the spine straight, and repeat 3 times (Figure 2–37). ② Then move the feet apart (The distance between the feet is about 33 cm.), keep the position of the hands, turn the palms outward, and repeat 7 times (Figure 2–38). ③ After a while, move the feet apart (The distance between the feet is about 66 cm.), fully bend the upper body to press the ground with the hands, and repeat 3 times (Figure 2–39). This exercise can help treat deficiency of the tendons and joints, as well as oppressive pain in the bones. Stretch and lift the hands to grasp the toes of both feet and pinch them. At this time, do not exert any force, in order to allow heart qi to flow towards the feet. Use both hands and feet together to exert force and then relax, and repeat 21 times (Figure 2–40). This exercise can help treat pain in the heels, hips and lower back, as well as tightness or discomfort in the point Jiexi (ST 41), and prevent gradual decrease in body weight.

［操作要领与注意事项］① 动作一：完成此动作过程中，舒展全身，如同伸懒腰。② 动作二：手掌外翻，有利于放松腰背部。③ 动作三：手向下按地，有利于放松肩膀与上肢；手指用力捏按脚趾时，须延展肌腱，忌收缩肌肉发力。

[Tips and notes] ① The first movement: During this movement, stretch the whole body. ② The second movement: Turning the palms outward helps to relax the whole back. ③ The third movement: Pressing the ground with the hands helps to relax the shoulders and upper limbs; when pinching the toes with the fingers, stretch the tendons and avoid contracting the muscles.

（5）坐式。凡是学习调息的人，首先须正坐，并拢膝盖和脚。初学时，先将脚趾相对，脚跟向外扒开，（臀部）坐于脚跟上，坐得安稳（图1-47）。再，将两脚跟向内相对，（臀部）坐于脚跟上，脚趾向外扒开（图1-48）；感觉闷痛后逐渐起身，然后再坐回脚跟上。（练习）直至上述两种坐姿都不觉得闷痛，才开始把两脚跟向上竖起，（臀部）坐于脚跟上，脚趾并拢，反方向朝外（图1-49）。以上三种坐姿就是正坐的一般练习方式。适用于膀胱内冷气、膝冷、双脚冷痛，喘息上气、腰疼这些病症。

(5) Take a sitting position. For those learning to regulate their breathing, it is important to sit upright and bring the knees and feet together. For beginners, start by positioning the toes facing each other and the heels turned outward, and sit on the heels for stability (Figure 1–47). Then, position the heels facing each other and the toes turned outward while sitting on the heels (Figure 1–48). Gradually stand up when experiencing oppressive pain, and then sit back on the heels. When there is no oppressive pain in the above-mentioned sitting positions, raise up the heels and sit on them with the toes together and facing outward (Figure 1–49). The above three postures are the typical practice methods of upright sitting. They can help eliminate cold in the bladder, knees and feet, and alleviate such symptoms as shortness of breath and lower back pain.

［操作要领与注意事项］学习此动作时，需循序渐进，按由易到难的顺序进行练习。

[Tips and notes] When learning this exercise, it is necessary to progress gradually and practice in order from easy to difficult.

2. 腰痛不得俯仰候提要

2. Pain and impaired bending forward and backward of the lower back

劳役损肾,伤其经络,又受风冷邪气侵袭,阴阳经脉俱病,致使腰痛不能俯仰自如。

The damage of the kidney meridian induced by overexertion combined with pathogenic wind and cold may influence yin, yang and meridians, and subsequently cause pain as well as impaired bending forward and backward of the lower back.

坐式。舒展伸直两脚,两手握两脚脚趾,做7次(图3–5,图3–6)。适用于腰部劳损不能俯仰、吐血、持久性的疼痛。

Take a sitting position. Stretch both legs forward, hold the toes of both feet with the hands and repeat 7 times (Figure 3–5 and Figure 3–6). This exercise can help treat lower back strain, inability to bend forward and backward, hemoptysis, and persistent pain.

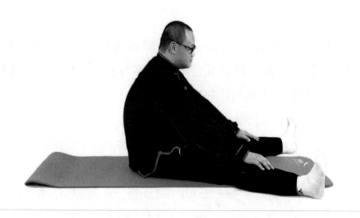

图3–5　Figure 3–5

Zhu Bing Yuan Hou Lun Dao Yin Shu (Explanations for the Daoyin Exercises in *Zhu Bing Yuan Hou Lun*) ● 《诸病源候论》导引术 ● 功法操作 ● Movements

191

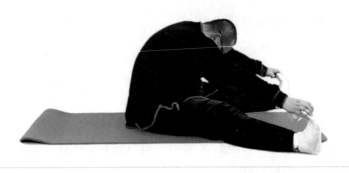

图3-6　Figure 3-6

［操作要领与注意事项］拔伸关节可强壮腰膝。

[Tips and notes] Stretching and extending the joints can strengthen the lower back and knees.

3. 胁痛候提要

3. Pain in the sub-costal region

外邪侵袭足少阳胆经的络脉，以致胁痛。

Pathogenic factors may invade the gallbladder meridian of foot-Shaoyang and subsequently cause pain in the sub-costal region.

（1）站式、坐式、卧式。左胁区突然疼痛的病症，可观想肝为青龙，左目的魂神导引五营的兵千乘万骑，在凌晨3点到5点进入左胁区驱除病邪（图3-7）。

(1) Take a standing, sitting or lying position. For sudden pain in the left side of the sub-costal region, visualize the liver as a green dragon, and the immortal of Ethereal Soul (*Hun*) living in the left eye leading ten thousand soldiers (transformed from *Wei*-defensive qi) to enter the left side of the sub-costal region between 3 and 5 o'clock in the morning to expel pathogenic

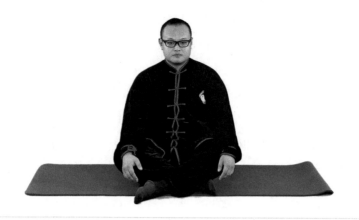

图3-7　Figure 3-7

factors (Figure 3–7).

［操作要领与注意事项］中医素有左肝右肺之议，肝生于左，故左为气机升发之处。寅时为肺经当令，取金克木之意，肝开窍于目，安魂以驱邪。完成此观想前，须先调整心意，忌操之过急。

[Tips and notes] TCM holds that the liver is on the left and the lung is on the right. The liver is responsible for promoting the free flow of qi, and during the time of the Tiger (3–5 am), the lung meridian is active, symbolizing the control of wood by metal. The liver opens into the eyes, and the immortal of Ethereal Soul (*Hun*) living in the left eye is able to expel pathogenic factors. Before doing this visualization exercise, one should first adjust the state of mind and avoid rushing through the process.

（2）站式、坐式、卧式。右胁区疼痛的病症，可观想肺为白虎，右目的魄神导引五营的兵千乘万骑，在下午15点到17点进入右胁区驱除病邪（图3-7）。

(2) Take a standing, sitting or lying position. For pain in the right side of the sub-costal region, visualize the lung as a white tiger, and the immortal of Corporeal Soul (*Po*) living in the right eye leading ten thousand soldiers (transformed from *Wei*-defensive qi) to enter the right side of the sub-costal region between 3 and 5 o'clock in the afternoon to expel pathogenic factors (Figure 3–7).

［操作要领与注意事项］中医素有左肝右肺之议，肺生于右，以肺魄之力，改善右侧气机运行。完成此观想前，须先调整心意，忌操之过急。

[Tips and notes] TCM holds that the liver is on the left and the lung is on the right. The immortal of Corporeal Soul (*Po*) living in the right eye can improve the circulation of qi on the right side. Before doing this visualization exercise, one should first adjust the state of mind and avoid rushing through the process.

（3）卧式（侧卧）。胁部着地，舒展伸直手脚，鼻纳气，口吐出，做7次这样的呼吸（图3–8）。有助于去除肋区的皮肤疼痛。

(3) Take a side-lying position. Rest the flank on the ground, stretch out the hands and feet, inhale through the nose and exhale through the mouth, and repeat this breathing pattern 7 times (Figure 3–8). This exercise can help relieve skin

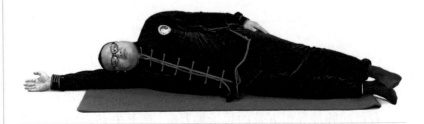

图3–8　Figure 3–8

pain in the rib area.

［操作要领与注意事项］完成此动作过程中，鼻纳气，以求饱满；用口吐出，以利疏泄；侧卧伸直四肢，以利少阳行气。

[Tips and notes] During the exercise, deeply inhale through the nose, exhale through the mouth to promote smooth circulation, and lie on one side with stretched out limbs to facilitate the qi circulation in the Shaoyang meridians.

（4）坐式（端坐）。舒展腰部，向右转头，两眼看右方，口缓缓纳气，咽气30口。有助于去除左胁区疼痛，使眼睛明亮（图3-9）。

(4) Take an upright sitting position. Stretch the waist, turn the head to the right, look to the right, slowly inhale through the mouth, and swallow qi 30 times. This exercise can help relieve pain in the left side of the sub-costal region and brighten the eyes (Figure 3-9).

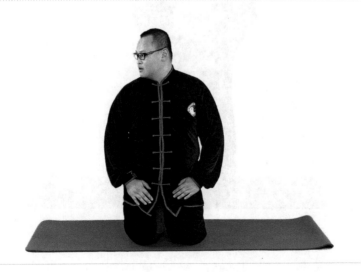

图3-9　Figure 3-9

［操作要领与注意事项］完成此动作过程中，双眼向右顾，同时左侧胸胁区慢慢舒张，以利左侧气血运行，可养肝明目。

[Tips and notes] During the exercise, look to the right, and slowly stretch the left chest and rib area to facilitate the circulation of qi and blood on the left side, nourish the liver and brighten the eyes.

（5）坐式。举起两手交于颈部上方，两手相握，尽力做到极势。适用于胁下疼痛。坐在地上，两手微微地握着，有牵拉之势。长期练此动作，可以使身体结实得像金刚一般，呼吸匀长，身内气机变化如风云转化且隐隐有雷音（图3-10）。

(5) Take a sitting position. Place both hands on the back of the head, and fully clasp them. This exercise can help relieve pain in the sub-costal region. Sit on the ground with both hands slightly clasped to stretch the body. Long-term practice can strengthen the immune system (Figure 3–10).

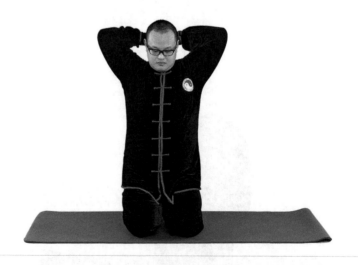

图3-10　Figure 3-10

［操作要领与注意事项］两手微微相握，使气机交融，阴阳相合。

[Tips and notes] Gently clasp the hands together to promote the qi activity and harmonize yin and yang.

四、消渴病诸候提要
Daoyin Exercises for Wasting and Thirst Disorders

本节论述消渴病诸候的导引术。消渴病的主要表现为口渴、饮水多而小便少。病因包括服用五石散等石药（古代有服食石药的风气），或过食肥腻甜的食物等，以致热毒留滞，血气不通，使人下焦虚热。

This chapter introduces the daoyin exercises for wasting and thirst disorders that are characterized by polydipsia, polyphagia and polyuria. Contributing factors include overeating of oily, sweet food, emotions, sexual indulgence, exposure to pathogenic warm heat or abuse of medicinal minerals. These factors may cause heat retention within the body, which may obstruct the circulation of qi and blood, and subsequently cause deficient heat in the lower jiao.

（1）卧式（仰卧）。闭眼，不吸不呼12次，适用于饮食不消化（图4-1）。

(1) Take a supine position. Close the eyes and passively hold the breath 12 times. This exercise can help treat indigestion (Figure 4–1).

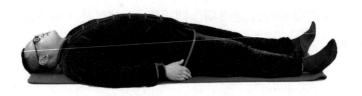

图4-1　Figure 4-1

[操作要领与注意事项]松静自然，不宜憋气。初学若掌握不好，可以减少操作的次数与时间。

[Tips and notes] Relax and breathe naturally. Beginners can reduce the frequency and duration of the exercise.

（2）卧式（仰卧）。松解衣服，松静自然，舒展腰部，做5次自然呼吸，使少腹抬起（图4-2）。引动肾气，有助于去除消渴，通利阴阳。

(2) Take a supine position. Loosen the clothes, relax the body, stretch the waist, and breathe naturally 5 times to lift the lower abdomen (Figure 4-2). This exercise can help stimulate kidney qi, treat wasting and thirst disorders and improve the balance of yin and yang.

练习这样的导引，要避开一些时辰或季节，如大饱、大饥时不宜练习，伤身体；如不好的日子和时节也要避开。导引完毕后，先走120步，多则可走上千步，然后再进食。饮食的法则：不宜大冷大热，五味宜调和。忌陈旧、腐败、隔夜食物和虫蝎。进食时须小口，多咀嚼，不要急咽。进食完毕不要立即睡觉。这称作谷药，饮食和气相调和，就是真正的良药。

When practicing this type of daoyin, it is important to avoid certain times or seasons. For example, it is not advisable to practice when you are overly full or excessively hungry, as it can be harmful to the body. Additionally, it is best to avoid

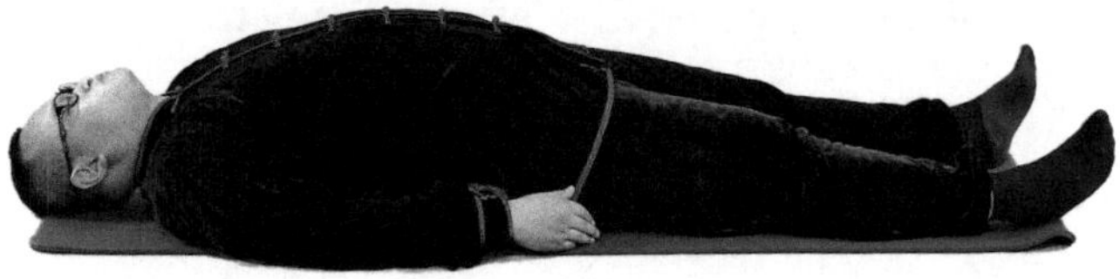

図4-2　Figure 4-2

practicing during unfavorable days or seasons. After the exercise and before eating, take a walk of 120 steps or a few thousand steps. Dietary rules: Avoid extremely hot or cold foods, and strive for a balance of the five flavors. Avoid stale, spoiled, leftover food, as well as insects or scorpions. During meals, it is important to take small bites and chew thoroughly. After finishing a meal, do not immediately go to sleep. This is known as the "grain medicine" principle, where diet and qi are harmonized, which is truly the best medicine.

[操作要领与注意事项] 松解衣服使身体没有挂碍，恬淡安卧，使心思专注不外驰，这样能够使气容易运行。舒展腰部，使肾区不受逼迫和紧压。尽量使气充满小腹，应该是腹部内后收摄牵动呼吸，同时使上面的气息下行，并止于此处。所谓引动肾气，就是把肾水导引到咽喉来，滋润上部。所谓通利阴阳，阴阳相合可以增加气力。

[Tips and notes] Loosening the clothes allows the body to be unobstructed, promoting a peaceful and relaxed state of mind, and preventing mental distractions. This helps to facilitate the smooth circulation of qi. Stretching the waist area helps to relieve pressure on the kidney. The goal is to fill the lower abdomen with qi by contracting the lower abdomen during inhalation and gently guiding the upward breath downward until it settles in this area. The concept of stimulating kidney qi refers to guiding the kidney water to the throat area, nourishing the upper part of the body. The idea of promoting the balance of yin and yang means that when yin and yang are in harmony, it can increase the body's energy and vitality.

五、伤寒病诸候提要
Daoyin Exercises for Cold Damage Disorders

本节论述伤寒病诸候的导引术。伤寒有狭义与广义之分。狭义的伤寒，指感受寒邪，即时发病。广义的伤寒，为一切外感疾病的统称。

This chapter introduces the daoyin exercises for cold damage disorders. In a narrow sense, they are a group of disorders caused by external cold. In a broader sense, they are used to encompass all externally contracted disorders.

（1）坐式（端坐）。舒展腰部，以鼻缓缓纳气，右手捏鼻，闭眼吐气（图5-1）。适用于伤寒所致阵阵头痛。练习以出汗为度。

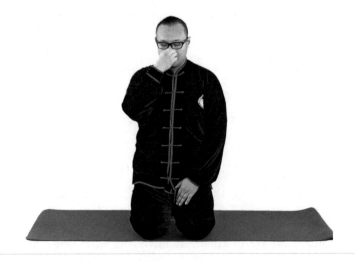

图5-1　Figure 5-1

(1) Take an upright sitting position. Stretch the waist, inhale slowly through the nose, pinch the nose with the right hand, close the eyes and exhale (Figure 5–1). This exercise can help treat intermittent headache caused by cold damage. Practice until sweating is present.

[操作要领与注意事项] 鼻纳气以开清窍，利头痛；右手捏鼻，有升阳祛寒之效；闭眼可安神，口吐气以驱邪，可舒缓头痛。

[Tips and notes] Inhaling through the nose can open the mind and relieve headache, while pinching the nose with the right hand can promote the ascending of clear yang qi and dispel cold. Closing the eyes can calm the mind, and exhaling through the mouth can expel pathogenic factors and thus relieve headache.

（2）站式。举左手，用左脚踩地，仰掌向上，持续到鼻纳气40次为止（图5-2）。有助于去除身体发热，脊背疼痛。

(2) Take a standing position. Raise the left hand, stomp the left foot, turn the palm upward, and inhale through the nose 40 times (Figure 5–2). This exercise can help alleviate feverish sensations in the body, and back pain.

[操作要领与注意事项] 举左手仰掌更利于合胸，火气向下行；左脚踩地，可退火。练习时要求含胸，左侧身躯放松；踩脚时，须全脚掌着地，忌脚跟或脚趾先着地。

[Tips and notes] Raising the left hand with the palm facing upward is beneficial for harmonizing the chest and directing the fire downward. Stomping the left foot can help clear away excessive fire. During practice, sink the chest and relax the left side

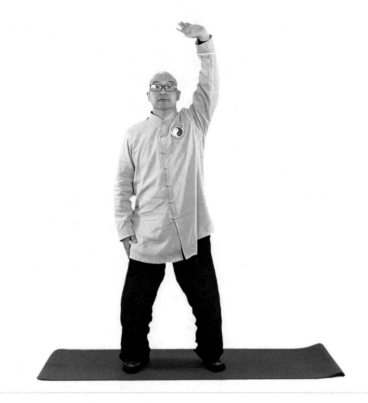

图5-2　Figure 5-2

of the body. When stomping the foot, touch the ground with the entire sole of the foot, and avoid landing on the heel or toes first.

六、时气病诸候提要
Daoyin Exercises for Disorders Induced by Non-seasonal Pathogens

本节论述时气病诸候的导引术。时气病，指时春应暖反寒，逢夏应热却冷，处秋应凉反热，临冬应寒又暖。当令的季节却出现反季的气候，使人致病，称时气病。

This chapter introduces the daoyin exercises for disorders induced by non-seasonal pathogens. Non-seasonal pathogens may occur when the weather is contrary to the expected climate during a particular season, including cold weather in spring and summer and hot weather in summer and winter.

站式、坐式、卧式。清晨，两手交叉从头上牵拉两耳向上，牵引至鬓发，气血就能流通（图6-1）。可使头发不白、耳不聋。两手相互摩擦，手掌温热后，以此热气摩面，从上到下，14次（图6-2）。有助于去除汗气，使面部有光泽。两手相互摩擦，手掌温热后，以此热气从上至下导引身体，名为干浴。有助于抵御风寒时气、治疗寒热头痛等。

Take a standing, sitting or lying position. In the morning, pull both ears upward to circulate qi and blood (Figure 6-1). This exercise can prevent gray hair and deafness. Rub the hands to generate heat, and then use the warm palms to massage the face from top to bottom 14 times. This exercise can remove sweat and make the face lustrous. Rub the hands to generate heat, and then use the warm palms to guide the body movements from top to bottom, known as "dry bathing". This exercise can help the body resist wind and cold, and treat varying disorders such as headache caused by cold or heat.

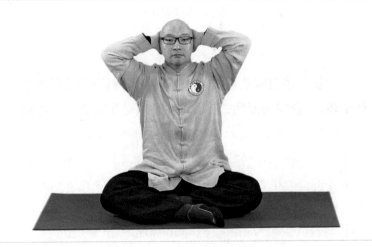

图6-1　Figure 6-1

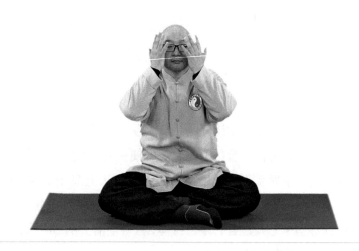

图6-2　Figure 6-2

［操作要领与注意事项］两手交叉牵拉两耳向上，可疏通少阳经，以鼓动肾气；手掌摩热，打开劳宫穴，摩面摸身，可疏通厥阴经，以助卫阳。

[Tips and notes] Pulling the ears upward can unblock the Shaoyang meridians and stimulate kidney qi. Rubbing the palms to generate heat and massaging the face and body can unblock the Jueyin meridians and support the defensive qi.

七、温病诸候提要
Daoyin Exercises for Warm Diseases

本节论述温病诸候的导引术。此温病指的是伏气温病，冬伤于寒，至春发为温病；不是指冬时感受非时之暖的冬温。

This chapter introduces the daoyin exercises for warm diseases. Warm diseases here refer to hidden warm diseases, which occur in spring after the body has been affected by pathogenic cold in winter, rather than referring to warm diseases caused by non-seasonal warmth in winter.

（1）站式、坐式、卧式。观想心气红色，肝气青色，肺气白色，脾气黄色，肾气黑色，在身体四周围绕并辟邪（图7-1）。

(1) Take a standing, sitting or lying position. Visualize the red heart qi, green liver qi, white lung qi, yellow spleen qi and black kidney qi surrounding the body and warding off pathogenic factors (Figure 7-1).

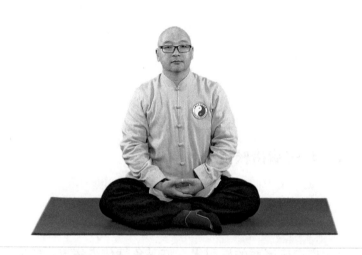

图7-1　Figure 7-1

[操作要领与注意事项] 完成此观想前，须先调整心意，松静自然。观想五行五色，可调和脏腑，祛邪扶正。

[Tips and notes] Before starting this visualization, it is necessary to adjust the mind and relax naturally. Visualizing the five elements and five colors can harmonize the zang-fu organs, and reinforce healthy qi to eliminate pathogenic factors.

（2）站式、坐式、卧式。想要辟邪驱鬼，应当常常诚意观想心（气）炎火如斗，煌煌光明。这样各种邪气就不敢侵犯，可以进入瘟疫地区之中（图7-1）。

(2) Take a standing, sitting or lying position. To expel pathogenic factors, visualize the heart (qi) as a blazing fire. In

this way, all kinds of pathogenic factors will not dare to invade the body, and one can enter the areas affected by epidemics with confidence (Figure 7-1).

[操作要领与注意事项] 完成此观想前,须先调整心意,松静自然。观想五行之火,红色应心阳,可祛邪扶正。

[Tips and notes] Before this visualization, it is necessary to keep a peaceful mind and relax the body. Visualize the element of fire. The color red corresponds to heart yang, which can dispel pathogenic factors and reinforce healthy qi.

八、疫疠病诸候提要
Daoyin Exercises for Epidemic Pestilence

论述疫疠病诸候的导引术。疫是急性传染病流行的通称,疠指病邪强烈,病势凶险。疫疠病指一年之中,由于节气不和、毒疫流行或瘴气所致的急性、烈性传染病。

This chapter introduces the daoyin exercises for epidemic pestilence. Epidemic pestilence refers to a group of contagious epidemic diseases caused by direct contact with virulent scourge or epidemic toxin and subsequent human-to-human or animal-to-human transmission.

（1）站式、坐式、卧式。延年益寿的方法,观想心气红色,肝气青色,肺气白色,脾气黄色,肾气黑色,在身体四周围绕并辟邪（图7-1）。

(1) Take a standing, sitting or lying position. To achieve longevity, visualize the red heart qi, green liver qi, white lung qi,

yellow spleen qi and black kidney qi surrounding the body and warding off pathogenic factors (Figure 7–1).

[操作要领与注意事项] 完成此观想前，须先调整心意，松静自然。观想五行五色，可调和脏腑，祛邪扶正。

[Tips and notes] Before starting this visualization, it is necessary to adjust the mind and relax naturally. Visualizing the five elements and five colors can harmonize the zang-fu organs, and reinforce healthy qi to eliminate pathogenic factors.

（2）站式、坐式、卧式。想要辟邪驱鬼，应当常常诚意观想心（气）炎火如斗，煌煌光明。这样各种邪气就不敢侵犯，可以进入瘟疫地区之中（图7–1）。

(2) Take a standing, sitting or lying position. To expel pathogenic factors, visualize the heart (qi) as a blazing fire. In this way, all kinds of pathogenic factors will not dare to invade the body, and one can enter the areas affected by epidemics with confidence (Figure 7–1).

[操作要领与注意事项] 完成此观想前，须先调整心意，松静自然。观想五行之火，红色应心阳，可祛邪扶正。

[Tips and notes] Before this visualization, it is necessary to keep a peaceful mind and relax the body. Visualize the element of fire. The color red corresponds to heart yang, which can dispel pathogenic factors and reinforce healthy qi.

九、冷热病诸候提要

Daoyin Exercises for Disorders Induced by Cold or Heat

本节论述冷热病诸候的导引术。冷热病主要由于阴阳失调，寒热偏胜所致。其中厥为气机逆乱的病证，阴气衰竭于下则发为热厥，阳气衰竭于下则发为寒厥。

This chapter introduces the daoyin exercises for disorders induced by cold or heat. Among these disorders, syncope is a group of critical conditions caused by disorder of qi. Exhaustion of yin qi in the lower part of the body may cause a heat syncope, while exhaustion of yang qi in the lower part of the body may cause a cold syncope.

（1）卧式（仰卧）。两膝靠拢，翻起两脚，舒展腰部，口纳气，使腹部胀满至极，做7次这样的呼吸（图1–15）。适用于大热疼痛、两腿动作不便。

(1) Take a supine position. Close the knees, lift both feet up, stretch the waist, inhale through the mouth until the abdomen is completely full, and repeat this breathing 7 times (Figure 1–15). This exercise can help relieve fever, pain, and impaired leg movements.

［操作要领与注意事项］完成此动作过程中，翻起两脚更利腰部舒展；口纳气，引气入腰腹，利于周身气血运行。

[Tips and notes] During the exercise, lift the legs to stretch the waist area; breathing in through the mouth allows qi to go into the waist and abdomen, facilitating the circulation of qi and blood throughout the body.

（2）卧式（俯卧）。去掉枕头，竖起两脚，鼻纳气40多次，再以鼻呼出。要令吸入鼻中的气极其微细，以至鼻子无法觉察的程度（图9-1）。有助于去除身中发热、脊背痛。

(2) Take a prone position. Remove the pillow, raise both feet, subtly inhale through the nose more than 40 times, and then subtly exhale through the nose (Figure 9–1). This exercise can help alleviate feverish sensations in the body and relieve back pain.

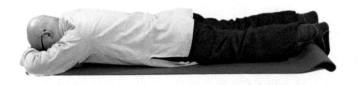

图9-1　Figure 9–1

［操作要领与注意事项］完成此动作过程中，鼻纳气40多次，须微细、迅速、连贯。

[Tips and notes] During this exercise, inhale through the nose more than 40 times in a subtle, rapid and continuous manner.

（3）坐式（正坐）。两手向后，手掌撑地，仰头面向太阳，以口纳气，因循着阳光咽下，做数十次（图9-2）。有助于去除发热、身体内伤、死肌。

(3) Take an upright sitting position. Place both hands behind to support the body with the palms, raise the head to face the sun, inhale deeply through the mouth, and swallow dozens of times (Figure 9–2). This exercise can help alleviate fever, internal injuries and necrosis.

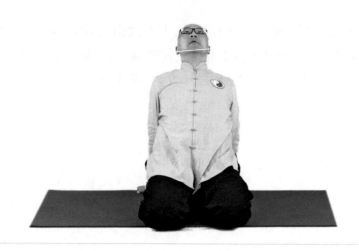

图9-2　Figure 9-2

[操作要领与注意事项] 遵循中医天人相应的规律。以太阳精华去除身体虚热,亦能活血化瘀生肌。

[Tips and notes] This exercise follows the principle of the correspondence between man and nature in TCM. By absorbing the essence of sunlight, it can help eliminate deficient heat in the body, promote blood circulation, resolve stasis, and regenerate tissues.

（4）站式。一脚踏地,另一脚向前,尽力舒展,手掌向四方回转。左右脚互换再做上述动作28次(图9-3)。有助于去除肠冷、腰背紧闷、骨头痛,并能使气血上下分布滋润全身。

(4) Take a standing position. Place one foot on the ground, fully lift the other foot forward, and rotate the palms. Change the position of the feet and repeat this movement 28 times on each side (Figure 9-3). This exercise can help relieve cold in the intestines, stiffness and tightness in the lower back, and bone pain, and can also circulate qi and blood to nourish the whole body.

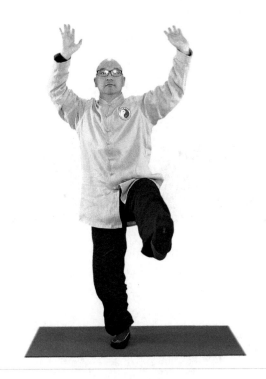

图9–3　Figure 9–3

［操作要领与注意事项］完成此动作过程中，单脚站立，在平衡稳定的基础上完成。缓缓转动手掌，有疏通经络，化瘀消结之效。

[Tips and notes] During the exercise, stand on one foot and complete it on the basis of balance and stability. Slowly rotate the palm to unblock the meridians and dissipate blood stasis.

（5）坐式。两脚相合（脚趾相对），两手紧握两脚脚趾，向上牵拉，头向后振动，尽力做到极势，21次（图9–4）。两脚继续尽力合住，两手向两侧舒展，全身与手脚尽力做到极势，14次（图9–5）。有助于去除身体各窍的病症及下身虚冷。

(5) Take a sitting position. Place the feet (soles) together, lift the feet with both hands, fully shake the head backward, and repeat 21 times (Figure 9–4). Keep the feet together, fully

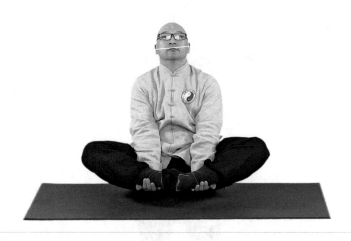

图9-4　Figure 9-4

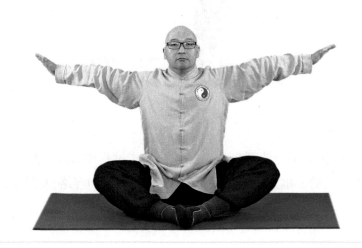

图9-5　Figure 9-5

extend both arms to the sides, and repeat 14 times (Figure 9-5). This exercise can help treat disorders involving the orifices, and alleviate cold in the lower part of the body.

［操作要领与注意事项］完成此动作过程中，若能使两腿持续离开地面，效果更好。体质虚弱的人，完成过程中可阶段性地使两腿暂离地面。

[Tips and notes] For better results, keep both legs off the ground. Those with a weak physical constitution can intermittently lift the legs off the ground during the exercise.

（6）坐式。两手交叉，反向撑地，身体慢慢向后仰。这个过程中脐腹自然用力，腰部向前散气，尽力做到极势时放松。上下来回做14次（图9-6）。有助于去除脐下寒冷、脚疼、五脏六腑不和。

(6) Take a sitting position. Cross both hands to support the body, and slowly and fully lean backward. During this process, exert force with the abdomen, and dissipate qi with the waist. Repeat this exercise 14 times (Figure 9–6). This exercise can help alleviate cold in the lower abdomen, foot pain, and disharmony between the zang organs and fu organs.

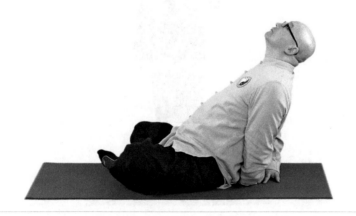

图9-6　Figure 9–6

［操作要领与注意事项］完成此动作过程中，身体缓缓后仰，使腰部慢慢贴向脐部，以助肾阳温化关元气海。

[Tips and notes] During the exercise, slowly lean backward to bring the waist close to the navel, which can help kidney yang warm the points Guanyuan (CV 4) and Qihai (CV 6).

（7）站式。两手向后托腰，尽力缩紧两肩，左右转身，来回做21次（图9-7）。有助于去除腹肚脐冷、肩胛发紧、胸部和腋下不适。

(7) Take a standing position. Place both hands on the lower back to hold it, fully close the shoulders, rotate the body left and right, and repeat 21 times (Figure 9-7). This exercise can help alleviate cold in the abdomen, tightness in the shoulders and scapula, and discomfort in the chest and armpits.

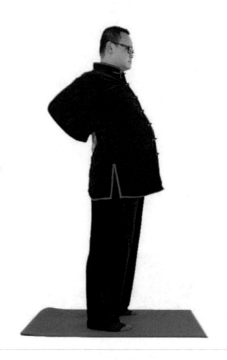

图9-7　Figure 9-7

［操作要领与注意事项］完成此动作过程中，肩部夹紧，以放松腰脊；两手向后托腰，以助肾阳温化关元气海；转身时，以手托腰转，腰部不主动用力转。忌用虎口掐腰。

[Tips and notes] During the exercise, close the shoulders to relax the spine. Place both hands behind the waist to help kidney yang warm the points Guanyuan (CV 4) and Qihai (CV 6). When rotating the body, use the hands to hold and turn the waist instead of actively using force in the waist. Avoid using the part of the hand between the thumb and the index finger to hold the waist.

（8）跪式（互跪）。两手向后，手掌撑地，鼻出气向下；然后腰腹逐渐向后下，当觉得腰脊部气息滞胀时，腰腹再恢复向上，上下来回做14次（图2–54）。身体正直，左右散气，转腰21次。有助于去除脐下冷闷、膝头冷、解溪内疼痛。

(8) Take a kneeling position. Kneel by placing the right knee on the ground, erecting the left knee and sitting on the right heel, almost like getting down on one knee. Place both hands behind the body to support the body weight, exhale through the nose, gradually bend backward until a distending sensation is present in the waist, return to the starting position, and repeat 14 times (Figure 2–54). Stand upright, relax the body, and rotate the waist 21 times. This exercise can help treat oppression and cold in the lower abdomen, cold in the knees, and pain in the point Jiexi (ST 41).

[操作要领与注意事项] 完成此动作过程中，腰腹逐渐向后下，可松解腰脊；配合鼻出气，小腹微微向腰部收，可温化关元气海。

[Tips and notes] Gradually bend backward to relax the back. Exhale through the nose and slightly tuck in the lower abdomen to warm the points Guanyuan (CV 4) and Qihai (CV 6).

（9）卧式（仰卧）。舒展两脚，鼻纳气，至满，脚掌转动30次（图1–34）。有助于去除脚寒、厥逆。

(9) Take a supine position. Extend the arms and legs, inhale through the nose deeply, and rotate the soles of the feet

功法操作 · Movements

30 times (Figure 1–34). This exercise can help alleviate cold in the feet, and syncope.

［操作要领与注意事项］伸展两脚，膝关节可微微放松，以脚趾带动脚掌转动，使鼻自然纳气。

[Tips and notes] Extend both feet and slightly relax the knee joints. Use the toes to drive the rotation of the feet and inhale through the nose naturally.

十、气病诸候提要
Daoyin Exercises for Qi Disorders

本节论述气病诸候的导引术。很多疾病是由于气机变化而发生的。如怒则气上，喜则气缓，思则气结，悲则气消，恐则气下，愁则气乱，寒则气收，热则气泄，劳则气散等。九气所引起的疾病各不相同。

This chapter introduces the daoyin exercises for qi disorders. Varying disorders can be induced by qi disorders, since anger causes qi to rise, joy causes qi to slack, overthinking causes qi to stagnate, sadness consumes qi, fear causes qi to descend, fright causes qi to become chaotic, cold causes qi to contract, heat causes qi to disperse, and overexertion causes qi to scatter.

1. 上气候提要
1. Disorders induced by the rising of qi

所谓上气，气上而不下，升而不降，痞满膈中，气道壅塞，肺气不得宣肃，喘息急且有声。

The rising of qi may cause fullness and stuffiness in the chest, impair the dispersing of lung qi, and subsequently lead to panting and rapid breathing.

（1）站式、坐式。两手向后，合手托腰尽力向上，全身振摇带动臂肘振摇，做7次（图10-1）。然后手不移位，身体直上直下反复14次。有助于去除脊、心、肺气的壅闷，使之消散。

（1）Take a standing or sitting position, place both hands on the lower back to support it, shake the whole body, and repeat 7 times (Figure 10-1). Without moving the hands, vertically lower the body and then stand up 14 times. This exercise can help eliminate stagnation and stuffiness in the spine, heart and lung.

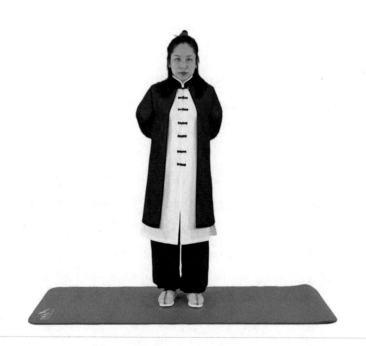

图10-1　Figure 10-1

［操作要领与注意事项］手托腰，更利于腰部放松，以腰胯为中心带动全身运动。

[Tips and notes] Placing the hands on the waist to support it is more conducive to relaxing the waist. Use the waist as the center to drive the movement of the entire body.

（2）坐式。凡是学习调息的人，首先须正坐，并拢膝盖和脚。初学时，先将脚趾相对，脚跟向外扒开，（臀部）坐于脚跟上，坐得安稳（图1-47）。再将两脚跟向内相对，（臀部）坐于脚跟上，脚趾向外扒开（图1-48）；感觉闷痛后逐渐起身，然后再坐回脚跟上。（练习）直至上述两种坐姿都不觉得闷痛，才开始把两脚跟向上竖起，（臀部）坐于脚跟上，脚趾并拢，反方向朝外（图1-49）。以上三种坐姿就是正坐的一般练习方式。有助于去除膀胱内冷气、膝冷、双脚冷痛、喘息上气、腰疼。

(2) Take a sitting position. For those learning to regulate their breathing, it is important to sit upright and bring the knees and feet together. For beginners, start by positioning the toes facing each other and the heels turned outward, and sit on the heels for stability (Figure 1–55). Then, position the heels facing each other and the toes turned outward while sitting on the heels (Figure 1–56). Gradually stand up when experiencing oppressive pain, and then sit back on the heels. When there is no oppressive pain in the above-mentioned sitting positions, raise up the heels and sit on them with the toes together and facing outward (Figure 1–57). The above three postures are the typical practice methods of upright sitting. They can help eliminate cold in the bladder, knees and feet, and alleviate such symptoms as shortness of breath and lower back pain.

［操作要领与注意事项］学习此动作时，需循序渐进，按由

易到难的顺序进行练习。

[Tips and notes] When learning this exercise, it is necessary to progress gradually and practice in order from easy to difficult.

（3）坐式。两脚脚趾相对，做5次呼吸，可以引动心肺气向下，适用于咳逆上气（图10-2）。继续用力使脚趾相对，心意放松，则肺中气出。然后通过辗转屈伸使肺内外得到舒张，觉得协调舒适，没有不舒服的感觉就好了。

(3) Take a sitting position. Bring the soles together and breathe 5 times to guide lung qi and heart qi downward. This exercise can help relieve cough and qi reversal (Figure 10-2). Continue to exert force to make the toes face each other and relax the mind to make lung qi go out. Then, do extension and flexion movements to comfort the lung.

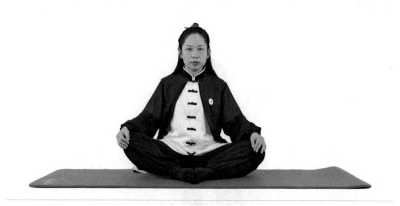

图10-2　Figure 10-2

［操作要领与注意事项］下颌微微上抬（下眼睑碰上眼睑），肺叶舒张，空气自然入肺。

[Tips and notes] Slightly lift the chin to expand the lung lobes and allow air to enter the lung naturally.

2. 卒上气候提要

2. Disorders induced by sudden counterflow of qi

肺失宣肃，或风邪突袭，或突然愤怒，皆可导致气机突然上逆。

Such factors as the failure of the lung to disperse qi, the invasion of pathogenic wind and sudden anger may cause sudden counterflow of qi.

站式。两手交叉放于下颌，身体松沉到极点，可补肺气，治疗突然气逆咳嗽。两手放于下颌，轻抚两侧颈动脉（图10-3），以下颌尽力向胸中勾，极速牵拉至喉骨，尽力做3次，补气充足（图10-4）。适用于暴气上气、失音等病。令气息调和匀长，声音洪亮。

Take a standing position. Cross the hands, place them under the jaw, and totally relax the body. This exercise can

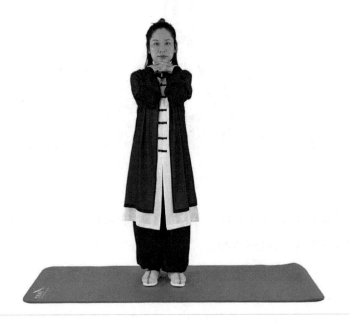

图10-3　Figure 10-3

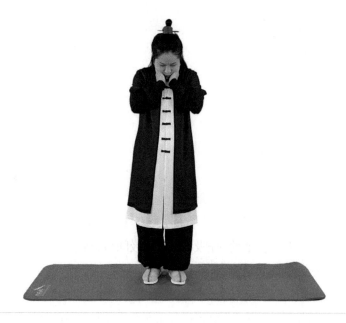

图10-4　Figure 10-4

supplement lung qi and treat sudden coughing induced by the counterflow of qi. Place the hands under the chin, gently massage the carotid arteries on both sides (Figure 10–3), fully bring the chin close to the chest, and repeat 3 times to tonify qi (Figure 10–4). This exercise can help treat disorders such as counterflow of qi and aphonia. It can regulate the breath and make the voice loud and clear.

［操作要领与注意事项］完成此动作过程中，两手交叉放于下颌，用于固定头部，人向下松沉，使气机向下。下颌尽力向胸中勾，颈椎胸椎配合动作，使胸椎打开。

[Tips and notes] During this exercise, cross the hands under the chin to stabilize the head, relax the body and sink qi downward. Fully bring the chin close to the chest with the help of cervical and thoracic vertebrae to open up the chest.

3. 结气候提要

3. Disorders induced by qi stagnation

思则气结。

Overthinking causes qi to stagnate.

（1）坐式（端坐）。舒展腰部，举左手，仰掌向上，右手后下，掌心向下，鼻纳气，至满，呼吸7次。呼吸间可稍顿右手（图10-5）。有助于去除手臂及背的疼痛、结气。

（1）Take an upright sitting position. Stretch the waist, raise the left hand, turn the palm upward, lower the right hand with the palm facing downward, deeply inhale through the nose, and breathe 7 times (Figure 10–5). This exercise can help relieve pain in the arms and back, and alleviate qi stagnation.

［操作要领与注意事项］完成此动作时，举左手，利于气机疏通；右手后下，指尖可朝下或朝前，利于鼻纳气。右手手指忌指尖朝后。

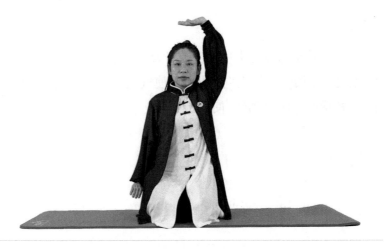

图10-5　Figure 10-5

[Tips and notes] During this exercise, lifting the left hand helps to regulate the flow of qi, while pressing down the right hand with the fingertips pointing downward or forward facilitates the inhalation through the nose. Avoid pointing the fingertips of the right hand backward.

（2）坐式（端坐）。舒展腰部，举左手，仰掌向上，右手托右胁，鼻纳气，至满，呼吸7次（图10-6）。有助于去除结气。

(2) Take an upright sitting position. Stretch the waist, lift the left hand, turn the palm upward, place the right hand on the right flank, deeply inhale through the nose, and breathe 7 times (Figure 10-6). This exercise can help alleviate qi stagnation.

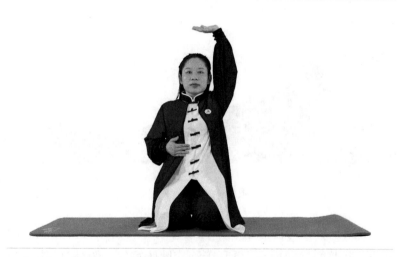

图10-6　Figure 10-6

［操作要领与注意事项］完成此动作时，举左手，利于气机疏通；右手后下，指尖可朝下或朝前，利于鼻纳气。右手手指忌指尖朝后。

[Tips and notes] During this exercise, lifting the left hand helps to regulate the flow of qi, while pressing down the right hand with the fingertips pointing downward or forward facilitates the inhalation through the nose. Avoid pointing the fingertips of the right hand backward.

（3）卧式。两手以肘头撑地，向上撑肚腹，尽力做到极势，当感到闷胀时，肚腹放松，上下来回做35次（图10-7）。有助于去除脊背体内疼、骨节拘急强直、肚肠宿气。练习这个动作不能吃太饱，也不能用肚编束缚腰腹。

(3) Take a lying position. Support the body with the elbows, fully lift the abdomen until an oppressive sensation is present, then relax the abdomen and repeat 35 times (Figure 10-7). This exercise can help alleviate back pain, joint stiffness, and intestinal qi retention. It is important to avoid practicing it when you are full and avoid wearing tight clothing that restricts the waist and abdomen.

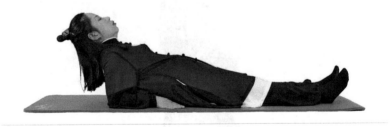

图10-7　Figure 10-7

［操作要领与注意事项］此动作可以仰卧或俯卧完成。仰卧时，肚脐微微向前顶，更利于治疗肚肠宿气。俯卧时，头微微举起，更利于治疗脊背体内疼、骨节拘急强直。

[Tips and notes] This exercise can be done in a supine position or prone position. When taking a supine position, pushing the navel forward slightly is more effective for intestinal qi retention. When taking a prone position, raising the head slightly is more effective for back pain and joint stiffness.

4. 逆气候提要
4. Disorders induced by counterflow of qi

逆气,有因大怒而致,又有因胃气不得下行,或因肺络不顺,或因肾虚水气上犯所致。

Such factors as rage, inability of stomach qi to descend, obstruction of the lung meridian, and ascending of water retention due to kidney deficiency may cause counterflow of qi.

卧式(仰卧)。以左脚跟勾住右脚拇指,鼻纳气,至满,做7次这样的呼吸(图1-31)。有助于去除气结气逆。

Take a supine position. Hook the left heel around the right big toe, inhale through the nose deeply, and repeat this breathing 7 times (Figure 1–31). This exercise can help treat qi stagnation and counterflow of qi.

[操作要领与注意事项] 完成此动作过程中,通过鼻纳气至满来舒展腰膝。勿用拙力。可补气行气,利气机下行。

[Tips and notes] During the exercise, inhale deeply through the nose to stretch the waist and knees. Do not use brute force. This exercise can tonify and circulate qi, and facilitate the downward movement of qi.

十一、脚气病诸候提要
Daoyin Exercises for Beriberi

本节论述脚气病诸候的导引术。脚气病由于感受风毒之邪所致。脚气痹弱、挛急、疼痛、麻木不仁为常见症状。脚气上气、心腹胀急、惊悸，是脚气病的危重证候。

This chapter introduces the daoyin exercises for beriberi. Beriberi is caused by the contraction of pathogenic wind and toxins. It is characterized by leg weakness, spasm, pain, numbness and insensitivity. Beriberi accompanied by counterflow of qi, abdominal distension or fright palpitations is a critical condition.

（1）坐式。两脚自然舒展，放松身心，纳气向下，内心柔和惬意（图1-40）。然后屈一脚，放于另一侧膝下；伸展的脚五趾尽力上翘，然后躺下仰卧，在头部还未接触地面时，两手臂立即尽力向前伸展，头部亦向上拉起，这一刻全身皆处于拉伸状态，这样做14次（图1-41）。左右脚互换再做上述动作。适用于脚疼、腰背肩臂冷、血冷、日渐亏损之病。

(1) Take a sitting position. Naturally extend the feet, relax the body, keep a peaceful mind, and inhale deeply (Figure 1–48). Then bend one leg and place it under the knee of the other leg. Raise the toes of the extended foot as high as possible and lie down on the back. Before the head touches the ground, immediately extend the arms forward and pull the head up to stretch the whole body. Repeat these movements 14 times (Figure 1–49). Change the position of the feet and repeat the above movements. This exercise can help relieve foot pain, cold sensation and blood stasis in the lower back and shoulders, and chronic consumptive conditions.

［操作要领与注意事项］动作外形与仰卧起坐相似，但此动作更注重身体内在气血运行，身体更为轻便。

[Tips and notes] The movement is similar to sit-ups, but

focuses more on the internal circulation of qi and blood in the body, making the body more relaxed.

（2）卧式（俯卧）。侧视，脚趾撑地脚跟向上，舒展腰部，鼻纳气，至满，呼吸7次（图11-1）。有助于去除脚中弦痛、转筋、脚酸疼、脚痹弱。

(2) Take a prone position. Turn the head to one side, lift the heels to support the ground with the toes, stretch the waist, deeply inhale through the nose, and breathe 7 times (Figure 11-1). This exercise can help relieve foot pain, leg cramps, and foot soreness and weakness.

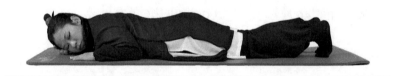

图11-1　Figure 11-1

［操作要领与注意事项］完成此动作时，侧视更利于脊柱延展；脚趾伸向下用力以助伸腰，上半身不用力。

[Tips and notes] During the exercise, turning the head to one side can help stretch the spine. Supporting the ground with the toes assists in stretching the waist, while the upper body should not use force.

（3）坐式。舒展两脚，散气到涌泉穴，3次。气彻底到了涌泉穴后，收屈右脚，两手握住涌泉穴向上拉，同时脚向下踏，这一刻手脚同时用力，尽力做到极势，送气至涌泉穴，做21次（图2-45）。完成上述动作的过程中，不要没有气的运行。有助于去除肾内冷气、膝冷、脚疼。

(3) Take a sitting position. Extend both legs and disperse qi to the point Yongquan (KI 1) 3 times. After qi has thoroughly reached the point, lift the right leg, and grip the point with both hands to fully pull upward while stepping down with the foot. Repeat 21 times (Figure 2–45). During the exercise, circulate qi. This exercise can help treat cold in the kidney and knees and can also treat foot pain.

［操作要领与注意事项］完成此动作过程中，自然放松地坐着，心气自然向下行至涌泉穴；两手抱脚向上牵拉时，须使大腿竖抱于腹前，不可横抱。

[Tips and notes] During this exercise, sit naturally and relax the body to make heart qi go downward naturally to the point Yongquan (KI 1). When pulling the foot upwards with the hands, keep the thighs vertical and close to the abdomen.

（4）坐式。一脚屈膝脚趾尽力向上翘，另一只脚放于膝头，心意放松，自然向两脚跟下出气。一手向下急按膝头，另一手向后按地，尽力做到最大幅度左右手脚互换做上述动作，各14次（图11-2）。有助于去除膝部、大腿的疼痛拘急。

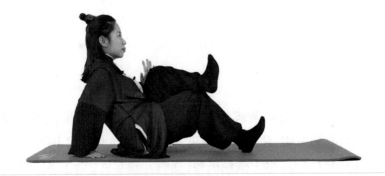

图11-2　Figure 11-2

(4) Take a sitting position. Bend one knee and fully lift the toes, place the other foot on the other knee, relax the mind and naturally make qi go out through the heels. Fully press down on the knee with one hand, and press down on the ground with the other hand to achieve the maximum range of motion. Repeat 14 times on each side (Figure 11-2). This exercise can help alleviate pain in the knees and thighs.

［操作要领与注意事项］完成此动作时，坐椅子上更易完成；整个动作把脚跟、跟腱做拔伸；整个动作有利于髋关节和骶髂关节打开。

[Tips and notes] It is much easier to do this exercise sitting in a chair. The entire movement involves stretching the heels and Achilles tendons. This movement is beneficial for opening up the hip and sacroiliac joints.

（5）站式。一脚踏地，另一脚向后，将解溪穴（脚背踝关节部位）安放在踏地一脚的脚跟上。侧身，两手从一侧向后伸展，尽力做到最大幅度。左右手脚互换做上述动作，各14次（图11-3）。有助于去除脚疼痛、痹急、腰痛。

(5) Take a standing position. Place one foot on the ground and the other foot behind, with the point Jiexi (ST 41) (located on the ankle joint on the top of the foot) resting on the heel of the foot on the ground. Stand sideways, extend both hands backward from one side, and strive to achieve the maximum range of motion. Repeat 14 times on each side (Figure 11-3). This exercise can help alleviate foot pain, acute *Bi*-impediment symptoms and lower back pain.

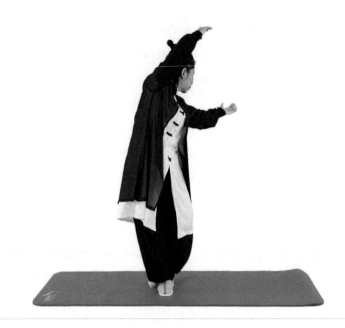

图11-3　Figure 11-3

［操作要领与注意事项］完成此动作过程中，另一脚不接触地面；转身要慢；站立稳定。

[Tips and notes] During this exercise, do not touch the ground with the other foot; turn the body slowly and stand steadily.

十二、咳嗽病诸候提要
Daoyin Exercises for Cough

本节论述咳嗽病诸候的导引术。咳嗽是由于肺脏首先感受外邪所引起，有新咳久咳、脏腑咳之分，虚证、实证之辨。

This chapter introduces the daoyin exercises for cough. Cough is caused by contraction of external pathogenic factors in the lung, and can be classified into newly contracted cough, chronic cough, as well as cough caused by disorders of the zang-fu organs. The nature of cough includes deficiency and excess.

（1）站式、坐式、卧式。先以鼻纳气，然后闭起嘴巴，再咳嗽，最后再以鼻纳气（图12-1）。适用于咳嗽。

(1) Take a standing, sitting or lying position. Inhale through the nose, close the mouth, cough, and then inhale again through the nose (Figure 12-1). This exercise can help treat cough.

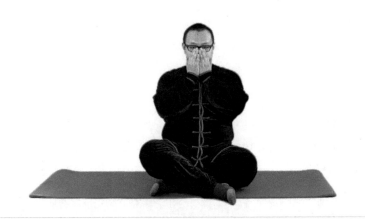

图12-1　Figure 12-1

［操作要领与注意事项］完成此动作时，可以两手辅助捂住嘴鼻；咳嗽时，忌气从嘴漏出。

[Tips and notes] During this exercise, use the hands to cover the mouth and nose. When coughing, do not let the air leak out of the mouth.

（2）卧式（仰卧）。清晨，去掉枕头，舒展手脚，闭起眼睛和嘴巴，闭气，尽力做到极限，当腹部和两脚有撑胀感时，休息片刻，再次吸起腹部，蹺起两脚约两个拳头的高度；待呼吸稍稍平复后，再次练习（图12-2）。春天做3次（3的倍数）、夏天做5次（5的倍数）、秋天做7次（7的倍数）、冬天做9次（9的倍数）。可以荡涤五脏，滋润六腑。

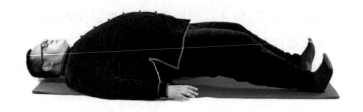

图12-2　Figure 12-2

(2) Take a supine position. In the morning, remove the pillow, stretch the arms and legs, close the eyes and mouth, fully hold the breath until an extending sensation in the abdomen and feet is present, then take a break, and raise the feet to a height of about two fists. Calm down the breath, and do the exercise again (Figure 12-2). In spring, do this exercise 3 or multiples of 3 times; in summer, do this exercise 5 or multiples of 5 times; in autumn, do this exercise 7 or multiples of 7 times; in winter, do this exercise 9 or multiples of 9 times. This exercise can cleanse the five zang organs and nourish the six fu organs.

［操作要领与注意事项］完成此动作过程中，略撑脚趾，有利于腹部产生撑胀感；迅速吸气则两脚自然跷起。此动作腰胯部的舒张，有助吸气，吸气后有助于腰胯部舒张。闭气至极限，建议医护人员在旁看护。

[Tips and notes] During this exercise, slightly extend the toes to help extend the abdomen, and inhale quickly to lift the feet naturally. Extending the lower back and hips helps with inhalation, and inhalation helps further extend the lower back and hips. Since this exercise requires fully holding the breath, it is recommended to do this exercise under the watchful eye of a person.

（3）站式。立正，转身向后看，然后不呼不吸7次（图1-83）。适用于咳逆、胸中病、寒热。

(3) Take a standing position. Stand upright, turn the head to look back, and passively hold the breath 7 times (Figure 1–83). This exercise can help treat cough, chest disorders, chills and fever.

［操作要领与注意事项］完成此动作过程中，以眼神带动整个脊柱运动，低头向后看，做连续动作。动作似狼顾，眼光内敛不外露，从下往上做下弦线弧度运动。

[Tips and notes] During this exercise, use the movement of the eyes to drive the movement of the spine, and keep the movements continuous and smooth.

十三、淋病诸候提要
Daoyin Exercises for Strangury

本节论述淋病诸候的导引术。淋病是由于肾虚膀胱热所引起的。膀胱为津液之府，过热则气化失常，水道不畅；津液上不能输送入血脉，下不能由前阴排出，而贮积于尿胞。虚则小便增多。尿频数，解又淋沥不畅，故为淋病。

This chapter introduces the daoyin exercises for strangury. Strangury is caused by kidney deficiency and damp heat affecting the bladder. The bladder is the reservoir of body fluids. Excessive damp heat in the bladder may disturb qi transformation, and subsequently cause water retention. Kidney deficiency may lead to frequent and hesitant urination.

1. 诸淋候提要
1. Strangury

淋病是由于肾虚而膀胱有热，气化失常所致。

Strangury is caused by kidney deficiency and damp heat affecting the bladder. The bladder is the reservoir of body fluids. Excessive damp heat in the bladder may disturb qi transformation.

（1）卧式（仰卧）。屈膝，脚跟放于臀部下，两手轻放于两膝头，口纳气，使腹部快速舒张，至极，鼻出气，做7次（图2-56）。有助于去除淋症、小便数。

(1) Take a supine position. Bend the knees with the heels placed under the buttocks, place both hands on the knees, inhale quickly through the mouth to fully extend the abdomen, and then exhale through the nose. Repeat 7 times (Figure 2–56). This exercise can help treat strangury and frequent urination.

［操作要领与注意事项］口纳气至腰腹，有利脾胃气血运化，土生金，又利于疏通肺部与大脑清窍。

[Tips and notes] Inhale through the mouth to guide qi to the lower back and abdomen, which helps circulate qi and blood in the spleen and stomach, and also clear the lung and mind.

（2）蹲式（下蹲）。臀部离地一尺左右，两手从大腿外侧经膝内弯入，放于脚背，迅速握两脚脚趾，令脚趾背曲，尽力做到极势，1次（图13-1）。可以通利腰部和髋部，适用于淋症。

(2) Take a squatting position. Squat down (The distance between the buttocks and the ground is about 30 centimeters.), place the hands on the insteps, quickly and fully grasp the toes until the toes are bent, and hold for a few seconds. Do this exercise once (Figure 13–1). It can help unblock the lower back and hips, and treat strangury.

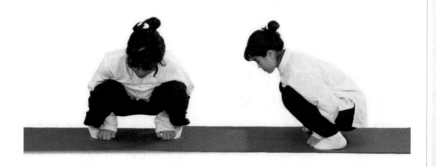

图13-1　Figure 13–1

［操作要领与注意事项］此动作有利于打开骶胯关节，配合纳气腰胯部舒张，更利腰髋部气血运行。

[Tips and notes] This posture can help open the sacroiliac joints. Together with inhalation and extending the lower back and hips, it promotes the circulation of qi and blood in the lower back and hips.

2. 石淋候提要
2. Stone strangury

石淋指小便淋痛而排出砂石。

Stone strangury is characterized by painful and dripping urination as well as the discharge of stones.

卧式（仰卧）。屈膝，脚跟放于臀部下，两手轻放于两膝头，口纳气，使腹部快速舒张，至极，鼻出气，做7次（图2-56）。有助于去除淋症、生殖器痛。

Take a supine position. Bend the knees with the heels placed under the buttocks, place both hands on the knees, inhale quickly through the mouth to fully extend the abdomen, and then exhale through the nose. Repeat 7 times (Figure 2-56). This exercise can help treat strangury and genital pain.

［操作要领与注意事项］口纳气至腰腹，有利脾胃气血运化，土生金，又利于疏通肺部与大脑清窍。

[Tips and notes] Inhale through the mouth to guide qi to the lower back and abdomen, which helps circulate qi and blood in the spleen and stomach, and also clear the lung and mind.

3. 气淋候提要
3. Qi strangury

气淋是由于肾虚膀胱热，胞内气胀所致。

Kidney deficiency and damp heat affecting the bladder may cause distension in the bladder, and subsequently lead to qi strangury.

（1）坐式。两脚跟放于对侧膝盖上（图13-2）。适用于癃症。

(1) Take a sitting position. Cross the lower legs and place the heels on the knees (Figure 13-2). This posture can help alleviate urinary retention.

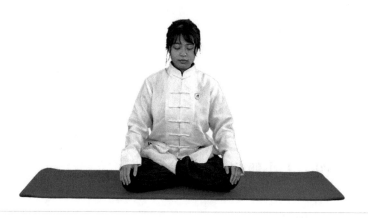

图13-2　Figure 13-2

［操作要领与注意事项］动作外形类似于双盘,有利于打开骶胯关节。此动作难度稍大易受伤,忌拙力,宜循序渐进。

[Tips and notes] Similar to full-lotus posture, this posture can help open the sacroiliac joints. This posture is more challenging and can cause injury. It is advisable to gradually progress and avoid using brute force.

（2）卧式（仰卧）。屈膝,脚跟放于臀部下,两手轻放于两膝头,口纳气,使腹部快速舒张,至极,鼻出气,做7次(图2-56)。适用于癃病、小便数、生殖器痛、阴下湿证、小腹痛、膝冷不灵活。

(2) Take a supine position. Bend the knees with the heels placed under the buttocks, place both hands on the knees, inhale quickly through the mouth to fully extend the abdomen, and then exhale through the nose. Repeat 7 times (Figure 2–56). This exercise can help treat urinary retention, genital pain, wet genitals, lower abdominal pain, cold in the knees and knee joint inflexibility.

［操作要领与注意事项］口纳气至腰腹,有利脾胃气血运化,土生金,又利于疏通肺部与大脑清窍。

[Tips and notes] Inhale through the mouth to guide qi to the lower back and abdomen, which helps circulate qi and blood in the spleen and stomach, and also clear the lung and mind.

十四、大小便病诸候提要
Daoyin Exercises for Disorders Involving Bowel/ Bladder Movements

本节论述大小便病诸候的导引术。大便病，是由于五脏不能调和，使三焦气化失利，冷热搏结所致。小便病的病源在肾与膀胱，或为虚寒，或为有热所致。

This chapter introduces the daoyin exercises for disorders involving bowel/bladder movements. Disharmony of the five zang organs may affect the qi transformation of the sanjiao and cause the retention of cold and heat in the sanjiao, thus leading to disorders involving bowel movements. Heat or deficient cold in the kidney and bladder may cause disorders involving bladder movements.

（1）坐式。两脚跟放于对侧膝盖上（图13-2）。有助于去除癃症。

(1) Take a sitting position. Cross the lower legs and place the heels on the knees (Figure 13-2). This posture can alleviate urinary retention.

［操作要领与注意事项］动作外形类似于双盘，有利于打开骶胯关节。此动作难度稍大易受伤，忌拙力，宜循序渐进。

[Tips and notes] Similar to full-lotus posture, this posture can help open the sacroiliac joints. This posture is more challenging and can cause injury. It is advisable to gradually progress and avoid using brute force.

（2）卧式（仰卧）。屈膝，脚跟放于臀部下，两手轻放于两膝头，口纳气，使腹部快速舒张，至极，鼻出气，做7次（图2-56）。适用于小便数。

(2) Take a supine position. Bend the knees with the heels placed under the buttocks, place both hands on the knees, inhale quickly through the mouth to fully extend the abdomen, and then exhale through the nose. Repeat 7 times (Figure 2–56). This exercise can help treat frequent urination.

［操作要领与注意事项］口纳气至腰腹，有利脾胃气血运化，土生金，又利于疏通肺部与大脑清窍。

[Tips and notes] Inhale through the mouth to guide qi to the lower back and abdomen, which helps circulate qi and blood in the spleen and stomach, and also clear the lung and mind.

（3）蹲式（下蹲）。臀部离地一尺左右，两手从大腿外侧经膝内弯入，放于脚背，迅速握两脚脚趾，令脚趾背曲，尽力做到极势，1次（图13-1）。可以通利腰部和髋部，适用于淋症。

(3) Take a squatting position. Squat down (The distance between the buttocks and the ground is about 30 centimeters.), place the hands on the insteps, quickly and fully grasp the toes until the toes are bent, and hold for a few seconds. Do this exercise once (Figure 13–1). It can help unblock the lower back

and hips, and treat strangury.

［操作要领与注意事项］此动作有利于打开骶胯关节，配合纳气腰胯部舒张，更利腰髋部气血运行。

[Tips and notes] This posture can help open the sacroiliac joints. Together with inhalation and extending the lower back and hips, it promotes the circulation of qi and blood in the lower back and hips.

（4）卧式（仰卧）。嘴纳气，鼻出气，当气温暖后，将气咽下，同时舒展伸直两手，小幅度旋转左右肋部（图14-1）。去除大便困难、腹痛、腹部中的寒气，这样做几十次，有助于疾病的恢复。

(4) Take a supine position. Inhale through the mouth and exhale through the nose. Once the air in the mouth is warm, swallow it while extending both arms and swinging the flanks slightly (Figure 14-1). To treat the difficulty in bowel movements, abdominal pain and cold in the abdomen, do this exercise dozens of times.

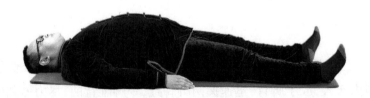

图14-1　Figure 14-1

［操作要领与注意事项］完成此动作时，口纳气有助腹部气机运化；左右转肋可松解两胁肋区，有助于排便。

[Tips and notes] Inhaling through the mouth can facilitate the transformation of qi in the abdomen. Swinging the flanks can release tension in the sub-costal region, and promote bowel movements.

（5）卧式（仰卧）。龟行气。藏身在衣被中，覆盖口鼻头面，不吸不呼，期间以鼻微微出气纳气，做9次这样的呼吸（图14-2）。适用于大便闭塞不通。

(5) Take a supine position. Assume the posture of a turtle to circulate qi, lie on the back covered by clothes, cover the mouth, nose, head and face, and breathe slowly 9 times (Figure 14-2). This exercise can help alleviate constipation.

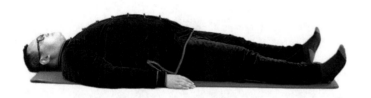

图14-2　Figure 14-2

［操作要领与注意事项］完成此动作过程中，松静自然，呼吸缓慢，渐渐深长，不宜憋气。初学若掌握不好，可以减少操作的次数与时间。

[Tips and notes] During the exercise, remain relaxed and calm, breathe slowly, gradually deepen the breath, and avoid holding the breath. Beginners can reduce the frequency and duration of the exercise.

（6）坐式（正坐）。两手交叉于后背（图14-3）。此动作称"带便"，适用于便秘，通利腹部气血，也适用于虚劳羸弱。跽坐。反叉两手放在背上，两手往上推至与心脏相平的位置（图14-4），头身后仰，做9次（图14-5）。适用于便秘、癃闭，通利腹部气血，也适用于虚劳羸弱。

Zhu Bing Yuan Hou Lun Dao Yin Shu (Explanations
for the Daoyin Exercises in *Zhu Bing Yuan Hou Lun*)

·

《诸 病 源 候 论》 导 引 术

242

功 法 操 作

·

Movements

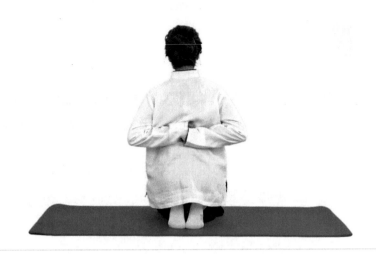

图14-3　　Figure 14-3

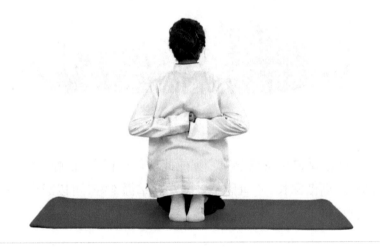

图14-4　　Figure 14-4

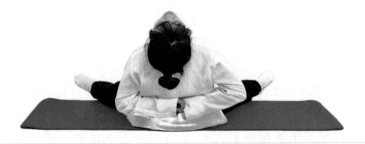

图14-5　　Figure 14-5

(6) Take an upright sitting position. Place the hands on the back and cross them (Figure 14–3). This exercise can help treat constipation, promote the circulation of qi and blood in the abdomen, and alleviate consumptive conditions and debility. Sit by stretching out and separating the legs like a winnowing pan, place the hands on the back and cross them, and push the hands upward until they are level with the heart (Figure 14–4). Then lean back, and repeat 9 times (Figure 14–5). This exercise can help treat constipation and urinary retention, promote the circulation of qi and blood in the abdomen, and alleviate consumptive conditions and debility.

[操作要领与注意事项] 完成此动作时,十指交叉(指尖朝下)放于骶骨位置配合正坐,更利于大便。初学应循序渐进,不宜逞强,以免拉伤背部肌肉。

[Tips and notes] During the exercise, cross the ten fingers with the fingertips facing downward and place them at the sacrum to assist in sitting upright and promoting bowel movements. Beginners should do the exercise step by step to prevent injury to the muscles in the back.

十五、五脏六腑病诸候提要
Daoyin Exercises for Disorders Involving the Zang-Fu Organs

本节论述五脏六腑病诸候的导引术。对藏象、虚实、病情发展、脉象等进行系统论述。

This chapter introduces the daoyin exercises for disorders involving the zang-fu organs. It provides a systematic analysis from the perspectives of *zang-xiang* (visceral manifestations), deficiency & excess, disease progression, and pulse conditions.

（1）站式、坐式、卧式。有肝病的人，容易忧愁不快乐，有悲伤、思虑、不满、恼怒的情绪，也会有头晕眼痛的症状。用"呵"字音出气，有助于疾病恢复（图15-1）。

(1) Take a standing, sitting or lying position. People with a liver disorder are prone to feeling unhappy and have emotional symptoms such as sadness, worry, dissatisfaction and anger, as well as symptoms such as dizziness and eye pain. Exhale with the sound "he" to help recover from the disorder (Figure 15–1).

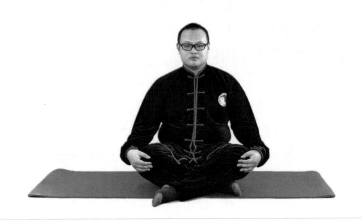

图15-1　Figure 15-1

［操作要领与注意事项］"呵"字音应火，应心。口发"呵"字音治肝病，为泻心火，母病泻子。凡字音"出气"须出声念，下同。

[Tips and notes] The sound "he" corresponds to the fire element and the heart. Since the liver is the mother of the heart in TCM theories, exhaling with the sound "he" can help treat liver disorders by draining excessive heart fire. This is in line with the principle of treating the mother organ to heal the child organ.

（2）站式、坐式、卧式。有心病的人，身体有发冷发热的症状。如果身体发冷，用"呼"字音吸气（图15-2）；如果发热，用"吹"字音出气（图15-3）。

(2) Take a standing, sitting or lying position. People with a heart disorder may experience symptoms such as chills and fever. For chills, inhale with the sound "hu". For fever, exhale with the sound "ci" (Figure 15-3).

［操作要领与注意事项］"呼"字音应土，应脾。口吸"呼"字音治寒证，为补脾土。"吹"字音应水，应肾，口发"吹"字音治热证，为泻肾之虚火。

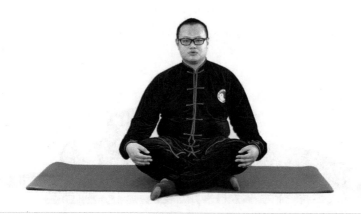

图15-2　Figure 15-2

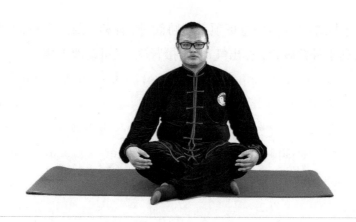

图15-3　Figure 15-3

[Tips and notes] The sound "hu" corresponds to the earth element and the spleen. Inhaling with the sound "hu" can help treat cold patterns via nourishing the spleen. The sound "ci" corresponds to the water element and the kidney. Exhaling with the sound "ci" can help treat heat patterns by eliminating the deficient fire of the kidney.

（3）卧式（侧卧）。左胁着地，伸直手脚，口纳气，鼻出气，周而复始不断练习（图15-4），有助于去除积聚和心下不适。

(3) Take a side-lying position. Place the left flank on the ground, stretch out the arms and legs, inhale through the mouth and exhale through the nose. Regular practice (Figure 15-4) can help remove accumulation and discomfort in the chest.

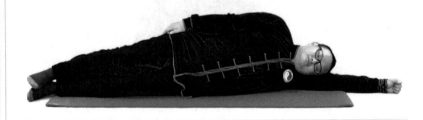

图15-4　Figure 15-4

[操作要领与注意事项] 左胁侧卧，有利于疏通上焦；口纳气，利于补益脾胃；鼻出气，既固摄肾气，又可疏泄上焦。

[Tips and notes] Lying on the left side can help unblock the upper jiao. Inhaling through the mouth is beneficial for nourishing the spleen and stomach. Exhaling through the nose can both consolidate and gather kidney qi, and also disperse the upper jiao.

（4）站式、坐式、卧式。有脾病的人,体表有游动风微微作痛、身体痒和烦闷疼痛的症状,用"嘻"字音出气(图15-5)。

(4) Take a standing, sitting or lying position. People with a spleen disorder may experience mild pain, itching and discomfort on the body surface. To address these symptoms, exhale with the sound "xi" (Figure 15-5).

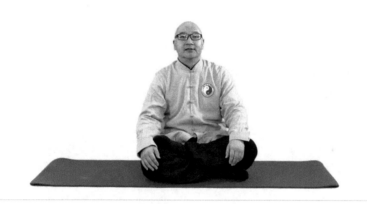

图15-5　Figure 15-5

［操作要领与注意事项］"嘻"字音应三焦。体表有风、火之邪,口发"嘻"字音以泻少阳。须出声念。

[Tips and notes]　The sound "xi" corresponds to the sanjiao organ. When there is pathogenic wind or fire affecting the body surface, exhale with the sound "xi" to disperse the Shaoyang meridians.

（5）站式、坐式、卧式。有肺病的人,躯体、胸背有疼痛胀满的症状,四肢感到烦闷不适,用"嘘"字音出气(图15-6)。

(5) Take a standing, sitting or lying position. People with a lung disorder may experience distending pain in the upper body and discomfort in the limbs. To alleviate these symptoms, exhale with the sound "xu" (Figure 15-6).

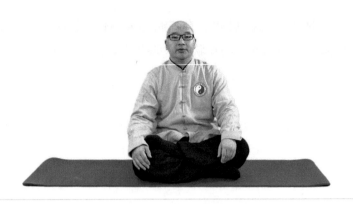

图15-6　Figure 15-6

操作要领与注意事项："嘘"字音应木，应肝。口发"嘘"字音以泻肝实。

[Tips and notes] The sound "xu" corresponds to the wood element and the liver. Exhaling with the sound "xu" can reduce liver excess.

（6）卧式（俯卧）。两手撑地伏身向下，口纳气，鼻出气（图15-7）。有助于去除胸中肺中诸病。

(6) Take a prone position. Place both hands on the ground, lower the body, inhale through the mouth and exhale through the nose (Figure 15-7). This exercise helps alleviate varying disorders involving the chest and lung.

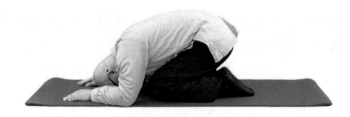

图15-7　Figure 15-7

［操作要领与注意事项］口纳气，可调脾胃；鼻出气，以泻肺邪。

[Tips and notes] Inhaling through the mouth can regulate the spleen and stomach, while exhaling through the nose helps dispel pathogenic factors from the lung.

（7）站式、坐式、卧式。有肾病的人，有咽喉阻塞、腹部胀满、耳聋不聪的症状，用"呬"字音出气（图15-8）。

(7) Take a standing, sitting or lying position. For those with a kidney disorder experiencing such symptoms as a foreign body sensation in the throat, abdominal fullness, impaired hearing and even deafness, exhale with the sound "hei" (Figure 15-8).

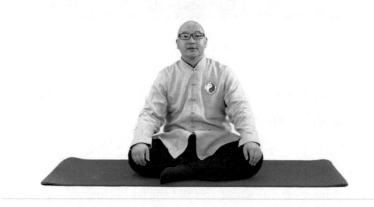

图15-8　Figure 15-8

［操作要领与注意事项］肾气亏虚，上窍受邪，口发"呬"字音以补肾祛邪。须出声念。

[Tips and notes] Exhaling with the sound "hei" can help treat kidney qi deficiency and pathogenic factors in the upper orifices.

（8）坐式。两脚相交而坐，两手握两脚解溪穴，两手向后牵拉，头向后仰，尽力做到极势，来回做7次（图15-9）。有助于去除肾气壅塞。

(8) Take a sitting position. Cross the feet, hold the points Jiexi (ST 41) on both sides with both hands, pull the feet backward, lean the head backward and repeat 7 times (Figure 15-9). This exercise helps relieve the stagnation of kidney qi.

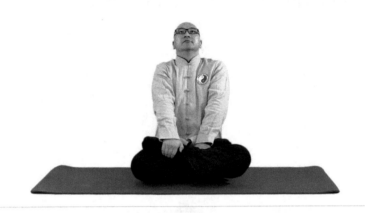

图15-9　Figure 15-9

［操作要领与注意事项］完成此动作过程中，脚尽量放松，后仰头部，有助松解脊骨，疏泄腰府气滞。

[Tips and notes] During the exercise, totally relax the feet and lean the head backward to release tension in the spine and alleviate the stagnation of qi in the lumbar region.

（9）蹲式（蹲坐）。侧身，两手尽力向前伸展，仰掌，做到极势，左右转动身体和腰部，21次（图15-10）。有助于去除膀胱内冷、血（虚动）风、骨节拘强。

(9) Take a squatting position. Turn the upper body to the side, extend both hands forward, turn the palms upward, and turn the body and waist to both sides 21 times (Figure

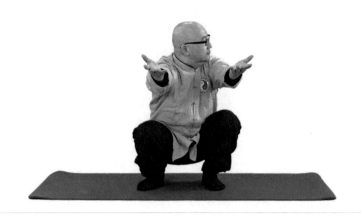

图15-10　Figure 15-10

15-10). This exercise helps alleviate cold in the bladder, blood deficiency stirring wind, as well as joint stiffness and rigidity.

［操作要领与注意事项］完成此动作过程中，蹲坐，限制下肢活动；侧身，打开腰胯活动度；两手向前，仰掌，有固定肩膀之意。

[Tips and notes] During the exercise, taking a squatting position can restrict the movement of the lower limbs. Turning the upper body to the side can open up the waist and hips. Extending both hands forward and turning the palms upward can stabilize the shoulders.

（10）跪式（互跪）。调和心气，气向下到脚。观想气一索一索地流布到身体各处，然后慢慢平展身体，匍匐至地；手舒展地放于两肋旁，手掌好像会不停地吸气呼气；当脸上觉得有点紧与闷时，就挺起背脊，（过一会）再向下至地，如此上下起伏做21次（图2-44）。有助于去除膝关节冷、膀胱宿病、腰脊僵硬、脐下冷闷。

(10) Take a kneeling position. Kneel by placing the right knee on the ground, erecting the left knee and sitting on the

right heel, almost like getting down on one knee. Harmonize heart qi and direct it downwards to the feet. Visualize the flow of qi spreading smoothly throughout the body, and then slowly bend the body forward. Extend and place the hands on the sides of the ribcage, and imagine continuously inhaling and exhaling through the palms. When oppressive and tight sensations are present, return to the starting posture and hold the position for a moment. Repeat 21 times (Figure 2–44). This exercise can help treat cold in the knees, chronic bladder disorders, stiff waist and back, as well as oppression and cold in the lower abdomen.

［操作要领与注意事项］完成此动作过程中，松静自然，心气自然向下。气行各处，观之即可，勿忘勿助。

[Tips and notes] During this exercise, keep a peaceful mind to descend heart qi naturally.

（11）站式、坐式、卧式。自膝部以下有病，当观想脐下有红光，红光里外相连周遍全身。自膝部以上至腰部有病，当观想脾有黄光。从腰部以上至头部有病，当观想心中有红光。病在皮肤有寒热，当观想肝内有青绿光。上述都要观想（各色）光里外相连周遍全身，同时通过闭气来收敛光芒向内照（病所）（图15-11）。

(11) Take a standing, sitting or lying position. For disorders below the knees, visualize a red light below the navel. For disorders between the knees and the waist, visualize a yellow light in the spleen. For disorders between the waist and the head, visualize a red light in the heart. For skin disorders accompanied by cold or heat symptoms, visualize a green light in the liver. In all cases, visualize the respective colored light

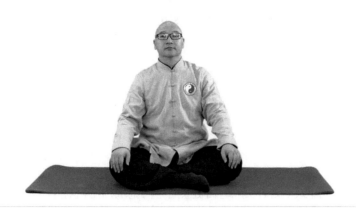

图15-11　　Figure 15-11

illuminating the entire body, while simultaneously holding the breath to draw the radiance inward towards the affected area (Figure 15–11).

［操作要领与注意事项］存想五色光，以感应五脏气机；通过闭气，加强气机运化；练习需要坚定、专注、细致。

[Tips and notes] Visualize the lights to perceive the qi activity of the five zang organs. Hold the breath to enhance the circulation of qi. Focus the mind on the practice.

十六、腹病诸候提要
Daoyin Exercises for Abdominal Disorders

本节论述腹病诸候的导引术。包括腹痛、腹胀。腹痛是由于脏腑虚弱，寒冷之气留着于肠胃募原之间，以致正邪对抗，故作痛。腹胀多为脾病，脾阳虚，阴气内积所致。

This chapter introduces the daoyin exercises for such abdominal disorders as abdominal pain and distention. Weakness of the zang-fu organs and the retention of cold qi between the intestines and the stomach may lead to a struggle between anti-pathogenic qi and pathogenic factors and subsequently result in pain. Abdominal distention is mostly due to a spleen disorder. Yang deficiency of the spleen may allow yin qi to accumulate in the spleen.

（1）卧式（侧卧）。蹲曲健侧手脚，患侧手脚自然伸直，鼻纳气，而后闭气，以意推至腹部令腹部鼓起，观想气达患病处，感到有温热感即可（图16-1）。适用于四肢疼痛。

(1) Take a side-lying position. Flex the leg and arm on the healthy side, extend the leg and arm on the affected side, inhale through the nose, hold the breath, use the mind to push qi to the abdomen in order to make the abdomen bulge, and visualize qi reaching the affected area until a warm sensation is present (Figure 16-1). This exercise can help treat pain in the limbs.

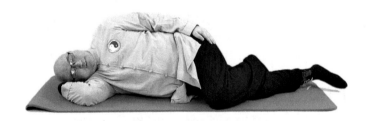

图16-1　Figure 16-1

［操作要领与注意事项］侧卧使健侧于下、患侧于上，可利患侧气血运行；鼻纳气后闭气，以利腰腹气血运行；微微用意，可助患侧气血运行。

[Tips and notes] Lying on the healthy side can facilitate the circulation of qi and blood on the affected side. After inhaling through the nose, holding the breath can facilitate the circulation of qi and blood in the waist and abdomen. Using the mind slightly can also help with the circulation of qi and blood on the affected side.

（2）卧式（仰卧）。舒展手脚，脚趾向上，鼻纳气，至满，做7次这样的呼吸（图16-2）。适用于腹中拘急剧痛。

(2) Take a supine position. Extend both legs and arms with the heels outward, inhale through the nose deeply, and repeat this breathing pattern 7 times (Figure 16-2). This exercise can help relieve severe abdominal pain and contracture.

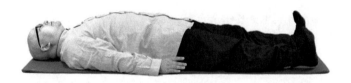

图16-2　Figure 16-2

［操作要领与注意事项］舒展四肢，鼻纳气可拔伸脊骨，以缓解腹中拘急。

[Tips and notes] Stretching out all four limbs and inhaling through the nose can help stretch the spine and relieve contracture.

（3）卧式（仰卧）。口缓缓纳气，鼻出气（图2-25，图2-26）。有助于去除腹内拘急疼痛、饱食不消化。然后小咽气几十口，起到温中的效果。如果受寒邪，使人干呕腹痛，以口纳气70次，腹部充盈则可扶正祛邪。再小咽气几十口，两手掌摩擦，温热后摩腹，令气下行（图2-27）。

(3) Take a supine position. Inhale slowly through the mouth and exhale through the nose (Figure 2-25 and Figure 2-26). This exercise can help treat abdominal cramps and pain,

as well as indigestion. Then, swallow the air dozens of times to warm the stomach. For retching and abdominal pain caused by contraction of pathogenic cold, inhaling through the mouth 70 times to make the abdomen full can reinforce healthy qi to eliminate pathogenic factors. Then, swallow the air dozens of times, rub the hands to generate warmth and knead the abdomen in order to promote the downward movement of qi (Figure 2–27).

［操作要领与注意事项］完成此导引动作时，空气要优良，气温不能过低。

[Tips and notes] During the exercise, the air quality should be excellent and the temperature should not be too low.

（4）卧式（仰卧）。仰起两脚两手，鼻纳气，至满，做7次这样的呼吸（图16-3）。有助于去除腹中拘急剧痛。

(4) Take a supine position. Lift both legs and arms up, inhale through the nose deeply, and repeat this breathing pattern 7 times (Figure 16–3). This exercise can help relieve severe abdominal pain and contracture.

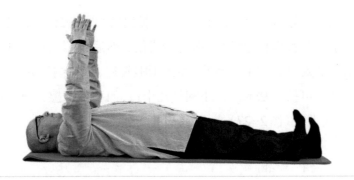

图16-3　Figure 16-3

[操作要领与注意事项] 舒展四肢，鼻纳气可拔伸脊骨，以缓解腹中拘急。

[Tips and notes] Stretching out all four limbs and inhaling through the nose can help stretch the spine and relieve contracture.

（5）蹲式（蹲坐）。定心安神，卷曲两手从心向下（图16-4），左右摇动两臂，交替侧斜身体，两肩尽量舒展，低头向肚，两手沿冲脉到脐下，上下来回做21次。有助于去除腹胀、肚腹拘挛、闷痛、食积不消化。

(5) Take a squatting position. Calm the mind, curl both hands down from the front of the chest (Figure 16-4), swing both arms from side to side while tilting the body alternately, fully stretch the shoulders, lower the head towards the abdomen, move both hands along the *Chong* meridian to the lower abdomen, and repeat 21 times. This exercise can help relieve abdominal distension, contracture, oppressive pain and indigestion.

[操作要领与注意事项] 练习时，静心宁神，低头向肚，助松解脊骨；两手缓缓沿冲脉，从心向下至脐下，同时左右摇动两

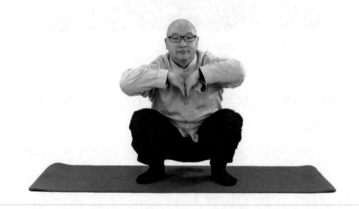

图16-4　Figure 16-4

臂,交替侧斜身体,两肩尽量舒展,以利肚腹部气血运行。

[Tips and notes] During the exercise, maintain a tranquil and focused mind and lower the head towards the abdomen to relax the spine. Tilt the body to both sides, fully stretch the shoulders, lower the head towards the abdomen, and move both hands along the *Chong* meridian to the lower abdomen in order to facilitate the circulation of qi and blood in the abdominal region.

(6) 站式、坐式、卧式。腹中苦于发胀且有寒气,用"呼"字音出气,做30次(图16-5)。

(6) Take a standing, sitting or lying position. For abdominal distention, and cold in the abdomen, exhale with the sound "hu" 30 times (Figure 16-5).

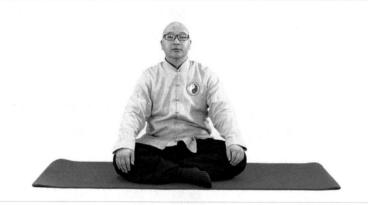

图16-5　Figure 16-5

[操作要领与注意事项]"呼"字音应土,应脾,口发"呼"字音可泻腹实。

[Tips and notes] The sound "hu" corresponds to the earth element and the spleen. Exhaling with the sound "hu" can help relieve excess in the abdomen.

（7）坐式（端坐）。舒展腰部，以口纳气数十次，胀满则吐，以舒适为度。可调理腹中胀满，饮食以后更觉饱胀。如果腹中仍觉得不舒服，可以反复操作（图16-6）。腹中有寒气，腹部不舒服，也可以用这个方法。

(7) Take an upright sitting position. Extend the waist, inhale through the mouth dozens of times, and exhale when the abdomen is full. This exercise can relieve abdominal distension and fullness after meals (Figure 16-6). This exercise can also be used for cold in the abdomen.

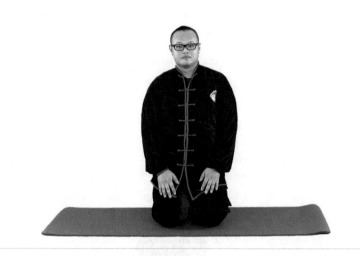

图16-6　Figure 16-6

［操作要领与注意事项］此为复合方法，伸腰鼓动肾气，进而促进脾胃运化。

[Tips and notes] This is a compound method. Stretching the waist can stimulate kidney qi, thus promoting the transformation and transportation of the spleen and stomach.

（8）站式。两手向同一侧伸展，身体同向侧转，尽力做到极势；头顶好像悬挂起来，使气自然散下，如同腐烂的东西从上往下松解散开，十指舒展伸直（图16-7）。左右两个方向都做上述导引动作,21次。然后正身直立,前后转动肩部和腰部,7次(图16-8)。有助于去除腹肚胀满、膀胱腰脊手臂寒冷、血脉拘急强硬、心悸。

(8) Take a standing position. Stretch both hands to the same side, fully turn the upper body in the same direction, imagine that the top of your head is being suspended, descend qi naturally as if the decaying things are loosening and dissolving from top to bottom, and extend all fingers (Figure 16-7). Perform the above movements on both sides (left and right), and repeat 21 times on each side. Then stand straight and swing the shoulders and waist back and forth 7 times (Figure 16-8). This exercise can help relieve abdominal distension, treat cold in the bladder, lower back, spine and arms, and also relieve muscle/tendon spasm and stiffness, as well as palpitations.

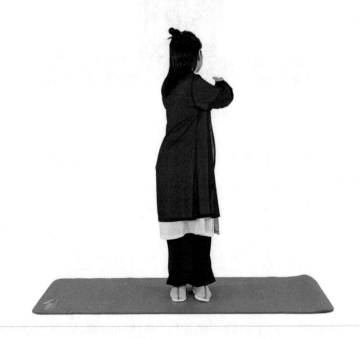

图16-7　Figure 16-7

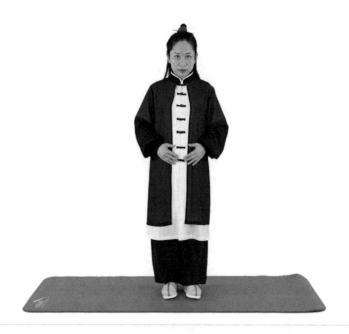

图16-8　Figure 16-8

[操作要领与注意事项]"发顶足，气散下"为下降浊阴的方法。正身直立，腰背脊柱放松，以眼神带动肩胛和腰部运动。

[Tips and notes] Imagining that the top of the head is being suspended, and descending qi naturally can descend turbid yin. Stand upright, relax the waist, back and spine, and use the eyes to guide the movement of the scapulae and waist.

（9）站式、坐式。脾主土，主肌肉，人身暖和则可以发汗，去除风冷邪气。如果腹部胀气，必须先使脚暖和，肚脐与气海穴上下按摩，不限次数，以多为好，左回右转21次（图1-84）。中和之气发挥作用的原则是，用身内一百一十三法，回转三百六十骨节，经脉畅行筋骨活动，气血布散润泽，二十四脉气和润，脏腑协调。中和之气具体运用的方法是，活动、旋转、摇摆、振动头部，手气上行、心气下行，清楚察觉气的去和来。无论是平手、侧腰、转身、摩气、屈转、回缩、转动各种动作结束后，心气向下散，送至涌泉穴，每一步骤和动作都遵循气的运行规律，运用得好则有益身心。不懂运用气的原则和方法，反而导致气紊乱。

(9) Take a standing or sitting position. The spleen governs muscles. When the body is warm, sweating can help dispel pathogenic wind and cold. For abdominal distension, warm up the feet first and massage the area around the navel and the point Qihai (CV 6) up and down. There is no limit to the number of massage but more is better (Figure 1–93). To facilitate the functions of harmonious qi, adopt the 113 internal methods within the body to unblock the meridians, promote the circulation of qi and blood, and harmonize the zang-fu organs. The specific methods for utilizing the harmonious qi include moving, rotating, shaking and vibrating the head, ascending hand qi, descending heart qi, and keeping a clear mind on the coming and going of qi. At the end, descend heart qi to the point Yongquan (KI 1). Each step and movement should follow the rules of qi circulation, and using it properly can be beneficial to the body and mind. Not understanding the principles or methods of using qi can lead to qi disorders.

［操作要领与注意事项］用身内一百一十三法（三十六天罡，七十二地煞，统以五行），意在以天人相应的规律引导气机运行。

[Tips and notes] Adopting the 113 internal methods within the body is to guide the flow of qi according to man-nature correspondence.

（10）卧式（仰卧）。践行养生大道，常常根据日月星辰运行的规律。在凌晨1～3点间内心清净纯澈，身体安卧，漱液满口分3次咽下（图16-9）。可以调和五脏，杀蛊虫，令人长寿，也适用于心腹痛。

(10) Take a lying position. To practice health preservation,

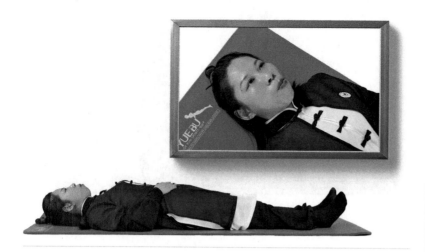

図16-9 Figure 16-9

it is important to follow the rules of the movement of the sun, moon, and stars. Between 1 am and 3 am, with a clear and calm mind and a relaxed body, produce some saliva in the mouth and swallow it in 3 times (Figure 16–9). This exercise can help regulate the five zang organs, treat schistosomiasis, promote longevity, and also alleviate abdominal pain.

［操作要领与注意事项］依照时辰练习此法，遵循中医天人相应的规律。凌晨1-3点为肝经循行，肝为将军之官，能调和诸脏。

[Tips and notes] Practice this method in accordance with the law of man-nature correspondence and specific timing. The liver meridian circulates between 1 am and 3 am. The liver is a general in charge of harmonizing the zang organs.

（11）坐式。伸右小腿，屈左膝，压在臀部下，做5次自然呼吸，引动脾的气机（图16-10）。有助于去除心腹寒热，胸中邪气闷胀。

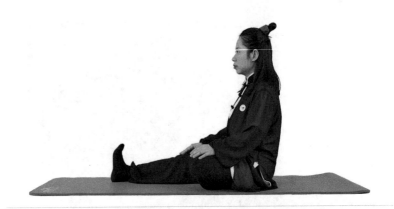

图16–10   Figure 16–10

(11) Take a sitting position. Extend the right leg, flex the left leg, and breathe 5 times to induce the qi activity in the spleen (Figure 16–10). This exercise can help eliminate cold and heat in the chest and relieve the stagnation of pathogenic qi in the chest.

［操作要领与注意事项］在这个姿势上自然呼吸，内心宁静后可引动右侧气机；做5次呼吸，中医"5"与脾土相应，为取类比象。

[Tips and notes] In this posture, breathe naturally and stay calm to stimulate the qi activity on the right side of the body. Breathe 5 times to correspond to the earth element and the spleen.

十七、痢病诸候提要
Daoyin Exercise for Dysentery

本节论述痢病诸候的导引术。痢病主要由于血气虚，无力抵御外邪。邪气入里，以致脾气不能运化水谷，大肠无力吸收精微,糟粕不能结聚,成为痢疾。

This chapter introduces the daoyin exercise for dysentery. Deficiency of blood and qi weakens the body's ability to resist external pathogenic factors. When pathogenic factors invade the body, the spleen cannot transform or transport water and food, and the large intestine cannot absorb essence or gather the waste, subsequently resulting in dysentery.

站式、坐式、卧式。泄利有寒的人,腹纳气,微微引动气息,然后以"吹"字音缓缓出气(图17-1)。想要吸气时再以鼻纳气,至满,重复上述方法就可以治愈(寒泄)。泄利有热的人,以"呼"字音缓缓出气(图17-2)。

Take a standing, sitting or lying position. For diarrhea accompanied by cold symptoms, inhale and slightly activate qi, and then exhale slowly with the sound "ci" (Figure 17-1). Deeply inhale through the nose, and repeat the exercise. For diarrhea accompanied by heat symptoms, slowly exhale with the sound "hu" (Figure 17-2).

[操作要领与注意事项] 此法遵循中医五行相克理论。"吹"字音应肾,口发"吹"字音可调节肾之气机;"呼"字音应

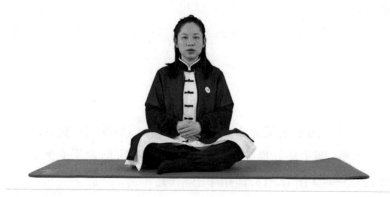

图17-1　Figure 17-1

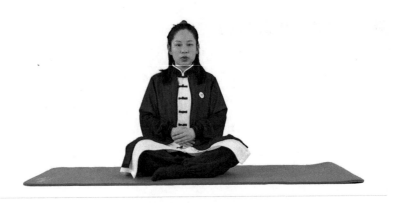

图17-2　Figure 17-2

脾，口发"呼"字音可调节脾胃气血运行。

[Tips and notes] This exercise follows the TCM theory of the five elements and their mutual restraint. The sound "ci" corresponds to the kidney, and thus regulates the qi activity of the kidney. The sound "hu" corresponds to the spleen, and thus regulates the qi and blood circulation of the spleen and stomach.

十八、九虫病诸候提要
Daoyin Exercise for Parasitic Diseases

本节论述九虫病诸候的导引术。九虫是中医对肠道寄生虫概称。

This chapter introduces the daoyin exercise for parasitic diseases.

坐式。两手相叉放于头部，长吸气，然后吐气：坐地，慢慢舒展两脚，两手从外抱膝，迅速低头放入两膝间，两手交叉头上，做12次呼吸（图18-1），适用于三尸病。

Take a sitting position. Cross the hands and place them on

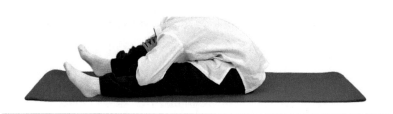

图18-1　Figure 18-1

the head, take a long breath and then exhale, slowly stretch the legs, hold the knees with the hands, quickly lower the head into the knees, cross the hands on the top of the head, and breathe 12 times (Figure 18–1). This exercise can help treat parasitic diseases induced by the Three Corpses.

［操作要领与注意事项］松解打开脊骨、胯骨，有利于督脉气血运行。此动作难度大，易受伤。初学者完成此动作时忌幅度大、速度快，宜循序渐进。

[Tips and notes] Relax and open the spine and hips to circulate qi and blood within the Governor Vessel. This exercise is difficult and can easily cause injury. Beginners should start slowly and gradually increase the range of motion.

"三尸"亦称"三虫"，一说指"长虫、赤虫、蛲虫"。另据道教经典，人身之中有三虫，上尸"彭琚"，中尸"彭踬"，下尸"彭蹻"分驻人体头、胸、腹，"三尸之为物，虽无形而实魂魄鬼神之属也。"

The term "Three Corpses," also known as "Three Worms," refers to "long worms, red worms, and pinworms." According to Taoist classics, there are three corpses in the human body, with the upper corpse named "*Peng Ju*," the middle corpse named "*Peng Zhi*," and the lower corpse named "*Peng Qiao*," residing in the head, chest, and abdomen respectively. It is stated that

"Although the three corpses are invisible, they are actually related to Ethereal Soul (*Hun*), Corporeal Soul (*Po*), ghosts, and immortals."

十九、积聚病诸候提要
Daoyin Exercises for Abdominal Masses

本节论述积聚病诸候的导引术。积聚之病，是阴阳之气不和，脏腑虚弱，感受风邪，邪气乘虚侵入所致。积病属阴，生于五脏，病变部位比较固定，可触到包块状。聚病属阳，生于六腑，病变部位并不固定，疼痛也没用一定的位置。

This chapter introduces the daoyin exercises for abdominal masses. Disharmony between yin and yang, and weakness of the zang-fu organs may allow pathogenic wind to invade the body, and subsequently cause abdominal masses. The nature of tangible masses is yin while that of intangible masses is yang. Tangible masses originate from the five zang organs while intangible masses originate from the six fu organs. Tangible masses are immobile and can cause abdominal distension and pain in fixed positions, while intangible masses are mobile and can cause migratory pain.

（1）卧式（仰卧）。以左脚踏在右脚上（图19-1）。有助于去除心下积。

(1) Take a supine position. Place the left foot on the top of the right foot (Figure 19-1). This exercise can help treat abdominal masses.

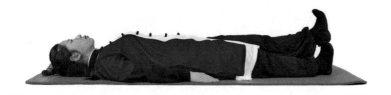

图19-1　Figure 19-1

［操作要领与注意事项］此动作可补气行气，利气机下行。

[Tips and notes] This exercise can tonify and circulate qi, facilitating the downward flow of qi.

（2）坐式（端坐）。患心下积聚之病，舒展腰部，仰头面向太阳，以口缓缓纳气，因循着阳光咽下，超过30次就可以停止，睁开眼睛（图19-2）。

(2) Take an upright sitting position. For abdominal masses, stretch the waist, raise the head to face the sun, inhale slowly through the mouth, swallow qi 30 times, and open the eyes (Figure 19-2).

［操作要领与注意事项］遵循中医天人相应的规律，吸收太阳精华。

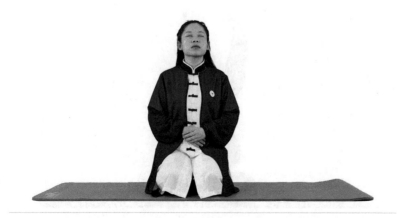

图19-2　Figure 19-2

[Tips and notes] Follow the rule of man-nature correspondence, and absorb the essence of the sun.

（3）卧式（侧卧）。左胁着地，伸直手脚，口纳气，鼻出气，周而复始不断练习（图15-4），有助于去除积聚和心下不适。

(3) Take a side-lying position. Place the left flank on the ground, stretch out the arms and legs, inhale through the mouth and exhale through the nose. Regular practice (Figure 15–4) can help treat abdominal masses and discomfort.

［操作要领与注意事项］左胁侧卧，有利于疏通上焦；口纳气，利于补益脾胃；鼻出气，既固摄肾气，又可疏泄上焦。

[Tips and notes] Lying on the left side can help unblock the upper jiao. Inhaling through the mouth is beneficial for nourishing the spleen and stomach. Exhaling through the nose can both consolidate and gather kidney qi, and also disperse the upper jiao.

（4）站式、坐式。以左手按右胁，尽力举起右手（图19-3）。有助于去除积病及老血。

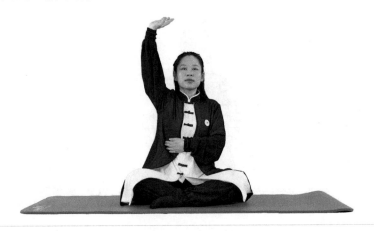

图19-3　Figure 19-3

(4) Take a standing or sitting position. Press the right flank with the left hand and fully raise the right hand (Figure 19–3). This exercise can help treat abdominal masses and blood stasis.

［操作要领与注意事项］举右手可养精血活气血。

[Tips and notes] Raising the right hand can nourish the essence, activate blood circulation and vitalize qi.

（5）坐式（正坐）。向东而坐。鼻微微纳气，闭起嘴巴，迫气下行，留置脐下，然后以口微微出气，分12次吐出（图19-4）。有助于去除结聚。低头不呼不吸，12次（图19-5）。可助饮食消化、身轻体强。长期练习可使人冬天不怕冷。

(5) Take an upright sitting position. Sit facing east. Inhale slightly through the nose, close the mouth, force the breath downward to the navel, and then exhale through the mouth in 12 parts (Figure 19–4). This exercise can help treat abdominal masses. Lower the head, passively hold the breath, and repeat 12 times (Figure 19–5). This exercise can help digest and strengthen the immune system. Long-term practice can make

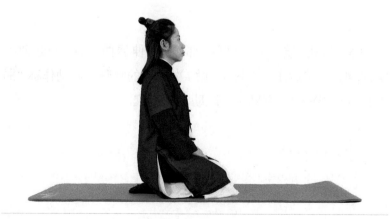

图19-4　Figure 19-4

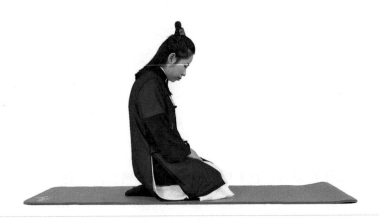

图19-5　Figure 19-5

people less susceptible to cold in winter.

［操作要领与注意事项］此法是有为法渐入无为法。"闭口，迫气下行，留置脐下"是有为法；"低头不呼吸"是无为法，清静自然则发生。

[Tips and notes] This method starts with an intentional action, but gradually leads to a state of effortless action. "Closing the mouth and forcing the breath downward to the navel" is an intentional action, while "lowering the head and passively holding the breath" is an effortless action, which arises naturally from a state of calmness and stillness.

（6）坐式（端坐）。舒展腰部，向上伸展两手臂，仰起两手掌，鼻纳气，然后闭气至极限，做7次这样的呼吸。此动作称"蜀王乔"（图19-6）。有助于去除肋下的积聚。

(6) Take an upright sitting position. Extend the waist, lift the arms, turn the palms upward, inhale through the nose, fully hold the breath, and repeat this breathing pattern 7 times. This exercise can help treat abdominal masses.

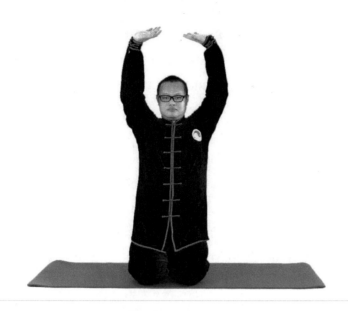

图19-6   Figure 19-6

［操作要领与注意事项］完成此动作过程中，鼻纳气配合仰掌，打开手三阴经，疏通三阳经，使积聚自然消散。闭气至极限，建议医护人员在旁看护。

[Tips and notes] During the exercise, inhaling through the nose while raising the palms upward helps open the three yin meridians of hand, unblock the three yang meridians of hand, and thus eliminate abdominal masses. Since this exercise needs to fully hold the breath, it is recommended to do this exercise under the watchful eye of a person.

（7）卧式（仰卧）。清晨，去掉枕头，舒展手脚，闭起眼睛和嘴巴，闭气，尽力做到极限，当腹部和两脚有撑胀感时，休息片刻，再次吸起腹部，跷起两脚约两个拳头的高度；待呼吸稍稍平复后，再次练习（图12-2）。春天做3次（3的倍数）、夏天做5次（5的倍数）、秋天做7次（7的倍数）、冬天做9次（9的倍数）。可以荡涤五脏，滋润六腑。上述练习的方法做到（腹部）有温热感就可以停止，癥瘕散破，病就好了。

(7) Take a supine position. In the morning, remove the

pillow, stretch the arms and legs, close the eyes and mouth, fully hold the breath until an extending sensation in the abdomen and feet is present, then take a break, and raise the feet to a height of about two fists. Calm down the breath, and do the exercise again (Figure 12–2). In spring, do this exercise 3 or multiples of 3 times; in summer, do this exercise 5 or multiples of 5 times; in autumn, do this exercise 7 or multiples of 7 times; in winter, do this exercise 9 or multiples of 9 times. This exercise can cleanse the five zang organs and nourish the six fu organs. Do this exercise and stop when a warm sensation is present in the abdomen.

功 法 操 作 · Movements

［操作要领与注意事项］完成此动作过程中，略撑脚趾，有利于腹部产生撑胀感；迅速吸气则两脚自然跷起。此动作腰胯部的舒张，有助吸气，吸气后有助于腰胯部舒张。闭气至极限，建议医护人员在旁看护。

[Tips and notes] During this exercise, slightly extend the toes to help extend the abdomen, and inhale quickly to lift the feet naturally. Extending the lower back and hips helps with inhalation, and inhalation helps further extend the lower back and hips. Since this exercise requires fully holding the breath, it is recommended to do this exercise under the watchful eye of a person.

二十、癥瘕病诸候提要
Daoyin Exercises for Masses

本节论述癥瘕病诸候的导引术。在积聚病候之外，复立癥瘕病候，指出癥瘕病因在于寒温失调，饮食不化，病邪与脏气相搏结而生。包块固定不移动为癥，包块不固定能移动为瘕。癥系于血，瘕系于气。

This chapter introduces the daoyin exercises for masses. The symptoms of masses are similar to those of abdominal masses. Imbalance of cold and warmth coupled with indigestion may cause a struggle between anti-pathogenic qi and pathogenic factors, and subsequently cause masses. Tangible masses are immobile and can cause abdominal distension and pain in fixed positions, while intangible masses are mobile and can cause migratory pain.

卧式（仰卧）。清晨，去掉枕头，舒展手脚，闭起眼睛和嘴巴，闭气，尽力做到极限，当腹部和两脚有撑胀感时，休息片刻，再次吸起腹部，蹺起两脚约两个拳头的高度；待呼吸稍稍平复后，再次练习（图12-2）。春天做3次（3的倍数）、夏天做5次（5的倍数）、秋天做7次（7的倍数）、冬天做9次（9的倍数）。可以荡涤五脏，滋润六腑。腹部有积聚，上述练习的方法做到（腹部）有温热感就可以停止。

Take a supine position. In the morning, remove the pillow, stretch the arms and legs, close the eyes and mouth, fully hold the breath until an extending sensation in the abdomen and feet is present, then take a break, and raise the feet to a height of about two fists. Calm down the breath, and do the exercise again (Figure 12–2). In spring, do this exercise 3 or multiples of 3 times; in summer, do this exercise 5 or multiples of 5 times; in fall, do this exercise 7 or multiples of 7 times; in winter, do this exercise 9 or multiples of 9 times. This exercise can cleanse the five zang organs and nourish the six fu organs. To treat abdominal masses, do this exercise and stop when a warm sensation is present in the abdomen.

［操作要领与注意事项］完成此动作过程中，略撑脚趾，有利于腹部产生撑胀感；迅速吸气则两脚自然跷起。此动作腰胯部的舒张，有助吸气，吸气后有助于腰胯部舒张。闭气至极限，建议医护人员在旁看护。

[Tips and notes] During this exercise, slightly extend the toes to help extend the abdomen, and inhale quickly to lift the feet naturally. Extending the lower back and hips helps with inhalation, and inhalation helps further extend the lower back and hips. Since this exercise requires fully holding the breath, it is recommended to do this exercise under the watchful eye of a person.

二十一、疝病诸候提要
Daoyin Exercises for Hernia

本节论述疝病诸候的导引术。疝病是由于阴寒内积，又加外寒侵袭，致使荣卫不调，气血虚弱，风冷入腹所致。疝，指痛病。这与后世"疝气病"含义不尽相同。

This chapter introduces the daoyin exercises for hernia. The accumulation of yin-cold in the body coupled with the invasion of external cold may lead to stagnation of qi and blood, and subsequently cause hernia. Here the term "hernia" refers to pain disorders, which is not entirely the same as the modern meaning of "hernia."

（1）蹲式（蹲踞）。两手举起两脚，使两脚极力横向打开。适用于气冲穴气血不调所致的肿痛、寒疝腹痛，补肾气。两手握两脚脚趾，脚趾离地，脚跟放低，使两脚极力横开，尽力牵拉，做1次自然呼吸（图21-1）。适用于荣卫不和所致的腹痛。

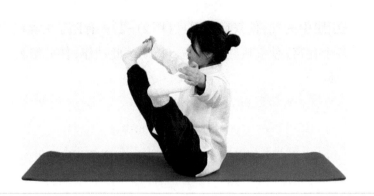

图21-1 Figure 21-1

(1) Take a squatting position. Lift both legs with both hands to fully open them. This exercise can help treat swelling and pain in the point Qichong (ST 30) due to disharmony between qi and blood, and abdominal pain caused by hernia, and can also tonify kidney qi. Grasp the toes of both feet with both hands, lift the toes off the ground, fully open the legs, fully pull the feet and take one natural breath (Figure 21–1). This exercise can help treat abdominal pain caused by disharmony between the *Ying*-nutrients and *Wei*-defense.

[操作要领与注意事项] 松解打开胯骨,有利于疏通全身气血,调和荣卫。此动作难度大,易受伤。初学者完成此动作时忌幅度大、速度快,宜循序渐进。

[Tips and notes] Relax and open the hips to circulate qi and blood within the Governor Vessel. This exercise is difficult and can easily cause injury. Beginners should start slowly and gradually increase the range of motion.

(2) 坐式。两手牵拉两脚脚趾,做5次自然呼吸,引动腹中气机。有助于去除疝瘕,通利孔窍。舒展两脚,两手握住两脚脚趾,使脚在头上,头在脚下,牵拉尽力做到极势,做5次自然呼吸，导引腹中的气，使气行遍周身（图21-2）。有助于去除疝瘕，通利各个孔窍，使气机往来顺畅。长期练此动作，使人精爽、聪明、长寿。

(2) Take a sitting position. Pull the toes of both feet with both hands and breathe naturally 5 times to induce the qi activity in the abdomen. This exercise helps treat hernia and unblock the orifices. Stretch out both legs, grasp both feet with both hands to make the legs over the head, fully pull the feet and breathe naturally 5 times to induce the qi activity in the abdomen and to circulate qi throughout the body (Figure 21–2). This exercise can help treat hernia, unblock the orifices, and facilitate the circulation of qi throughout the body. Long-term practice can make a person energetic and sharp-minded, and achieve longevity.

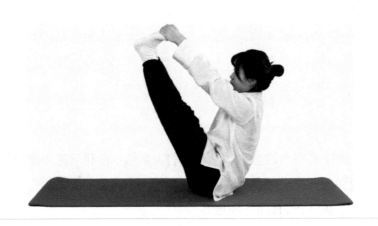

图21-2　Figure 21-2

［操作要领与注意事项］此动作难度大，易受伤。初学者完成此动作时忌幅度大、速度快，宜循序渐进。身体柔软，慢慢做到气遍行身体五脏。

[Tips and notes] This exercise is difficult and can easily cause injury. Beginners should start slowly and gradually increase the range of motion.

二十二、痰饮病诸候提要

Daoyin Exercises for Disorders Induced by Phlegm-Fluid Retention

本节论述痰饮病诸候的导引术。痰饮是由于阳气虚弱，气道闭塞，津液运行不畅，水饮之气停留在胸府，凝结而成痰。水液流走肠间，辘辘有声，即为痰饮。

This chapter introduces the daoyin exercises for disorders induced by phlegm-fluid retention. Weakness of yang qi and obstruction of the airway may impair the circulation of body fluids, and make them obstruct in the chest, subsequently causing disorders.

（1）卧式（侧卧）。不吸不呼12次。有助于治疗痰饮不消。右侧有痰饮，则右侧着地（图22-1），左侧有痰饮，则左侧着地（图22-2）。如果还有痰饮没有消除的情况，可用调整呼吸的方法来排除痰饮。不呼不吸12次，适用于痰饮。

(1) Take a side-lying position. Passively hold the breath 12 times. This exercise can help treat disorders induced by phlegm-fluid retention. For phlegm-fluid retention on the right side, lie on the right side (Figure 22–1). For phlegm-fluid retention on the left side, lie on the left side (Figure 22–2). For phlegm-fluid retention after doing the exercise, adjust the

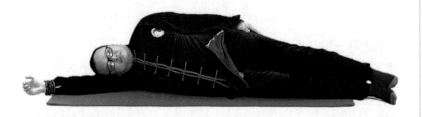

图22-1　Figure 22-1

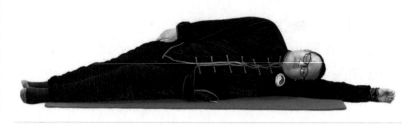

图22-2　Figure 22-2

breathing to help with expectoration. Passively holding the breath 12 times can help treat phlegm-fluid retention.

［操作要领与注意事项］侧卧调畅少阳经，疏通肝胆气机，以利豁痰开窍。

[Tips and notes] Taking a side-lying position can regulate the Shaoyang meridians, unblock the qi activity of the liver and gallbladder, and open the orifices.

（2）站式、坐式。鹜行气。低头靠墙，不吸不呼12次，心意放松，浊气自然下降。痰饮和宿食向下排出就能痊愈。鹜行气时，身正（脊柱正），头颈部如鸭子一般上下伸缩运动，气向下行排出，做12次（图22-3）。适用于宿食。长期练此动作，不需要借助另外的通塞方法。

(2) Take a standing or sitting position. Assume the posture of a duck to circulate qi. Lower the head, lean against a wall, passively hold the breath 12 times, relax the mind and descend turbid qi naturally. To treat phlegm-fluid retention and food retention, it is important to expel them downward. When assuming the posture of a duck to circulate qi, keep the body upright, and move the head and neck up and down like a duck, allowing qi to flow downward and out. Repeat this exercise 12 times (Figure 22-3). This exercise can help treat food retention.

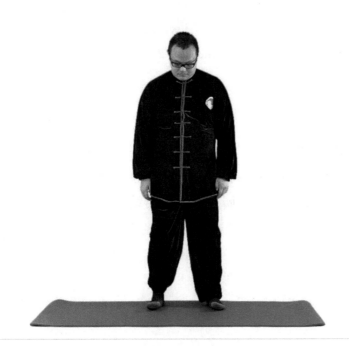

图22-3　Figure 22-3

［操作要领与注意事项］完成此动作时，靠墙可放松脊柱，有利于头颈上下伸缩运动。

[Tips and notes] Leaning against a wall during this exercise can help relax the spine and facilitate the up-and-down movement of the neck.

二十三、癖病诸候提要
Daoyin Exercise for Masses in the Sub-costal Region

本节论述癖病诸候的导引术。癖病指肠胃运化不畅的情况下，饮水过多，停留不化，又外受寒邪，水寒之气搏结，留着于两胁偏僻处，时而作痛的病证。

This chapter introduces the daoyin exercise for masses in the sub-costal region. The failure of the intestines and stomach to transport may cause water fluid retention in the sub-costal region. This condition coupled with the contraction of external cold may lead to pain in the sub-costal region that comes and goes.

蹲式（蹲坐）。两手撑地，两膝竖起，夹住两侧脸颊，成俯身姿势（图23–1）。适用于宿痈。长期练此动作，适用于伏梁。长期练此动作，肠可化为筋，骨头可变得结实。

Take a squatting position. Place both hands on the ground, raise both knees up, and clamp both cheeks to form a forward-bending posture (Figure 23–1). This exercise can help treat *Su Yong*. Long-term practice can help treat *Fu Liang* and strengthen the bones.

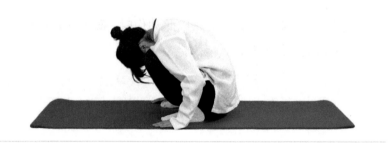

图23–1　Figure 23–1

［操作要领与注意事项］伏梁，指宿食不消化形成癖积，癖积形如杯子或和盘子。宿痈，指由于宿水宿气导致的癖积不消，进而成痈。

[Tips and notes] *Fu Liang* refers to the masses in the upper abdomen. The masses are shaped like cups or plates. They often result from accumulation of foul turbidity and stagnant qi and blood. *Su Yong* refers to abscess disorders. Stagnant water and qi may cause masses. Over time, the masses transform into abscesses.

二十四、否噎病诸候提要
Daoyin exercises for Stuffiness and Dysphagia

本节论述否噎病诸候的导引术。痞病指由于气机痞塞,而致腹内气结、痞塞胀满,并常伴高热的病证。噎指因三焦气化失常,津液运行不畅,以致食物堵住咽喉不得下咽的病证。

This chapter introduces the daoyin exercises for stuffiness and dysphagia. Stuffiness refers to the condition where qi stagnates in the abdomen, causing bloating and fullness, and is often accompanied by high fever. Dysphagia refers to the condition where the transformation and the transportation of body fluids are disrupted due to the dysfunction of the sanjiao, leading to difficulty in swallowing food, as if something is stuck in the throat.

坐式(正坐)。尽力伸展腰部,挺胸抬头,两手手指相对,尽力向前推按地面(图24-1),身体向下低俯,头、胸一起向下向前(图24-2),在将要接触地面时,起身(图24-3),上下来回做14次。有助于去除胸肋的痞满、内脏寒冷、两臂痛闷、腰脊痛闷不适。

Take an upright sitting position. Fully stretch the waist, straighten the chest, lift the head, make the fingers of both

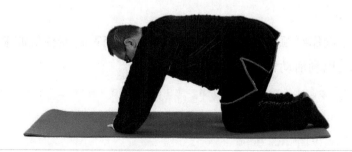

图24-1　Figure 24-1

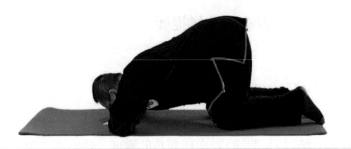

图24-2　Figure 24-2

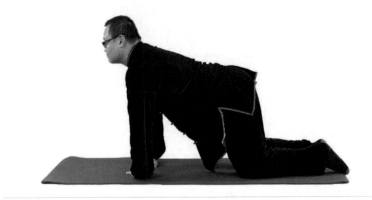

图24-3　Figure 24-3

功 法 操 作 · Movements

hands face each other and push the ground forward (Figure 24-1). Lower the body, with the head and chest moving down and forward together (Figure 24-2). When the body is about to touch the ground, lift the body (Figure 24-3). Repeat this movement 14 times. This exercise can help relieve fullness and discomfort in the chest and sub-costal region, cold in the internal organs, and oppressive pain in the arms, lower back and spine.

［操作要领与注意事项］完成此动作过程中，身体成波浪状运动，以利活动脊柱关节，调畅胸胁气机。

[Tips and notes] During the exercise, move the body like waves to facilitate the movement of the spine and regulate the qi activity in the chest.

二十五、脾胃气不和不能饮食候提要

Daoyin Exercise for Inability to Eat or Drink Due to Disharmony between Spleen Qi and Stomach Qi

本节论述脾胃气不和不能饮食候的导引术。脾为脏，胃为腑，两者合为表里，胃主纳谷，脾司运化。如果脾胃虚实不调，则水谷不能消化，而致腹中虚胀，或大便泄泻，不能饮食。

This chapter introduces the daoyin exercise for the inability to eat or drink due to disharmony between spleen qi and stomach qi. The spleen belongs to the zang organs, the stomach belongs to the fu organs, and together they form an interior-exterior relationship. The stomach receives grains, while the spleen governs transformation and transportation. Imbalance in the deficiency and excess of the spleen and stomach may cause the failure of the two organs to digest water and grains, leading to abdominal distension or diarrhea and inability to eat or drink.

站式。侧身，两手向同一侧伸展，然后快速挺身，舒展头和手，这个过程中两手相握，争相牵拉，慢慢尽力做到极势。(这个过程中)气和力须相互均匀融合。换另一侧也做上述动作，各21次(图25-1)。两手在头颈前后两侧慢慢舒展开，就好像是向外扒开的样子，放松身心，摇动21次，左右交替(图25-2)。有助于去除胃脘不和、臂部和腰部的虚闷不舒。

Take a standing position. Stand sideways, stretch both hands to the same side, then quickly straighten up the body and extend the head and hands. During this process, hold the hands together with the fingers intersecting, and fully pull each other. During this process, the breath and strength should be evenly integrated with each other. Do the above movements on

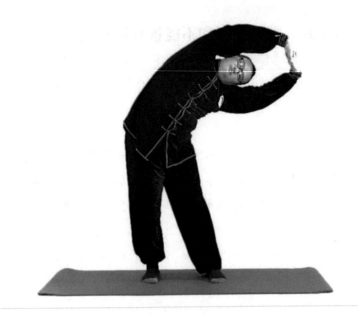

图25-1　Figure 25-1

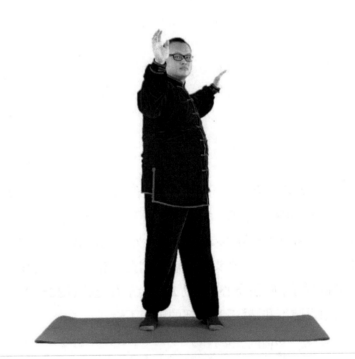

图25-2　Figure 25-2

the other side, and repeat 21 times on each side (Figure 25–1).
Slowly stretch both hands to the front and back of the neck,
relax the body and swing 21 times alternately from left to right

(Figure 25-2). This exercise can help relieve discomfort in the stomach area, arms and waist.

［操作要领与注意事项］完成此动作过程中,侧身落下时要慢,身体向远处拔伸;起身时需快,腿、腰、腹均用力。

[Tips and notes] During the exercise, lower the body slowly while leaning sideways, and stretch the body towards the far side. When returning to the neutral position, stand up quickly and utilize the strength in the legs, waist and abdomen.

二十六、呕吐候提要
Daoyin Exercises for Retching and Vomiting

本节论述呕吐病候的导引术。呕与吐皆是由于脾胃虚弱,又受风邪所致。胃气上逆则呕;胸膈间有停饮,或胃中有久寒,则呕且吐。

This chapter introduces the daoyin exercises for retching and vomiting. Both retching and vomiting are caused by deficiency of the spleen and stomach coupled with the invasion of pathogenic wind. When the stomach qi ascends upwards, it leads to retching. Water retention in the chest or chronic cold in the stomach can result in both retching and vomiting.

（1）坐式(正坐)。两手于身后,一侧手握另一侧手腕,(被握住手腕一侧的)手掌反向撑地,身体尽力后仰,使腹部绷紧,上下反复做7次(图1-46)。两手姿势互换重复刚才的动作。有助于减轻肚腹冷风、久宿气积、胃口冷、饮食反胃、呕吐不下。

(1) Take an upright sitting position. Place both hands

behind the body, grasp the wrist of one hand with the other, and invert the palm of the grasped wrist to support the body weight on the ground. Lean the body backward, tighten the abdominal muscles, and repeat the movements 7 times in an up-and-down motion (Figure 1–46). Change the position of the hands and repeat the movements. This exercise can help alleviate cold and wind in the abdomen, qi stagnation due to food retention, poor appetite, and stomach reflux.

[操作要领与注意事项] 身体尽力后仰时,头部保持前视、不后仰;初学动作过程注重腹部绷紧,腰部放松,利于减轻肚腹疾患。

[Tips and notes] When leaning the body backward, avoid bending the head backward. For beginners, it is important to focus on tightening the abdominal muscles while relaxing the lower back, as this can help alleviate abdominal disorders.

(2) 卧式(仰卧)。舒展手脚,双脚竖起脚跟,鼻纳气,至满,做7次(图26-1)。适用于胃脘病证、呕吐。

(2) Take a supine position. Stretch out the hands and feet, raise the heels, and deeply inhale through the nose. Repeat this movement 7 times (Figure 26–1). This exercise can help treat gastric disorders including retching and vomiting.

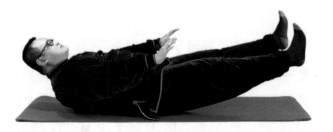

图26-1　Figure 26-1

[操作要领与注意事项] 此动作有利于打开骶胯关节，配合纳气腰胯部舒张，更利腰髋部气血运行。

[Tips and notes] This posture can help open the sacroiliac joints. Together with inhalation and extending the lower back and hips, it promotes the circulation of qi and blood in the lower back and hips.

（3）坐式。舒展两脚，两手牵拉两脚脚趾，尽力做到极势，做12次。适用于肠胃不纳食、吐逆。两手伸直攀两脚底，待两脚感到疼痛时，自然放松。将头放于膝上，尽力做到极势，做12次（图26-2）。适用于肠胃不纳食、吐逆。

(3) Take a sitting position. Extend both legs, grasp the toes of both feet with both hands to the maximum range of motion, and repeat 12 times. This exercise can alleviate indigestion, retching and vomiting. Extend the hands, grasp the soles of both feet until a feeling of pain is present in the feet, and then naturally relax. lower the head and place it on the knees to the maximum range of motion, and repeat 12 times (Figure 26–2). This exercise can help alleviate indigestion, retching and vomiting.

[操作要领与注意事项] 此动作有利于打开骶胯关节，配合纳气腰胯部舒张，更利腰髋部气血运行。

[Tips and notes] This posture can help open the sacroiliac joints. Together with inhalation and extending the lower back

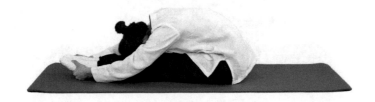

图26-2　Figure 26-2

and hips, it promotes the circulation of qi and blood in the lower back and hips.

二十七、宿食不消候提要
Daoyin Exercises for Food Retention (Indigestion)

本节论述宿食不消候的导引术。宿食不消是由于脏气虚弱,脾胃有寒,阳气不运,所以食入不易消化。

This chapter introduces the daoyin exercises for food retention (indigestion). Qi weakness of the zang organs coupled with cold in the spleen and stomach may block the circulation of yang qi, and subsequently cause food retention (indigestion).

(1)坐式。凡是饭后觉得腹内过饱,是由于肠内有宿气,应经常在吃饭前后,通过这样的动作来调理:两手抱两膝,向左右侧身(图27-1),腹部向前,腰部前挺使肚腹前凸,向左做21次,向右做14次(图27-2);然后转身并托按腰脊,尽力做到极势(图27-3)。适用于胃和腹内的宿气不化、脾痹、肠瘦、脏腑不和,可使腹部胀满日渐消除。

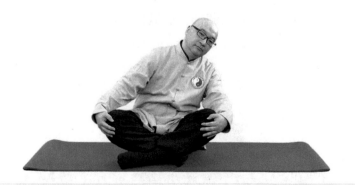

图27-1　Figure 27-1

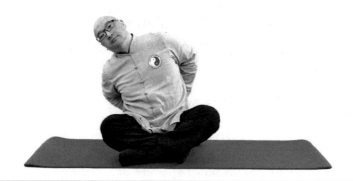

图27-2　　Figure 27-2

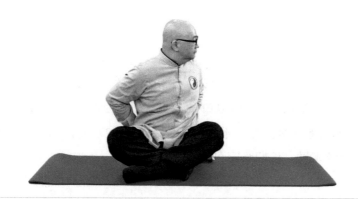

图27-3　　Figure 27-3

(1) Take a sitting position. Feeling excessively full after a meal is caused by qi retention in the intestines. It is recommended to do the following daoyin exercise regularly before and after meals to promote digestion: Hold both knees with both hands, tilt the body to the left and right sides (Figure 27–1), protrude the abdomen forward, and keep the waist straight to make the belly bulge forward. Repeat 21 times on the left side and 14 times on the right side (Figure 27–2); then turn around and support the waist with the hands to the maximum range of motion (Figure 27–3). This exercise can help alleviate qi retention in the stomach and abdomen, spleen *Bi*-impediment, intestinal disorders, disharmony between the zang and fu organs, and abdominal distension.

［操作要领与注意事项］此动作的坐姿有利放松骶胯部，促进下焦气血运行；运动过程中的挺腰就肚，动作须缓，以利中焦气血运行。

[Tips and notes] The sitting posture of this exercise is beneficial for relaxing the sacroiliac joints, promoting the circulation of qi and blood in the lower jiao. During the exercise, keep the waist straight and the belly protruding, and do the movements slowly to facilitate the circulation of qi and blood in the middle jiao.

（2）坐式（正坐）。向东而坐。鼻微微纳气，闭起嘴巴，迫气下行，留置脐下，然后以口微微出气，分12次吐出（图27-4）。有助于去除结聚。低头不呼不吸，12次（图27-5）。可助饮食消化、身轻体强。长期练习可使人冬天不怕冷。

（2）Take an upright sitting position and face east. Inhale slightly through the nose, close the mouth, force the breath downward to the navel, and then exhale through the mouth in 12 parts (Figure 27-4). This exercise can help eliminate accumulation and obstruction in the body. Lower the head, and passively hold the breath 12 times (Figure 27-5). This exercise can help digest and strengthen the immune system. Long-term

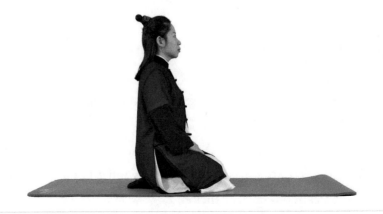

图27-4　Figure 27-4

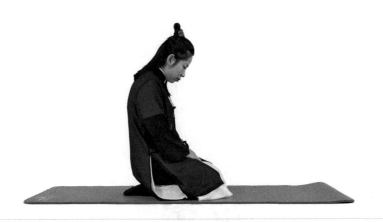

图27-5　Figure 27-5

practice can make people less susceptible to cold in winter.

［操作要领与注意事项］此法是有为法渐入无为法。"闭口，迫气下行，留置脐下"是有为法；"低头不呼吸"是无为法，清静自然则发生。

[Tips and notes] This method starts with an intentional action, but gradually leads to a state of effortless action. "Closing the mouth and forcing the breath downward to the navel" is an intentional action, while "lowering the head and passively holding the breath" is an effortless action, which arises naturally from a state of calmness and stillness.

（3）坐式（正坐）。舒展腰部，举右手，仰掌向上，以左手托左胁，鼻纳气，至满，呼吸7次（图27-6）。适用于胃寒、积食不化。

(3) Take an upright sitting position. Stretch the waist, raise the right hand with the palm facing upward, support the left side with the left hand, deeply breathe in through the nose, and then exhale. Repeat 7 times (Figure 27-6). This exercise can help alleviate cold in the stomach, and indigestion.

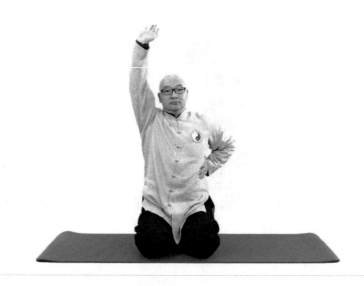

图27-6　Figure 27-6

［操作要领与注意事项］完成此动作时，举右手拔伸右侧肢体，利于壮精血，运化脾胃气机。

[Tips and notes] When doing this exercise, raise the right hand and stretch the right side of the body, which can invigorate the essence and blood, and promote the transformation of the spleen and stomach.

（4）站式、坐式。鹜行气。低头靠墙，不吸不呼12次，心意放松，浊气自然下降。痰饮和宿食向下排出就能痊愈。鹜行气时，身正（脊柱正），头颈部如鸭子一般上下伸缩运动，气向下行排出，做12次（图22-3）。适用于治疗宿食。

(4) Take a standing or sitting position. Assume the posture of a duck to circulate qi. Lower the head, lean against a wall, passively hold the breath 12 times, relax the mind and descend turbid qi naturally. To treat phlegm-fluid retention and food retention, it is important to expel them downward. When assuming the posture of a duck to circulate qi, keep the body upright, and move the head and neck up and down like a duck, allowing qi to flow downward and out. Repeat this exercise 12

times (Figure 22–3). This exercise can help treat food retention.

［操作要领与注意事项］完成此动作时，靠墙可放松脊柱，有利于头颈上下伸缩运动。

[Tips and notes] Leaning against a wall can help to relax the spine and facilitate the up and down movement of the neck.

（5）蹲式（蹲踞）。雁行气。低下胳臂推着膝盖，用绳捆绑左臂与左膝，低头，不呼不吸12次（图27-7）。有助于消化积食、轻健身体、增长精神，使恶气不得侵犯。

(5) Take a squatting position. Assume the posture of a wild goose to circulate qi. Push the knees with the lower arms, tie the left arm and left knee with a rope, lower the head, and passively hold the breath 12 times (Figure 27–7). This exercise can help treat food retention, strengthen the body, enhance mental spirit, and prevent pathogenic qi from invading the body.

［操作要领与注意事项］完成此动作过程中，内心宁静，不呼不吸，气机萌新。束缚左侧肢体，导引右侧精血，同时又利脾胃气血运行。

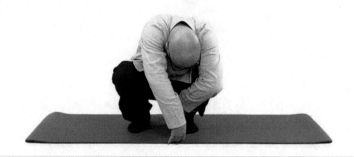

图27-7　Figure 27-7

[Tips and notes] During the exercise, keep a tranquil mind and passively hold the breath to promote the qi activity. Binding the left limbs can guide the essence and blood flow of the right side, and also promote the circulation of qi and blood in the spleen and stomach.

（6）坐式（正坐）。仰面向天，呼吸天之精华。可化解酒食胀饱。以口吐气，数十次，一会儿就有饥饿感，且有助于醒酒（图27-8）。夏天做此导引，令人感到清凉。

(6) Take an upright sitting position. Raise the head, and breathe in the essence of the heaven. This exercise can alleviate abdominal distension or fullness caused by overeating and drinking. Exhale through the mouth several times, and soon a feeling of hunger will be present, which can help to sober up (Figure 27–8). Doing this exercise in summer can provide a cooling sensation.

［操作要领与注意事项］遵循中医天人相应的规律，呼吸天之精华。宜口吸口呼，以助脾胃气血运化。

[Tips and notes] Follow the principles of man-nature

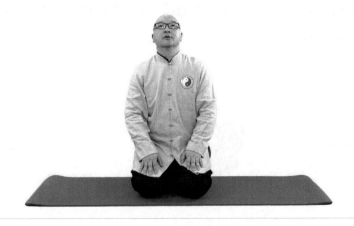

图27-8　Figure 27–8

correspondence in TCM. Breathe in the essence of the heaven. It is recommended to inhale and exhale through the mouth to promote digestion and the circulation of qi and blood in the spleen and stomach.

二十八、食伤饱候提要
Daoyin Exercises for Disorders due to Overeating

本节论述食伤饱候的导引术。食过饱，则脾气受伤更加不能运化食物，以致宿食停滞，使人气急烦闷，不得安卧。

This chapter introduces the daoyin exercises for disorders due to overeating. Damage of spleen qi due to overeating may impair the functions of the spleen in transporting and transforming food, and subsequently result in food stagnation, vexation, and restlessness.

坐式（端坐）。如果腹中胀满，饮食以后更觉饱胀，可以用这个方法调理：端坐。舒展腰部，以口纳气数十次，胀满则吐，以舒适为度；如果腹中仍觉得不舒服，可以反复操作（图16-6）。腹中有寒气，腹部不舒服，也可以用这个方法。

Take an upright sitting position. For abdominal distension or fullness after eating, sit upright, stretch the waist, deeply inhale through the mouth 10 times and exhale. Repeat the exercise until the disorder is relieved (Figure 16–6). This exercise can also be used for abdominal discomfort caused by cold.

［操作要领与注意事项］此为复合方法，伸腰鼓动肾气，进

而促进脾胃运化。

[Tips and notes] This is a compound exercise that stretches the waist and stimulates kidney qi, thereby promoting digestion, as well as the transportation and transformation of the spleen and stomach.

二十九、水肿候提要
Daoyin Exercise for Edema

本节论述水肿候的导引术。水肿与肾、脾、胃、三焦的关系密切。肾主水,肾阳虚弱则气化失调;胃腑虚弱则不能传化水气;脾病则不能制约于水;三焦气化不通利则水渗溢。以上均使水湿泛滥,浸渍脏腑,渗溢皮肤,发为水肿。

This chapter introduces the daoyin exercise for edema, a condition closely linked to the kidney, spleen, stomach, and sanjiao. The kidney governs water. Weakness of kidney yang may impair qi transformation. Weakness of the stomach may impair water and qi transportation. Disorders involving the spleen may cause the failure of the spleen to control water in the body. If the qi in sanjiao is not circulating well, water will accumulate and overflow, leading to water and dampness spreading throughout the body and causing edema.

坐式(正坐)。虾蟆行气。摇动两手臂,不吸不呼12次(图2-20)。适用于五劳七伤和水肿病。

Take an upright sitting position. Assume the posture of a toad to circulate qi. Shake the arms and passively hold the breath 12 times (Figure 2–20). This exercise can help treat the five exhaustions (Long- time observation damages blood; long-time lying damages qi; long-time sitting damages muscles; long-time standing damages bones; and long-time walking damages sinews) and seven damages (Refers to seven pathogenic factors that lead to deficiency and consumption, including improper diet, anxiety, drink, sex, hunger, over-exertion, and damage to meridians, collaterals, *Ying*-nutrients, *Wei*-defense and qi) as well as oedema.

[操作要领与注意事项] 完成此动作时, 通过摇动双臂带动腰背部的运动。忌憋气。

[Tips and notes] During this exercise, the movement of the waist and back should be driven by shaking the arms. Avoid holding the breath.

三十、转筋候提要
Daoyin Exercises for Leg Cramps

本节论述转筋候的导引术。转筋是由于荣卫气虚, 风冷邪气搏结于筋所致。

This chapter introduces the daoyin exercises for leg cramps. Qi deficiency of the *Ying*-nutrients and the *Wei*-defense coupled with the binding of pathogenic wind and cold in the tendons may result in leg cramps.

(1) 卧式 (仰卧)。伸展两腿两手, 脚跟向外, 脚趾相对, 鼻纳气, 至满, 做7次这样的呼吸 (图1-21)。有助于去除两膝寒凉、胫骨疼痛、转筋。

(1) Take a supine position. Extend both legs and arms

with the heels facing outward and the toes touching each other, inhale through the nose deeply, and repeat this breathing pattern 7 times (Figure 1–21). This exercise can help treat cold in the knees, shin bone pain, and leg cramps.

［操作要领与注意事项］完成此动作过程中，通过鼻纳气至满来舒展腰膝。

[Tips and notes] During this exercise, inhale deeply through the nose to stretch the waist and knees.

（2）坐式。舒展两小腿和脚趾，呼号5次，适用于转筋。尽力舒张脚掌，用力弯两脚脚趾，大声呼号（图30–1）。有助于去除筋膜骨节拘急挛缩和瘫痛。长期练此动作，能使肢体舒展。

(2) Take a sitting position. Stretch the lower legs and toes, take a deep breath and exhale with an "ah" sound loudly 5 times. This exercise can help relieve leg cramps. Try to stretch the soles of the feet, and bend the toes with force, while exhaling loudly (Figure 30–1). It can help relieve muscle/tendon spasm and pain. Long-term practice of this exercise can make the limbs more flexible.

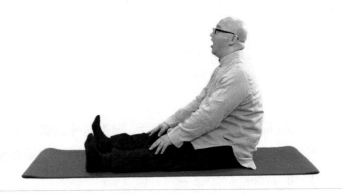

图30–1　Figure 30–1

Zhu Bing Yuan Hou Lun Dao Yin Shu (Explanations
for the Daoyin Exercises in Zhu Bing Yuan Hou Lun)

•

《诸病源候论》导引术

301

功法操作

•

Movements

［操作要领与注意事项］舒展两小腿及脚趾，用以导引气血运行；大声呼号，以壮筋骨。

[Tips and notes] Stretch the lower legs and toes to guide the circulation of qi and blood, and exhale loudly to strengthen the bones and tendons.

（3）卧式（俯卧）。侧视，脚趾撑地脚跟向上，舒展腰部，鼻纳气，至满，呼吸7次（图11-1）。适用于脚中弦痛、转筋、脚酸疼、脚弱。

(3) Take a prone position. Turn the head to one side, lift the heels to support the ground with the toes, stretch the waist, deeply inhale through the nose, and breathe 7 times (Figure 11-1). This exercise can help relieve foot pain, leg cramps, and foot soreness and weakness.

［操作要领与注意事项］完成此动作时，侧视更利于脊柱延展；脚趾伸向下用力以助伸腰，上半身不用力。

[Tips and notes] During the exercise, turning the head to one side can help stretch the spine. Supporting the ground with the toes assists in stretching the waist, while the upper body should not use force.

三十一、筋急候提要
Daoyin Exercises for Tendon Stiffness

本节论述筋急候的导引术。筋急是由于身体虚弱再中风寒，风寒所中的经筋就会挛急而不可屈伸。

This chapter introduces the daoyin exercises for tendon

stiffness. Physical weakness coupled with the invasion of wind and cold may cause tendon stiffness.

（1）坐式。两手抱两脚，头不动，使脚朝向脸面，但不要近到触及呼出之气，使全身骨节气散，如此反复做21次（图31-1）。两手握两脚，向左右侧身，皆用力牵拉，腰不动（图31-2）。适用于四肢、腰脊髓内冷、血脉冷、筋脉挛急。

(1) Take a sitting position. Lift both feet with the hands to make them close to the head, keep the head still, disperse qi throughout the bones and joints, and repeat this movement 21 times (Figure 31-1). Lift both feet with the hands, and turn the upper body to both sides while keeping the waist still (Figure

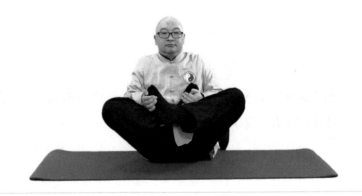

图31-1　Figure 31-1

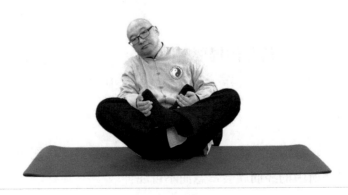

图31-2　Figure 31-2

31-2). This exercise can help relieve cold in the limbs and lower back, and muscle/tendon spasm.

［操作要领与注意事项］两手抱脚，尽力拔伸，使全身骨节松解开来，有利于周身气血运行，腰骨脊髓放松。

[Tips and notes] Lift the feet with both hands to the maximum range of motion in order to relax the joints and promote the circulation of qi and blood throughout the body.

（2）坐式。一脚向前跪地，身体尽力压在脚跟上；同侧手向前伸展，用力作上托的姿势；另一脚向后曲，同侧手握住解溪穴，用力牵拉，尽力做到极势；膝头贴地使腿绷紧，缓缓抬头，使气融化散开，从上至下流布全身。左右手脚互换做上述动作，各做21次（图31-3）。适用于腰部、伏兔穴和腋下闷痛，脊骨内筋拘急。

(2) Take a sitting position. Kneel with one leg and sit on the foot, lift and fully stretch the arm on the same side. Bend the other foot backward, grasp the point Jiexi (ST 41) with the hand on the same side and pull it to the maximum range of motion. Keep the knees close to the ground in order to tighten the

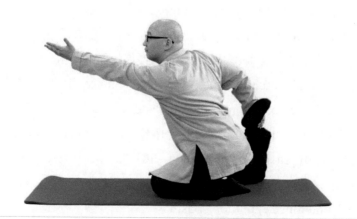

图31-3　Figure 31-3

legs. Slowly raise the head, and let qi flow from top to bottom, spreading throughout the body. Change the position of the hands and feet, and repeat this exercise 21 times (Figure 31–3). This exercise can help relieve oppressive pain in the lower back, the point Futu (ST 32) and armpits, as well as tendon spasm in the back.

［操作要领与注意事项］完成此动作过程中，单脚跪地，在平衡稳定的基础上，全身尽量舒展。初学宜有辅助人员看护。

[Tips and notes] During this exercise, kneel on one foot and fully stretch the entire body on the basis of balance and stability. For beginners, it is recommended to do this exercise under the watchful eye of a person.

（3）坐式（踞坐）。一脚舒展，一脚弯曲，两手牵拉足三里处，膝盖用力向前，身体后仰牵拉，这一刻全身皆处于拉伸状态，病气在内消散，就好像骨头完全松解散开一般。左右手脚互换做上述动作，各21次（图1-50）。适用于肩部脊背的风寒、血寒、筋脉拘急。

(3) Take a sitting position. Sit with the knees raised and the feet on the ground. Extend one leg and bend the other, put the hands on the point Zusanli (ST 36) to pull the leg, push the knee forward, and lean backward. At this moment, the whole body is in a stretching state, and illnesses are dissipated, just like the bones are completely relaxed and separated. Change the position of the hands and feet to do the exercise, and repeat 21 times on each side (Figure 1–50). This exercise can help eliminate wind and cold in the shoulders and spine, cold in blood, and muscle/tendon spasm.

［操作要领与注意事项］完成此动作过程中，膝盖向前顶，身体向后仰，两向用力，形成对拉劲，利于周身气机运行。

[Tips and notes] During the exercise, push the knee forward and lean the body backward, exerting force in both directions to create a stretching sensation, which facilitates the circulation of qi throughout the body.

（4）坐式。舒展两小腿和脚趾，呼号5次，适用于转筋。尽力舒张脚掌，用力弯两脚脚趾，大声呼号（图30-1）。有助于去除筋膜骨节拘急挛缩和瘸痛。长期练此动作，能使肢体舒展。

(4) Take a sitting position. Stretch the lower legs and toes, take a deep breath and exhale with an "ah" sound loudly 5 times. This exercise can help relieve leg cramps. Try to stretch the soles of the feet, and bend the toes with force, while exhaling loudly (Figure 30–1). It can help relieve muscle/tendon spasm and pain. Long-term practice of this exercise can make the limbs more flexible.

［操作要领与注意事项］舒展两小腿及脚趾，用以导引气血运行；大声呼号，以壮筋骨。

[Tips and notes] Stretch the lower legs and toes to guide the circulation of qi and blood, and exhale loudly to strengthen the bones and tendons.

（5）站式、坐式。两手反向托腰，尽力向后仰头，手托处不动，舒张两肘头，使其相对，尽力做到极势，21次（图31-4）。有助于去除两肩筋脉挛急、血冷、咽骨掘弱。

(5) Take a standing or sitting position. Place both hands on the lower back to support it, lean the head and upper body

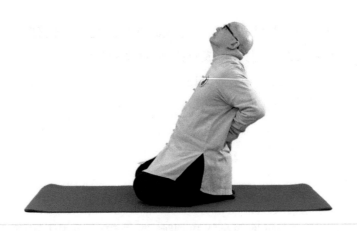

图31-4　　Figure 31-4

backwards, keep the hands still, and try your best to close the elbows. Repeat this movement 21 times (Figure 31-4). This exercise can help alleviate muscle/tendon spasm in the shoulders, and cold in blood.

［操作要领与注意事项］完成此动作过程中，仰头有利于纵向伸展脊柱；两肘背后相对有利于横向拉伸躯干。

[Tips and notes] During this exercise, raising the head is beneficial for stretching the spine, while closing the elbows is beneficial for horizontally stretching the torso.

（6）站式。一手尽力前推，另一手尽力向后舒展，使身体像"夫"字形。腰脊不能动。左右手交换做上述动作14次（图31-5）。适用于身体中八个关节的骨肉血冷、筋髓虚弱、颈肩部挛急。

(6) Take a standing position. Lift one hand and fully push forward, while fully lift and extend the other hand backward. Keep the lower back and spine still. Change the position of the hands to do the exercise, and repeat 14 times on each side (Figure 31-5). This exercise can help relieve cold in the eight

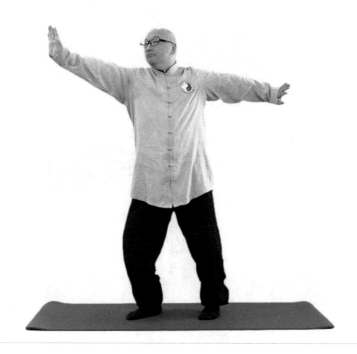

图31-5　Figure 31-5

major joints (two elbow joints, two shoulder joints, two hip joints and two knee joints) in the body, weakness of tendons, and muscle/tendon spasm in the neck and shoulders.

［操作要领与注意事项］完成此动作过程中，动作缓缓，逐渐拔伸到骶骨、两胯，才可能形如"夫"字。

[Tips and notes]　During this exercise, keep the movements slow and soft, and gradually stretch the sacrum and hips.

（7）站式。一脚踏地，一手向前舒展，另一脚尽量向后。这样舒展一手一脚，同时尽意快速振动14次（图31-6）。左右手脚互换都这样做。适用于骨髓痛、筋挛急、百脉不和。

（7）Take a standing position. Stand on one foot, lift and extend one hand forward, lift and extend the other leg backward, and vigorously shake the foot and the hand 14 times

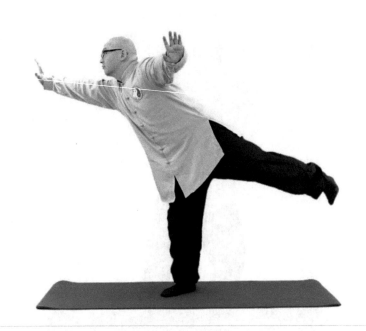

图31-6　Figure 31-6

(Figure 31-6). Change the position of the hands and feet to do the exercise. This exercise can help relieve bone pain, tendon spasm, and disharmony of the meridians.

[操作要领与注意事项] 完成此动作过程中, 单脚站立, 在平衡稳定的基础上, 全身尽量舒展。初学宜在医护人员辅助下完成。

[Tips and notes] During the exercise, stand on one foot and fully stretch the entire body on the basis of balance and stability. For beginners, it is recommended to do this exercise under the watchful eye of a person.

(8) 站式。① 两手掌反方向托于两肩前, 贴住两腋尽力做上下快速振摇, 反复做21次(图1-57)。完成后, 手不移动位, 两肘部用力向上举, 尽力做到极势, 上下振摇14次(图1-58)。两手握拳做7次(图1-59), 握拳后合拢做21次(图1-60)。有助于去除颈、肩部的筋脉拘急和劳损。② 一手握拳向左,另一手抓住对侧手肘,向内牵拉,尽力拔伸到极势(图1-61);握拳的手放松,舒展手指3次;然后换手做28次,尽力做到极势(图1-62)。可调理肘部和肩部的筋脉痉挛。③ 两手向上托起,尽力做到极势,上下做21次(图1-63)。手不动,肘部尽力向上做到极势,做7次。手、肘、臂都不动,尽力侧身,左右来回做21次(图1-64)。有助于去除颈椎的风寒、拘急不舒。

(8) Take a standing position. ① Place the palms of both hands in front of both shoulders in opposite directions, press against both armpits, and shake up and down 21 times (Figure 1–57). Keep the position of the hands, fully lift both elbows upward, and shake up and down 14 times (Figure 1–58). Clench the fists with both hands 7 times (Figure 1–59), and then close the hands 21 times (Figure 1–60). This exercise can help alleviate muscle/tendon spasm and strain in the neck and shoulders. ② Make a fist with one hand and stretch towards the left, while grab the elbow with the other hand and fully pull inward (Figure 1–61); relax the hand making a fist and stretch the fingers 3 times. Then change the position of the hands and repeat the exercise 28 times (Figure 1–62). This exercise can relieve muscle/tendon spasm in the elbows and shoulders. ③ Fully lift both hands up and stretch 21 times (Figure 1–63). Keep the hands still, and fully lift the elbows 7 times. Keep the hands, elbows and arms still, fully lean sideways and repeat 21 times on each side (Figure 1–64). This exercise can help alleviate wind, cold and muscle/tendon spasm in the cervical vertebrae.

[操作要领与注意事项] ① 动作一:手须贴住两腋做上下运动。② 动作二:肩胛与背脊在放松的前提下,以脊柱为中心做上下延展、左右延展。在极势时不用浊力,拔伸时肘部向后

向内卷。忌将肩胛骨夹紧。③ 动作三: 上臂尽量向脑后方向靠拢。

[Tips and notes] ① For the first movement, keep the hands close to the armpits and move them up and down. ② For the second movement, relax the shoulder blades and spine to extend up and down and left and right around the spine without using too much force. When extending, roll the elbows backward and inward. Avoid squeezing the shoulder blades too tightly. ③ For the third movement, try to bring the forearms as close as possible to the back of the head.

(9) 站式、坐式、卧式。拘魂门, 制魄户的方法叫作握固。大拇指弯曲, 其余四指向内握住大拇指, 日积月累积不停习练, 即使睡觉时也不松开, 可使人不被魅魇侵犯(图31-7)。

(9) Take a standing, sitting or lying position. Bend the thumb and grasp it tightly with the other four fingers. This hand posture is used to govern the Ethereal Soul (*Hun*) and control the Corporeal Soul (*Po*). Make this hand posture and practice it continuously for a long time, even when sleeping. Legend goes that this exercise can prevent being invaded by evil spirits (Figure 31-7).

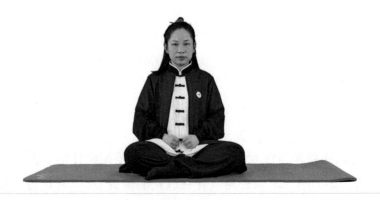

图31-7　Figure 31-7

［操作要领与注意事项］握固，以大拇指弯曲放于环指掌指关节处。可安心定意，固护精气。

[Tips and notes] In this exercise, bend the thumb and grasp it tightly with the other four fingers. Regular practice can calm the mind and preserve the essence. (Figure 31–7).

三十二、注病诸候提要
Daoyin Exercises for *Zhu*-Retention Disease

本节论述注病诸候的导引术。注，即住，邪气留着于体内故名"注"。注病是由于阴阳二气失司，劳倦又感外邪所致。此外，伤寒病未及时发汗或发汗未得真汗，使病邪传入阴经，深入五脏，以致病邪留着；或宿食冷热不调，以致邪气留着；或突然感受秽浊之气，均可导致此病。

This chapter introduces the daoyin exercises for *Zhu*-retention disease. *Zhu* refers to the retention of pathogenic qi in the body. The imbalance of yin qi and yang qi, coupled with fatigue and the invasion of external pathogenic factors may result in this condition. Additionally, if sweat-inducing therapy is not applied in time to cold damage, or if true sweat is not produced during the therapy, pathogenic factors may enter the yin meridians and affect the five zang organs, leading to the retention of pathogenic factors. Furthermore, food retention or sudden exposure to pathogenic qi can also cause this disease.

（1）站式、坐式、卧式。两手相交托于两肩与面部，两肘头尽力向上仰起，身正头仰，保持这样的姿势，肘头上下摇动21次（图32–1）。适用于肩肘风注、咽项拘急、血脉不通。

(1) Take a standing, sitting or lying position. Raise both

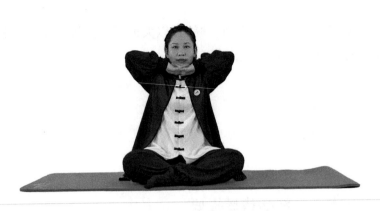

图32-1　Figure 32-1

hands and cross them beneath the chin, and then try your best to raise the elbows while keeping the body and head upright. Hold this posture and shake the elbows up and down 21 times (Figure 32–1). This exercise can help alleviate *Zhu*-retention disease involving the shoulders and elbows, and neck stiffness, and can also help promote blood circulation within the meridians.

［操作要领与注意事项］两手托于两肩与面部，肘头上仰，有利于头、颈、肩放松。

[Tips and notes] Raise both hands and cross them beneath the chin, and then try your best to raise the elbows in order to relax the head, neck and shoulders.

（2）站式。一手舒展打开，手掌向上；另一手握住下颌向外侧推拉。每次做到极势，左右手交换做上述动作14次。然后手不动，身体向两侧快速尽量转动，做14次（图1-19）。适用于颈椎活动障碍、头痛脑眩、喉痹、肩部冷痛、偏风的病症。

(2) Take a standing position. Fully extend and open one hand with the palm facing upward, grip the jaw and push and pull it outward with the other hand. Change the position of the

hands and do the above movement 14 times. Then, keep the hands still, and quickly rotate the body to both sides 14 times (Figure 1–19). This exercise can help treat impaired cervical movement, headache, dizziness, throat *Bi*-impediment, pain and cold in the shoulders, and hemiplegia.

［操作要领与注意事项］完成此动作过程中，容易导致颈椎小关节错位，宜缓做。忌爆发力。

[Tips and notes] Since this movement is easy to cause dislocation of the small joints in the cervical vertebrae, do it slowly and avoid using brute force.

三十三、蛊毒病诸候提要
Daoyin Exercises for Disorders Induced by Schistosomiasis

本节论述蛊毒病诸候的导引术。蛊毒有多种，都是变幻之气。

This chapter introduces the daoyin exercises for disorders caused by schistosomiasis, a type of parasitic toxin. The toxin of schistosomiasis has various types and is a transforming pathogen.

（1）坐式。两手相叉放于头部，长吸气，然后吐气：坐地，慢慢舒展两脚，两手从外抱膝，迅速低头放入两膝间，两手交叉头上，做12次呼吸（图18-1），适用于蛊毒、三尸毒、腰中大邪气。

(1) Take a sitting position. Cross the hands and place them on the head, take a long breath and then exhale, slowly stretch

the legs, hold the knees with the hands, quickly lower the head into the knees, cross the hands on the top of the head, and breathe 12 times (Figure 18-1). This exercise can help treat schistosomiasis, Three Corpses toxin, and strong pathogens in the lower back.

［操作要领与注意事项］松解打开脊骨、胯骨，有利于督脉气血运行。此动作难度大，易受伤。初学者完成此动作时忌幅度大、速度快，宜循序渐进。

[Tips and notes] Relax and open the spine and hip bones to circulate qi and blood within the Governor Vessel. This exercise is difficult and can easily cause injury. Beginners should start slowly and gradually increase the range of motion.

（2）卧式（仰卧）。践行养生大道，常常根据日月星辰运行的规律。在凌晨1～3点间内心清净纯澈，身体安卧，漱液满口分3次咽下（图16-10）。可以调和五脏，杀蛊虫，令人长寿，也适用于心腹痛。

(2) Take a supine position. To practice health preservation, it is important to follow the rules of the movement of the sun, moon, and stars. Between 1 am and 3 am, with a clear and calm mind and a relaxed body, produce some saliva in the mouth and swallow it in 3 times (Figure 16-10). This exercise can help regulate the five zang organs, treat schistosomiasis, promote longevity, and also alleviate abdominal pain.

［操作要领与注意事项］依照时辰练习此法，遵循中医天人相应的规律。凌晨1～3点为肝经循行，肝为将军之官，能调和诸脏。

[Tips and notes] Practice this method in accordance with the law of man-nature correspondence and specific timing. The liver meridian circulates between 1 am and 3 am. The liver is a general in charge of harmonizing the zang organs.

（3）站式、坐式、卧式。闭眼闭气，内视丹田，鼻缓缓纳气，令腹部胀满至极点，以口缓缓吐气，不要听到气息声，吸气多吐气少，气息轻柔（图1-85）。内视五脏，看到五脏的形色，再内视胃中，令神光充盈，鲜活明晰洁白如丝绢。做到疲倦至极并且出汗就可以停止了，用粉轻扑于身上，按摩身体。汗未出但感到疲倦的，也可以停止。待第二天再做。

(3) Taking a standing, sitting, or lying position, Close the eyes, hold the breath, focus on the *Dantian*, and inhale slowly through the nose to make the abdomen full. Then exhale slowly through the mouth without making any sound. The inhalation should be longer than the exhalation, and the breathing should be gentle and soft (Figure 1–85). Look at the five zang organs, and observe their forms and colors. Then look at the stomach, and make it bright, lively, clear and white as silk. Continue until exhaustion and sweating are present, then stop, lightly apply powders to the body, and massage the body. If exhaustion is felt but sweating has not yet occurred, stop and repeat the practice the following day.

［操作要领与注意事项］此导引动作中，闭气属有为法，然后纳气、吐气，气息须轻柔，再做观想。观想以丝绢形容白色的鲜活、流动、飘荡，不宜观想成实物。

[Tips and notes] In this daoyin exercise, holding the breath is considered an active method. After that, one should inhale and exhale gently, and the visualization should be done afterward.

The visualization should describe the vividness, fluidity, and fluttering of white silk instead of a real object.

（4）站式、坐式、卧式。存想巨雷闪电，雷鸣电闪，进入腹中。能这样坚持存想，有助于疾病痊愈。

(4) Take a standing, sitting or lying position. Visualize great thunder and lightning, with thunderbolts and flashes entering into the abdomen. Persistent visualization can help keep a peaceful mind.

［操作要领与注意事项］完成此动作时，实地观察巨雷闪电，更利于感同身受，帮助观想自然流出。

[Tips and notes] When practicing this exercise, observing the actual thunder and lightning in nature can help to feel more deeply and facilitate the visualization process.

三十四、饮酒中毒候提要
Daoyin Exercise for Alcoholism

本节论述饮酒中毒候的导引术。酒性有毒。人过度饮用后，自身不能消除，留着体内，便使人烦躁闷乱，毒害身心。

The chapter introduces the daoyin exercise for alcoholism. Alcohol has toxic properties, and excessive consumption may accumulate toxins within the body to damage the body both physically and mentally, and also result in such symptoms as vexation and restlessness.

正坐。仰面向天，（以口吐气）呼出酒食醉饱的浊气。吐气之后，立刻就有饥饿感，也觉得清醒了（图27-8）。

Take an upright sitting position. Raise the head, and breathe out the turbid qi through the mouth. After exhaling, you will immediately feel hunger and become sober (Figure 27-8).

［操作要领与注意事项］遵循中医天人相应的规律。呼吸天之精华。口呼气，身体更易放松。

[Tips and notes] Follow the principle of man-nature correspondence in TCM. Breathe in the essence of the heaven. Exhaling through the mouth helps relax the body.

三十五、血病诸候提要
Daoyin Exercise for Blood Disorders

本节论述血病诸候的导引术。血病，即出血诸病。

This chapter introduces the daoyin exercise for blood disorders. Blood disorders here refer to various bleeding disorders.

坐式。舒展伸直两脚，两手握两脚脚趾，做7次（图3-5，图3-6）。适用于腰部劳损不能俯仰、吐血、持久性的疼痛。经常练习这样的动作，身体可以变得柔软。

Take a sitting position. Stretch both legs forward, hold the toes of both feet with the hands and repeat 7 times (Figure 3-5 and Figure 3-6). This exercise can help treat lower back strain, inability to bend forward and backward, hemoptysis, and persistent pain. Regular practice of this exercise can make the body more flexible.

［操作要领与注意事项］拔伸关节可强壮腰膝。

[Tips and notes] Stretching and extending the joints can strengthen the lower back and knees.

三十六、毛发病诸候提要
Daoyin Exercises for Hair Disorders

本节论述毛发病诸候的导引术。毛发病主要与足少阳、足少阴、足阳明、手阳明等经脉的气血盛衰相关。

This chapter introduces the daoyin exercises for hair disorders. Hair disorders are mainly related to deficiency of qi and blood within the meridians of the gallbladder, kidney, stomach, and large intestine.

（1）坐式。解开发髻，握固，不吸不呼1次（图1-69）。然后向东而坐，从左右两侧举起手，掩住两耳（图1-70）。适用于头风，令头发不变白。用手反复梳头5次，使血脉流通（图1-71）。

(1) Take a sitting position. Untie the hair bun, bend the thumb, and grasp it tightly with the other four fingers. Passively hold the breath (Figure 1-69). Then sit facing east and raise the hands to cover the ears (Figure 1-70). This exercise can help treat head wind and prevent gray hair. Use the hands to comb the hair 5 times to promote blood circulation (Figure 1-71).

［操作要领与注意事项］向东而坐，以利气机生发。握固，

将大拇指弯曲,其余四指向内握住大拇指。完成此动作过程中,两手上举起时,心中不能缺少向下内敛之意。

[Tips and notes] Sit facing east to facilitate the generation of qi. For each hand, bend the thumb and grasp it with the other four fingers. When raising the hands, sink the intention.

（2）站式、坐式、卧式。清晨,两手交叉从头上牵拉两耳向上,牵引至鬓发,面部气血就能流通(图6-1)。

(2) Take a standing, sitting or lying position. In the morning, pull both ears upward to circulate qi and blood (Figure 6-1).

［操作要领与注意事项］两手交叉牵拉两耳向上,可疏通少阳经,以鼓动肾气,利于周身气血运行。

[Tips and notes] Pulling the ears upward can unblock the Shaoyang meridians, and thus stimulate kidney qi and promote the circulation of qi and blood throughout the body.

（3）坐式。坐地,伸直两脚,两脚相距一尺,两手指向两小腿,(身体向下低俯)使头低至地,做12次(图36-1)。可调整身体脊椎,利发根令头发乌黑顺柔。

(3) Take a sitting position. Extend and open the legs. The distance between the feet is about 33 cm. Bend the upper body and extend the hands forward to bring the head close to the ground, and do this exercise 12 times (Figure 36-1). This exercise can adjust the spine and nourish the hair roots to keep the hair dark, smooth and soft.

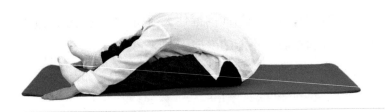

图36-1　Figure 36-1

　　[操作要领与注意事项]头低至地,调整身体脊椎,可强腰府,壮精血,故可令头发乌黑顺柔。初学者完成此动作时忌幅度大、速度快,宜循序渐进。如果头部不能弯曲至地,可由医护人员小心辅助。

　　[Tips and notes] Closing the head to the ground can strengthen the lower back and nourish the essence and blood, which can make the hair black, smooth, and soft. This exercise is difficult and can easily cause injury. Beginners should start slowly and gradually increase the range of motion. It is recommended to do this exercise under the watchful eye of a person.

　　(4) 蹲式(蹲踞)。两手举起两脚脚趾,低头,尽力做到极势,则气可遍行身体五脏(图21-2)。适用于耳朵听不到声音、眼睛看不清东西。长期练此动作,可以使白头发恢复乌黑。

　　(4) Take a sitting position. Pull the toes of both feet with both hands, and lower the head to the maximum range of motion. This exercise allows qi to circulate throughout the five zang organs (Figure 21-2). This exercise can help treat deafness and blurred vision. Long-term practice can restore gray hair to black.

　　[操作要领与注意事项]此动作难度大,易受伤。初学者完成此动作时忌幅度大、速度快,宜循序渐进。身体柔软,慢慢做

到气遍行身体五脏。

[Tips and notes] This exercise is difficult and can easily cause injury. Beginners should start slowly and gradually increase the range of motion. Make the body flexible in order to promote qi circulation in the five zang organs.

（5）站式、坐式、卧式。观想心气散布于身体上下，正赤色光芒四射通彻天地，自身高大（图36-2）。做这样的观想，有助于气力倍增、发白复黑、齿落再生。

(5) Take a standing, sitting or lying position. Visualize that the heart qi is spreading throughout the body, emitting a bright red light that penetrates the sky and earth, and correspondingly, the body is becoming tall and huge (Figure 36-2). Legend goes that this visualization exercise can make the person full of vigor and vitality, increase physical strength, make the grey hair turn into black, and promote tooth regeneration.

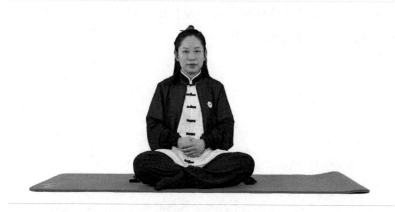

图36-2　Figure 36-2

［操作要领与注意事项］观想红色以沟通天气正气。先得正气，后有色相。忌先有色相，而无正气，徒耗心力。

[Tips and notes] Visualizing the red heart qi spreading throughout the body helps connect you with the healthy qi of the heaven. It is important to first cultivate healthy qi and then develop a healthy facial complexion. Avoid pursuing a healthy facial complexion without cultivating healthy qi first, as this can be a waste of effort.

三十七、目鼻耳齿唇口喉病诸候提要
Daoyin Exercises for Disorders Involving the Eyes, Nose, Ears, Teeth, Lips, Mouth and Throat

本节论述目鼻耳齿唇口喉病诸候的导引术。

This chapter introduces the daoyin exercises for disorders involving the eyes, nose, ears, teeth, lips and throat.

（1）坐式（踞坐）。伸出右脚，两手抱住左膝，鼻纳气，腰部自然舒展，做7次这样的呼吸，同时向外侧舒展右脚（图1-10）。适用于腿脚难以完成屈伸和跪站动作的症状、小腿痛痹的病症，以及风邪入目、耳聋的病症。

(1) Take a sitting position. Sit with the knees raised and the feet on the ground. Stretch out the right foot, hold the left knee with both hands, extend the waist naturally, breathe through the nose 7 times, and stretch the right foot outward at the same time (Figure 1–10). This exercise can help treat the difficulty of the legs and feet in flexion, extension, kneeling and standing, and can also treat pain in the lower legs, pathogenic wind invading the eyes, and deafness.

［操作要领与注意事项］呼吸与动作做到位后，腰部会自然舒展伸起。

[Tips and notes] Once the breathing and movements are done correctly, the waist will naturally stretch and extend.

（2）坐式（踞坐）。伸出左脚，两手抱住右膝，鼻纳气至满，腰部自然舒展，做7次这样的呼吸，同时向外舒展左脚（图1–13）。适用于腿脚难以完成屈伸和跪站动作的症状，以及小腿痛痹的病症。风邪入目、目暗耳聋的病症也可消除。

(2) Take a sitting position. Sit with the knees raised and the feet on the ground. Extend the left foot, hold the right knee with both hands, inhale through the nose deeply, and naturally extend the waist. Repeat this breathing pattern 7 times while extending the left foot outward (Figure1–13). This movement can help treat the difficulty of the legs and feet in flexion, extension, kneeling and standing, and can also help treat pain in the lower legs, pathogenic wind invading the eyes, blurred vision, and deafness.

［操作要领与注意事项］呼吸与动作做到位后，腰部会自然舒展伸起。

[Tips and notes] Once the breathing and movements are done correctly, the waist will naturally stretch and extend.

（3）坐式（端坐）。舒展腰部，以鼻缓缓纳气，右手捏鼻，缓缓闭眼吐气（图5-1）。有助于去除目暗、流泪、鼻息肉、耳聋；也适用于伤寒所致阵阵头痛。练习以出汗为度。

(3) Take an upright sitting position. Stretch the lower back, inhale slowly through the nose, pinch the nose with the right hand, close the eyes and exhale (Figure 5–1). This exercise can help treat blurred vision, watery eyes, nasal polyps, and

deafness, and can also help treat intermittent headache caused by cold damage. Practice until sweating occurs.

［操作要领与注意事项］鼻纳气以开清窍，利头痛；右手捏鼻，有升阳祛寒之效；闭眼可安神，口吐气以驱邪，可舒缓头痛。

[Tips and notes] Inhaling through the nose can open the mind and relieve headache. Pinching the nose with the right hand can lift yang and dispel cold. Closing the eyes can calm the mind, and exhaling through the mouth can expel pathogenic factors, and thus relieve headache.

（4）坐式。鼻纳气，左手捏鼻，适用于目暗、流泪（图37-1）。

(4) Take a sitting position. Inhale through the nose and pinch the nose with the left hand. This exercise can help treat blurred vision and watery eyes (Figure 37-1).

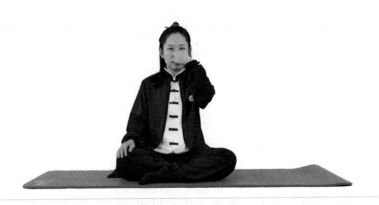

图37-1　Figure 37-1

［操作要领与注意事项］纳气以开清窍，利头痛；左手捏鼻，利于左侧气机运化，有舒畅肝木之效。

[Tips and notes] Inhaling through the nose can clear the mind and relieve headache. Pinching the nose with the left hand can facilitate the circulation of qi on the left side and promote the free flow of liver qi.

（5）站式、坐式。鼻纳气，嘴巴闭合，至满，做7次这样的呼吸（图37-2）。有助于去除两胁下瘀积的气和血。

(5) Take a standing or sitting position. Inhale through the nose deeply, and close the mouth. Breathe 7 times (Figure 37-2). This exercise can help eliminate qi stagnation and blood stasis in the sub-costal region.

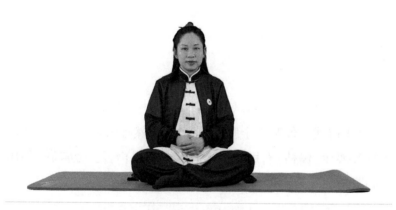

图37-2　Figure 37-2

［操作要领与注意事项］鼻纳气，吸足，气血自然会引向两胁，有和气化瘀之效。

[Tips and notes] Deeply inhale through the nose to make qi and blood naturally flow towards the sub-costal region, and thus harmonize qi and resolve stasis.

（6）蹲式（蹲踞）。两手举起两脚脚趾，低头，尽力做到极势，则气可遍行身体五脏（图21-2）。适用于耳朵听不到声音、眼睛看不清东西。长期练此动作，有助于白头发恢复乌黑。

(6) Take a squatting position. Pull the toes of both feet

with both hands, and lower the head to the maximum range of motion. This exercise allows qi to circulate throughout the five zang organs (Figure 21–2). This exercise can help treat deafness and blurred vision. Long-term practice can restore the gray hair to black.

[操作要领与注意事项] 此动作难度大，易受伤。初学者完成此动作时忌幅度大、速度快，宜循序渐进。身体柔软，慢慢做到气遍行身体五脏。

[Tips and notes] This exercise is difficult and can easily cause injury. Beginners should start slowly and gradually increase the range of motion. Make the body flexible in order to promote qi circulation in the five zang organs.

功法操作 · Movements

（7）卧式。勾起十个脚趾，做5次自然呼吸（图1-2）。适用于腰背痹症、偏枯，有助于让人耳朵听得见声音。经常做，不用担心眼睛和耳朵会得病。

(7) Take a supine position. Fully stretch the toes, naturally inhale and exhale 5 times (Figure 1–2). This exercise can help treat Bi-impediment involving the lower back, hemiplegia, and deafness. Regular practice can keep the eyes and ears clear and also prevent eye and ear disorders.

[操作要领与注意事项] 完成此动作时，脚趾要往上抬、往上勾，可助肾气强盛。

[Tips and notes] During the exercise, fully stretching the toes can strengthen kidney qi.

（8）坐式。伸左腿,屈曲右膝内压在臀部下,做5次呼吸（图2-62）。引气入肺,头微微上仰,去风虚,令人目明。依据经络循行的规则练习,引肺中气,适用于风虚病,也能令人目明。

(8) Take a sitting position. Extend the left leg, flex the right leg, and breathe 5 times (Figure 2–62). By following the pathways of meridians, guide qi into the lung and raise the head slightly. This exercise can help treat deficiency due to wind and brighten the eyes.

［操作要领与注意事项］上额微微抬起（眼睛上翻）,肺叶舒张,气向前走。

[Tips and notes] Raise the head slightly (roll the eyes upward), expand the lung lobes, and guide the breath forward.

（9）站式、坐式、卧式。在凌晨1～3点间,两手相互摩擦,手掌温热后,以此热气贴熨双眼,做3次（图37-3）；手指按压眼睛,观想双眼有神光（图37-4）。有助于眼睛明亮、不生病痛。

(9) Take a standing, sitting or lying position. Between 1 am and 3 am, rub the hands to generate heat, and then use the warm palms to cover the eyes 3 times (Figure 37–3). Press the eyes with the fingers and visualize a shining light (Figure

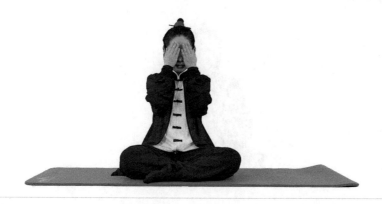

图37-3　Figure 37-3

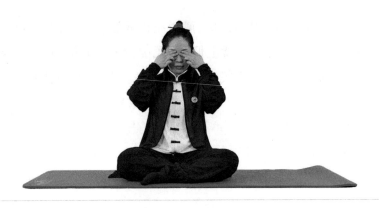

图37-4　Figure 37-4

37-4). This exercise can help brighten the eyes and prevent eye disorders.

［操作要领与注意事项］凌晨1～3点间为肝经气血循行时，两手互摩后贴熨双眼，可调节足厥阴肝经。

[Tips and notes] Between 1 am and 3 am, qi and blood in the liver meridian are circulating. During this period, rub both hands to produce warmth, and then use the warm hands to press the eyes, which can regulate the liver meridian of foot-Jueyin.

（10）坐式。向东而坐。不呼不吸14次（图37-5）。两手中指沾嘴巴里的唾液，按摩眼睛14次，有助于眼睛明亮（图37-6）。

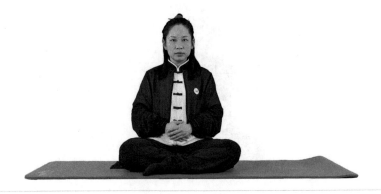

图37-5　Figure 37-5

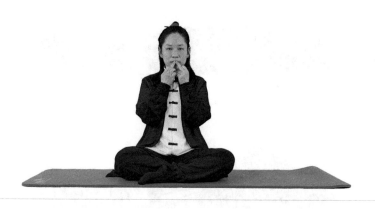

图37-6　Figure 37-6

(10) Take a sitting position facing east. Passively hold the breath 14 times (Figure 37-5). Apply some saliva to the middle fingers, and then use the middle fingers to massage the eyes 14 times. This exercise can help brighten the eyes (Figure 37-6).

[操作要领与注意事项] ① 动作一：向东而坐，以利气机生发；不呼不吸时自然萌动身体气机。此动作是用内气洁净身体，从而使眼睛洁净。② 动作二：漱液，以唾洗眼，有助于去除眼疾和尘垢，使眼睛清洁明亮。此动作是用外洗的方法，有助于去除眼睛的尘垢。

[Tips and notes] ① In the first movement, sit facing east to facilitate the generation of qi. Passively hold the breath to naturally promote the qi activity. This exercise purifies the body by boosting internal qi and thus brightens the eyes. ② In the second movement, massaging the eyes with saliva can help treat eye disorders, clean the eyes, and thus brighten the eyes.

(11) 卧式（仰卧）。下颌向下，使内心安静，这样引气下行3次（图37-7），两手按捏脖子两侧的大筋脉做5次（图37-8）。适用于视物不清。

(11) Take a supine position. Tuck in the chin to calm the

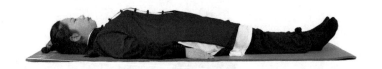

图37-7　Figure 37-7

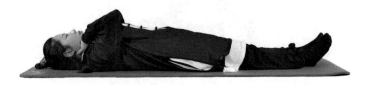

图37-8　Figure 37-8

mind, then guide qi downward 3 times (Figure 37-7) and massage the tendons on both sides of the neck 5 times (Figure 37-8). This exercise can help alleviate blurred vision.

［操作要领与注意事项］此动作类似中医推拿手法"推桥弓"，可清肝明目醒脑。推桥弓：从翳风穴到缺盆穴连成一直线，以指腹自上而下揉推。

[Tips and notes] This exercise is similar to the tuina manipulation called "pushing the point Qiaogong", which can clear the liver, brighten the eyes, and awaken the mind. Pushing the point Qiaogong involves rubbing and pushing the line connecting the points Yifeng (TE17) and Quepen (ST12) from top to bottom using the fingertips.

（12）站式、坐式、卧式。在凌晨1～3点间，漱液，弯曲左手示指摩擦另一手示指（图37-9），使之发热，然后着唾摩眼，这样做14次（图37-10，图37-11）。经常在凌晨1～3点间沾唾液摩眼睛，有助于去除眼睛模糊不清，使其内含精彩光明，彻视万里，遍见四方，不昏花。

（12）Take a standing, sitting or lying position. Between

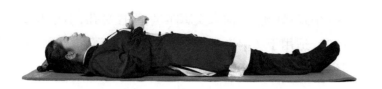

图37-9　Figure 37-9

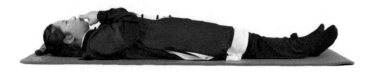

图37-10　Figure 37-10

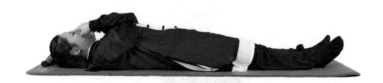

图37-11　Figure 37-11

1 am and 3 am, rinse the mouth with saliva, bend the index finger of one hand to rub the index finger of the other hand until it becomes warm (Figure 37-9), and then apply some saliva to the index fingers to massage the eyes 14 times (Figure 37-10 and Figure 37-11). Regular practice between 1 am and 3 am can help deal with blurred vision, and brighten the eyes.

［操作要领与注意事项］凌晨1～3点间为肝经气血循行时，两手互摩后贴熨双眼，可调节足厥阴肝经。

[Tips and notes] The circulation of qi and blood in the liver meridian is between 1 am and 3 am. Rubbing the hands to produce warmth and then using the warm hands to massage the eyes can regulate the liver meridian of foot-Jueyin.

（13）坐式（跂坐）。向东交脚跂坐，手捏鼻孔，不呼不吸3次（图37-12），适用于鼻中疾患，通利肺上痈疮，清除涕唾，使鼻道通畅闻到香臭。长期练此导引，可以闻到周围远近气味。

(13) Take a cross-legged sitting position, facing east. Pinch the nose with one hand and passively hold the breath 3 times (Figure 37–12). This exercise can help treat nasal disorders and lung abscesses, clear mucus, and unblock nasal passages to improve the sense of smell.

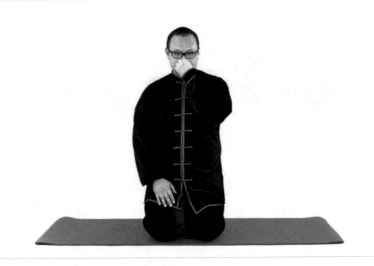

图37-12　Figure 37–12

［操作要领与注意事项］向东而坐，以利气机生发；手捏鼻孔，更有利于打开鼻窍与咽腔，能更好地促进这个部位的气血运行；不呼不吸，能更好地调整全身气机。

[Tips and notes] Sit facing east to facilitate the generation of qi. Pinching the nose can open the nasal passages and throat, promoting the circulation of qi and blood in these areas. Passively holding the breath can regulate the body's qi activity.

（14）坐式（踞坐）。两膝靠拢，两脚张开，不呼不吸5次（图37-13）。有助于去除鼻疮。

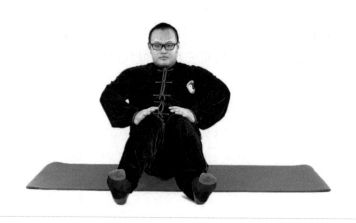

图37-13　Figure 37-13

(14) Take a sitting position. Sit with the knees raised and the feet on the ground. Bring the knees together and open the feet, and passively hold the breath 5 times (Figure 37–13). This exercise can help treat nasal sores.

［操作要领与注意事项］合两膝张两脚，有利于腰、脊、清窍的气机运行。

[Tips and notes] Bringing the knees together and opening the feet can help promote the circulation of qi in the lower back, spine and head.

（15）坐式（端坐）。舒展腰部，以鼻缓缓纳气，右手捏鼻，缓缓闭眼吐气（图5-1）。适用于目暗、流泪、鼻息肉、耳聋；也适用于伤寒所致阵阵头痛。练习以出汗为度。

(15) Take an upright sitting position. Stretch the lower back, inhale slowly through the nose, pinch the nose with the right hand, close the eyes and exhale (Figure 5–1). This exercise can help treat blurred vision, watery eyes, nasal polyps, and deafness, and can also help treat intermittent headache caused by cold damage. Practice until sweating occurs.

［操作要领与注意事项］鼻纳气以开清窍，利头痛；右手捏鼻，有升阳祛寒之效；闭眼可安神，口吐气以驱邪，可舒缓头痛。

[Tips and notes] Inhaling through the nose can open the mind and relieve headache. Pinching the nose with the right hand can lift yang and dispel cold. Closing the eyes can calm the mind, and exhaling through the mouth can expel pathogenic factors, and thus relieve headache.

（16）（坐式）向东而坐。手捏鼻孔，不呼不吸3次（图37-1），适用于鼻中息肉。

(16) Take a sitting position, facing east. Pinch the nose and passively hold the breath 3 times (Figure 37–1). This exercise can help treat nasal polyps.

［操作要领与注意事项］向东而坐，以利气机生发；手捏鼻孔，更有利于打开鼻窍与咽腔，能更好地促进这个部位的气血运行；不呼不吸，能更好地调整全身气机。

[Tips and notes] Sit facing east to facilitate the generation of qi. Pinching the nose can open the nasal passages and throat, promoting the circulation of qi and blood in these areas. Passively holding the breath can regulate the body's qi activity.

（17）坐式。坐在地上，交叉两脚，两手从脚弯处伸入，低头，再把手交叉于项后（图1-79）。适用于久寒自身无力变暖、耳朵听不到声音。

(17) Take a sitting position. Sit on the ground with the feet crossed, then lower the head and cross the hands behind the neck (Figure 1–79). This exercise can help treat chronic cold

sensations in the body and deafness.

［操作要领与注意事项］松解打开脊骨、胯骨，有利于督脉气血运行。此动作难度大，易受伤。初学者完成此动作时忌幅度大、速度快，宜循序渐进。

[Tips and notes] Relax and open the spine and hip bones to circulate qi and blood within the Governor Vessel. This exercise is difficult and can easily cause injury. Beginners should start slowly and gradually increase the range of motion.

（18）坐式。脚放于头上，不呼不吸12次（图1-80）。适用于身体大寒感觉不到暖热，顽固性冷疾、耳聋目眩。长期练此动作就能有效，每次做30次，不能改变。

(18) Take a sitting position. Place the feet on the top of the head and passively hold the breath 12 times (Figure 1-80). Persistent exercise can help treat extreme cold sensations in the body, intractable cold-related disorders, deafness and blurred vision. Do this exercise 30 times per session.

［操作要领与注意事项］松解打开脊骨、胯骨，有利于督脉气血运行。此动作难度大，易受伤。初学者完成此动作时忌幅度大、速度快，宜循序渐进，在医护人员辅助下完成。

[Tips and notes] Relax and open the spine and hip bones to circulate qi and blood within the Governor Vessel. This exercise is difficult and can easily cause injury. Beginners should start slowly and gradually increase the range of motion, and do this exercise under the watchful eye of a person.

（19）坐式。向东而坐。不呼不吸4次，叩齿14次（图37-14），适用于牙痛，使牙齿洁白不黑。一种解释是，张大嘴巴，叩齿14次，不呼不吸1次，这样重复做4次。另一种解释是，只要张大嘴巴叩齿，之后不必在乎次数，旨在消除疾病，不再疼痛，病症缓解就可以了。可使牙齿洁白不黑，也不会有间隙或脱落。长期这样练习，可以咬碎坚硬的东西。

(19) Take a sitting position facing east. Passively hold the breath 4 times and then click the teeth 14 times (Figure 37–14). This exercise can help relieve toothache and whiten teeth. There are two ways to do the exercise: Open the mouth, click the teeth 14 times and passively hold the breath. Repeat 4 times. Alternatively, open the mouth and click the teeth until the toothache is relieved. Regular practice can whiten teeth, prevent teeth from falling out, and improve the ability to bite and chew hard food.

［操作要领与注意事项］向东而坐，以利气机生发；不呼不吸，气机萌新；上下扣齿，促使齿部气血运行，使牙齿坚固。

[Tips and notes] Sit facing east to facilitate the generation

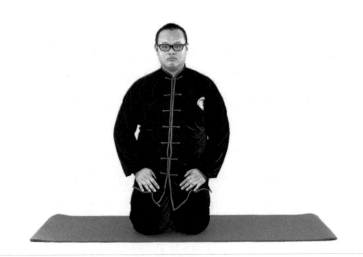

图37-14　Figure 37–14

of qi. Passively hold the breath to naturally promote the qi activity. Clicking the teeth can promote the circulation of qi and blood in the teeth, and make them stronger.

（20）（坐式）向东而坐。不呼不吸4次，上下叩齿36次（图37-14）。适用于齿痛。

(20) Take a sitting position facing east. Passively hold the breath 4 times and then click the teeth 36 times (Figure 37-14). This exercise can help treat toothache.

［操作要领与注意事项］向东而坐，以利气机生发；不呼不吸，气机萌新；上下扣齿，促使齿部气血运行，使牙齿坚固。

[Tips and notes] Sit facing east to facilitate the generation of qi. Passively hold the breath to naturally promote the qi activity. Clicking the teeth can promote the circulation of qi and blood in the teeth, and make them stronger.

（21）站式、坐式。有人觉得脊背僵紧不舒憋闷，无论什么时节，可以缩咽于肩（图1-36），仰面，肩胛骨上抬，头顺着左右两个方向移动，做21次（图1-37），然后稍停，待气血平复再做下一次。开始时要慢做再逐渐加快，不能先快后慢。如果是无病之人，可以在清晨3点至5点、中午11点至13点、下午17点至19点三个时间段操作，每个时段做14次。适用于寒热病、脊腰颈项痛、风痹、口内生疮、牙齿风、头眩。

(21) Take a standing or sitting position. For back rigidity, tuck in the throat (Figure 1-36), raise the head and scapula, and rotate the head to both sides 21 times (Figure 1-37). Then take a break to calm down qi and blood and do it again. Begin slowly and gradually increase the speed. Avoid starting fast and

then slowing down. People in good health can do this exercise 14 times during each of the three time periods: 3–5 am, 11 am–1 pm, and 5–7 pm. This exercise can help treat chills, fever, and pain in the lower back, neck and shoulders, and can also treat wind *Bi*-impediment, mouth ulcer, toothache, and dizziness.

［操作要领与注意事项］腰背脊柱放松，肩部自然打开。即，仰面带脊背肩胛向后固定，在此基础上再缩咽。

[Tips and notes] Relax the waist, back and spine, and open the shoulders naturally. Raise the head to fix the spine and scapula, and then tuck in the throat.

（22）站式、坐式、卧式。两手托两颊，手不动，两肘向内使筋绷紧，腰内随之绷紧，维持这个状态一段时间（图2-1）。两肘头向外放松，使肘、肩、腰内气缓缓散去，放松到极势，当身体感到憋闷时再重新开始做，反复做7次。两肘头向外放松，使肘、肩、腰内气缓缓散去，放松到极势，当身体感到憋闷时再重新开始做，反复做7次。有助于去除喉痹。

(22) Take a standing, sitting or lying position. Hold both cheeks with both hands, keep the hands still, pull the elbows inward to tighten the tendons, and tighten the waist accordingly. Maintain this posture for a period of time (Figure 2-1). Relax the elbows to dissipate qi within the elbows, shoulders and waist, totally relax the body until an oppressive feeling is present, and repeat 7 times. This exercise can help alleviate throat *Bi*-impediment.

［操作要领与注意事项］完成此动作过程中，阴（内）侧筋经延长产生紧促感，筋经鼓动肾气，故能治疗肘臂劳损。

Zhu Bing Yuan Hou Lun Dao Yin Shu (Explanations for the Daoyin Exercises in *Zhu Bing Yuan Hou Lun*) • 《诸 病 源 候 论》 导 引 术

339

功 法 操 作 • Movements

[Tips and notes] During the exercise, the stretching of the yin (inner) meridians produces a tightness sensation, and the stimulation of the meridians activates kidney qi, thus helping to treat elbow and arm strain.

（23）站式。一手舒展打开，手掌向上；另一手握住下颌向外侧推拉。每次做到极势，左右手交换做上述动作14次。然后手不动，身体向两侧快速尽量转动，做14次（图1-19）。适用于颈椎活动障碍、头痛脑眩、喉痹、肩部冷痛、偏风的病症。

(23) Take a standing position. Fully extend and open one hand with the palm facing upward, grip the jaw and push and pull it outward with the other hand. Change the position of the hands and do the above movement 14 times. Then, keep the hands still, and quickly rotate the body to both sides 14 times (Figure 1–19). This exercise can help treat impaired cervical movement, headache, dizziness, throat *Bi*-impediment, pain and cold in the shoulders, and hemiplegia.

［操作要领与注意事项］完成此动作过程中，容易导致颈椎小关节错位，宜缓做。忌爆发力。

[Tips and notes] Since this movement is easy to cause dislocation of the small joints in the cervical vertebrae, do it slowly and avoid using brute force.

三十八、胸痹候提要
Daoyin Exercise for Chest *Bi*-Impediment

本节论述胸痹候的导引术。寒气客于五脏六腑，脏气虚弱，气上冲胸间，形成胸痹。轻则胸中郁结满闷，咽喉间噎塞不畅，有痒感或哽涩干燥。重则心间急痛，不能俯仰，甚或痛连背脊，自汗出。若不及时救治则有生命危险。

This chapter introduces the daoyin exercise for chest *Bi*-impediment. When cold qi invades the five zang organs and six fu organs, the organs become weak and qi rises to the chest, causing chest *Bi*-impediment. Mild cases may experience chest tightness and fullness, and an itchy or a dry throat with a foreign body sensation. Severe cases may experience sudden chest pain that restricts the movements of the upper body and even radiates to the back, with spontaneous sweating. Without timely treatment, this condition is life-threatening.

卧式（仰卧）。右脚放于左脚上（图38-1）。适用于胸痹以及吃热食引起的呕吐。

Take a supine position. Place the right foot on the toes of the left foot (Figure 38–1). This exercise can help alleviate chest *Bi*-impediment, and retching and vomiting caused by consuming hot food.

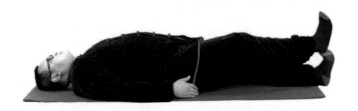

图38-1　Figure 38-1

［操作要领与注意事项］可养精血，改善胸痹、胃肠挛急。

[Tips and notes] This exercise can nourish essence and blood, and alleviate chest *Bi*-impediment and gastro spasm.

三十九、嗜眠候提要

Daoyin Exercises for Hypersomnia

本节论述嗜眠候的导引术。嗜睡是由于肠胃过大，以致皮肤肌肉之间荣血卫阳流行不利，卫阳困于阴分而致。

This chapter introduces the daoyin exercises for hypersomnia. Enlarged intestines and stomach may impair the circulation of yang qi and blood within the skin and muscles. This condition may trap yang qi in the yin phases and subsequently result in hypersomnia.

（1）坐式（跂踞）。两腿相交，其形如箕（图39–1），两手从弯曲的腿中伸入，两手交叉，用力牵引（图39–2）。适用于昏沉久寐、精气不清明。长期练此动作可减少嗜睡，增长精神。

(1) Take a sitting position with the legs crossed and shaped like a winnow (Figure 39–1). Insert both hands into the bent legs and cross them, and then pull them apart with force (Figure 39–2). This exercise can help alleviate drowsiness and mental cloudiness. Long-term practice of this exercise can help treat hypersomnia and improve bright spirit.

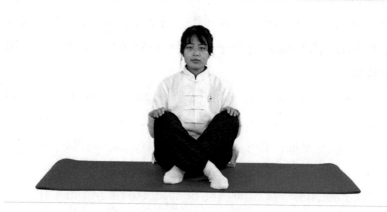

图39–1　Figure 39–1

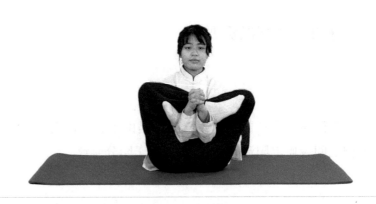

图39-2　Figure 39-2

　　［操作要领与注意事项］跂踞，两手从弯曲的腿中伸入。左手从右脚腕上方伸入左脚，随着空隙向下；右手从左脚腕上伸入右脚，随着空隙向下。两手伸出后抱住两脚，然后两手快速牵引2次。

　　[Tips and notes] Cross the legs and insert both hands into the bent legs. The left hand reaches into the right foot from above and goes down along the gap, while the right hand reaches into the left foot from above and goes down along the gap. After extending both hands, grab both feet and pull quickly twice.

　　（2）（站式）一手托住下颌，极力向上，另一手尽量用力向后舒展，手掌向四个方位转动，这一刻皆尽力做到极势，做28次（图1-67）。两手互换做上述动作。两手托住下颌，使身体侧身旋转14次（图1-68），有助于去除手、肩和头部的风邪，也适用于昏睡。

　　(2) Take a standing position. Hold the chin with one hand and fully lift it. Fully extend the other hand backward and rotate the palm 28 times (Figure 1-67). Then change the position of the hands and repeat the above movements. Hold the chin with both hands and rotate the body sideways 14 times (Figure 1-68). This exercise can help dispel pathogenic wind in the

hands, shoulders and head, and also treat lethargy.

[操作要领与注意事项] 此动作可舒展颈肩部的筋膜, 利于气血运行。

[Tips and notes] This exercise can stretch the fascia of the neck and shoulders, promoting the circulation of qi and blood.

四十、疽候提要
Daoyin Exercises for Deep-rooted Ulcers

本节论述疽候的导引术。疽, 即局部皮肤下发生的疮肿。中医指局部皮肤肿胀坚硬而皮色不变的毒疮。疽为五脏不调所引起, 如喜怒无常、饮食不节都会导致五脏不调。由于脏气行内主里, 所以疽生长在肌肉深层, 一旦发病时间较长, 则血肉腐败, 甚则伤骨烂筋, 引发生命危险。

This chapter introduces the daoyin exercises for deep-rooted ulcers. These ulcers refer to localized swellings and sores that occur beneath the skin. In TCM, they are toxic ulcers characterized by local skin swelling and hardening with no change in skin color. Deep-rooted ulcers are caused by disharmony of the five zang organs. Emotional disturbances, an irregular diet, and other factors may contribute to the disharmony. As qi of the five zang organs flows inside and governs the interior, these ulcers often grow deep in the muscles. Over time, the flesh may rot, and the bones and tendons may be damaged, leading to life-threatening conditions.

(1) 站式、坐式。立正或正坐。靠墙, 不呼不吸, 行气, 从头至脚（图1-1）。适用于疽。行气的意思是，鼻纳气，吸5次吐1次，这样作为1次。做满12次适用于疾病。

(1) Take a standing or sitting position. Stand straight or sit upright. Lean against a wall, passively hold the breath, and circulate qi from the head to the feet (Figure 1–1). This exercise can help treat ulcers. Circulating qi means inhaling through the nose, exhaling 5 times, and then inhaling once. Doing this 12 times can help alleviate the disorder.

［操作要领与注意事项］① 行气的原则：自然放松，气自然向下行。② 此动作站、坐皆可，靠墙完成，非常适用于体质虚弱的偏枯患者及平衡能力弱的人。

[Tips and notes] ① The principle of qi circulation: Relax the body and promote qi downward naturally. ② This movement can be done by leaning against a wall in a standing or sitting position. It is very suitable for hemiplegia patients with a weak constitution and for those with a weak balance ability.

（2）站式、坐式。立正或正坐。靠墙，不呼不吸，行气，从口部把气引至头部（图1-3）。适用于痈疽、风痹、大风病、偏枯等。

(2) Take a standing or sitting position. Stand straight or sit upright. Lean against a wall, passively hold the breath, and circulate qi from the mouth to the head (Figure 1–3). This exercise can help treat abscesses, wind *Bi*-impediment, blood deficiency stirring wind, and hemiplegia.

［操作要领与注意事项］这个导引动作如同打哈欠一般，引清气上入脑窍。

[Tips and notes] This movement is like yawning. It ascends clear qi to the brain.

四十一、瘰疬瘘候提要
Daoyin Exercise for Scrofula and Fistula Disorders

本节论述瘰疬瘘候的导引术。瘰疬瘘是由于风邪毒气侵入肌肉，随着人体虚处停留，进而结聚而成。瘰疬在皮肤之下，形似枣核大小，两三个连在一起，时而伴见寒热；病久则壅积化脓，溃破而成瘘。

This chapter introduces the daoyin exercise for scrofula and fistula disorders. Pathogenic wind may invade the muscles and accumulate in the weak parts of the body. This condition may result in scrofula and fistula disorders. Scrofula appears as small bumps under the skin, resembling the size of jujubes, and may be accompanied by chills and fever. Over time, it may develop into an abscess and eventually rupture, forming fistulas.

坐式（跂踞）。两个手从弯曲的大腿内伸入，然后手放在地上，弯曲的大腿放于手上，把臀部举起来（图41−1）。这个动作可以用来行气。适用于瘰疬、乳房疼痛。

Take a cross-legged sitting position. Insert both hands into the bent legs, then place both hands on the ground, place the thighs on the hands, and lift the buttocks with the hands (Figure 41−1). This exercise can circulate qi and help treat scrofula and breast pain.

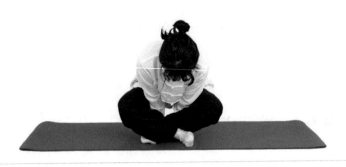

图41-1　Figure 41-1

［操作要领与注意事项］此动作可舒解改善胸胁部气血运行。此动作难度大，易受伤。初学者完成此动作时忌幅度大、速度快，宜循序渐进。

[Tips and notes] This exercise can improve the circulation of qi and blood in the chest and sub-costal region. This exercise is difficult and can easily cause injury. Beginners should start slowly and gradually increase the range of motion.

四十二、㿗瘘候提要
Daoyin Exercise for Testicular Swelling

本节论述㿗瘘候的导引术。㿗病症状为睾丸肿大。往往因强力劳动伤及少阴经气，以致肾气不能固护外阴，气胀不通，所以成㿗；久则溃破成瘘。

This chapter introduces the daoyin exercise for testicular swelling, a disorder characterized by enlarged testicles. Damage of the Shaoyin meridian due to overexertion may impair the function of kidney qi in protecting genitalia, leading to obstruction of qi in the testicles. Without proper treatment, this condition may result in ulceration and fistula formation over time.

卧式（仰卧）。舒展手脚，心中观想月亮犹如油囊裹着朱砂的颜色。适用于阴囊肿大、少腹重、便秘（图42-1）。腹中有热的情况，以口纳气，鼻出气，做几十次，不需要小咽气。腹中不热的情况，做7次小咽气，使气温暖后再咽下，做十几次。

Take a supine position. Stretch the limbs and visualize the moon in the mind, as if it were the color of cinnabar wrapped in an oil bag. This can help alleviate such conditions as swollen scrotum, lower abdomen heaviness, and constipation (Figure 42-1). To relieve a hot sensation in the abdomen, inhale through the mouth, exhale through the nose and repeat several tens of times. For those without a hot sensation in the abdomen, breathe 7 times, warm the air in the mouth, swallow the warm air, and repeat more than 10 times.

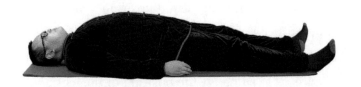

图42-1　Figure 42-1

［操作要领与注意事项］完成此观想前，须先调整心意，松静自然。观想月亮以利阴气，观想朱砂色以利水肿。

[Tips and notes] Before practicing this visualization, adjust the mind to keep a tranquil mind. Visualizing the moon is beneficial for nourishing yin qi, while visualizing the color of cinnabar can help alleviate edema.

四十三、诸痔候提要
Daoyin Exercises for Hemorrhoids

本节论述诸痔候的导引术。痔病有很多种。痔病的多因感受风邪,或房室不慎,或醉后入房,以致劳伤扰动血气,血不循经流溢于外,下注肛门所致。

This chapter introduces the daoyin exercises for hemorrhoids. There are many types of hemorrhoids. Sexual indulgence/sexual intercourse after drinking, coupled with the contraction of pathogenic wind may disturb blood and qi, in which blood may overflow outside the meridians and accumulate in the anus, resulting in hemorrhoids.

(1)站式、坐式。一脚踏地,另一腿屈膝,两手合抱在膝眼下,迅速用力向身体牵拉,尽力做到极势(图2-17)。左右脚交换做上述动作28次,有助于去除痔疾、五劳所伤、足三里的气机不得下行。

(1) Take a standing or sitting position. Place one foot on the ground, lift the other leg, with both hands clasped under the lifted knee, and quickly and fully pull the knee towards the body (Figure 2–17). Change the position of the legs and repeat the movements 28 times on each side. This exercise can help treat hemorrhoids, the five exhaustions, and qi stagnation in the point Zusanli (ST 36).

[操作要领与注意事项]完成此动作过程中,自然纳气,以利归元。

[Tips and notes] During the exercise, breathe naturally to guide qi into the *Dantian*.

(2)坐式(踞坐)。两膝靠拢,两脚张开,不呼不吸5次(图37-13)。适用于鼻疮。

(2) Take a sitting position. Sit with the knees raised and

the feet on the ground. Bring the knees together, open the feet, and passively hold the breath 5 times (Figure 37–13). This exercise can help treat nasal sores.

[操作要领与注意事项] 合两膝张两脚,有利于腰、脊、清窍的气机运行。

[Tips and notes] Bring the knees together and open the feet to promote the circulation of qi in the waist, spine and mind.

（3）坐式。两手抱两脚,头不动,使脚朝向脸面,但不要近到触及呼出之气,使全身骨节气散,如此反复做21次(图31-1)。两手握两脚,向左右侧身,皆用力牵拉,腰不动(图31-2)。有助于去除四肢、腰脊髓内冷、血脉冷、筋脉挛急、痔疮。

(3) Take a sitting position. Lift both feet with the hands to make them close to the head, keep the head still, disperse qi throughout the bones and joints, and repeat this movement 21 times (Figure 31–1). Lift both feet with the hands, and turn the upper body to both sides while keeping the waist still (Figure 31–2). This exercise can help relieve cold in the limbs and lower back, muscle/tendon spasm, and hemorrhoids.

[操作要领与注意事项] 两手抱脚,尽力拔伸,使全身骨节松解开来,有利于周身气血运行,腰骨脊髓放松。

[Tips and notes] Lift the feet with both hands to the maximum range of motion in order to relax the joints and promote the circulation of qi and blood throughout the body.

（4）坐式。两脚对踏,脚掌合拢,向会阴侧做快速的轻微收缩，两手捧膝头，朝两个方向用力到极致，按捺14次（图2-6）。然后身体尽力向两侧活动14次（图2-7），腰部前后活动7次（图2-8）。适用于心劳、痔病。

(4) Take a sitting position. Bring the soles together, quickly and slightly contract the pelvic muscles, hold both knees with both hands and pull the knees 14 times (Figure 2–6). Then fully bend the body to both sides 14 times (Figure 2–7), and move the waist forward and backward 7 times (Figure 2–8). This exercise can help treat heart deficiency, and hemorrhoids.

［操作要领与注意事项］完成此动作过程中，膝关节向下，背部向上，两向极势，提中气故能治心劳；腰腹打开，阳气升促进气血旺盛，腰腹强，肾气充足，故能治膝冷。

[Tips and notes] During this exercise, fully drop the knee joints and lift the back to regulate middle qi and thus treat heart deficiency. Open the waist and abdomen to promote the ascending of yang qi, tonify qi and blood, and strengthen the kidney, lower back and abdomen, thereby treating cold in the knees.

四十四、诸恶疮候提要
Daoyin Exercise for Intractable Ulcers

本节论述诸恶疮候的导引术。各种疮证多是由于体虚感受风热之邪，风热与血气搏结而引发。

This chapter introduces the daoyin exercise for various types of intractable ulcers. Physical weakness coupled with the invasion of pathogenic wind and heat into blood and qi may cause intractable ulcers.

跪式（跪伏）。龙行气。叩头，额头着地，眼睛向下看，不呼不吸12次（图44-1）。适用于风疥、恶疮，可使热邪不进入体内。

Take a kneeling position. Assume the posture of a dragon to circulate qi. Place the forehead on the ground, look downward, and passively hold the breath 12 times (Figure 44-1). This exercise can help treat scabies and intractable ulcers, and prevent the invasion of pathogenic heat into the body.

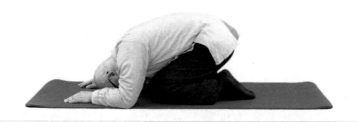

图44-1　Figure 44-1

［操作要领与注意事项］此动作外形上可使脊柱完全放松；不呼不吸的状态下可自然调节气机，可祛风邪，散热毒。

[Tips and notes] This exercise can relax the spine. Naturally regulate the qi movement under the state of passively holding the breath in order to dispel wind and disperse heat toxins.

四十五、疥候提要
Daoyin Exercise for Scabies

本节论述疥候的导引术。疥疮有很多种，都是有虫的。多因皮肤感受风邪热气而引起。

This chapter introduces the daoyin exercise for scabies. There are many types of scabies, all of which are caused by parasites. Mostly, this condition is caused by the invasion of pathogenic wind and heat into the skin.

跪式（跪伏）。龙行气。叩头，额头着地，眼睛向下看，不呼不吸12次（图44-1）。适用于风疥、恶疮，可使热邪不进入体内。

Take a kneeling position. Assume the posture of a dragon to circulate qi. Place the forehead on the ground, look downward, and passively hold the breath 12 times (Figure 44-1). This exercise can help treat scabies and intractable ulcers, and prevent the invasion of pathogenic heat into the body.

[操作要领与注意事项] 此动作外形上可使脊柱完全放松；不呼不吸的状态下可自然调节气机，可祛风邪，散热毒。

[Tips and notes] This exercise can relax the spine. Naturally regulate the qi movement under the state of passively holding the breath in order to dispel wind pathogens and disperse heat toxins.

四十六、卒被损瘀血候提要
Daoyin Exercises for Blood Stasis due to Traumatic Injury

本节论述卒被损瘀血候的导引术。因外伤而内有瘀血者，会有记忆力减退、害怕听到器物击动的声音、胸部满闷、唇口萎而少泽、舌色青紫、口干但只想漱口不欲喝水、腹部不胀满而自觉胀满的表现，这些是瘀血的症状。

This chapter introduces the daoyin exercises for blood

stasis due to traumatic injury. The manifestations of this condition include memory decrease, fear of hearing the sound of striking objects, chest tightness, lips without luster or moisture, a bluish-purple tongue, a dry mouth with the desire to rinse instead of drinking water, and a subjective sensation of abdominal fullness.

（1）坐式（端坐）。舒展腰部，举左手，仰掌向上，右手托右胁，鼻纳气，至满，呼吸7次（图10-6）。有助于去除瘀血、结气。

(1) Take an upright sitting position. Stretch the waist, lift the left hand, turn the palm upward, place the right hand on the right flank, deeply inhale through the nose, and breathe 7 times (Figure 10–6). This exercise can help alleviate blood stasis and qi stagnation.

［操作要领与注意事项］完成此动作时，举左手，利于气机疏通；右手后下，指尖可朝下或朝前，利于鼻纳气。右手手指忌指尖朝后。

[Tips and notes] During this exercise, lifting the left hand helps to regulate the flow of qi, while pressing down the right hand with the fingertips pointing downward or forward facilitates the inhalation through the nose. Avoid pointing the fingertips of the right hand backward.

（2）站式、坐式。鼻纳气，嘴巴闭合，至满，做7次这样的呼吸（图37-2）。有助于去除两胁下瘀积的气和血。

(2) Take a standing or sitting position. Inhale through the nose deeply, and close the mouth. Breathe 7 times (Figure 37–2). This exercise can help eliminate qi stagnation and blood

［操作要领与注意事项］鼻纳气，吸足，气血自然会引向两胁，有和气化瘀之效。

[Tips and notes] Deeply inhale through the nose to make qi and blood naturally flow towards the sub-costal region, and thus harmonize qi and resolve stasis.

（3）坐式（端坐）。右手放于腰部，鼻纳气7次，左右转头各30次（图46-1）。有助于去除体内瘀血、颈项部疼痛。

(3) Take an upright sitting position. Place the right hand on the waist, inhale through the nose 7 times, and turn the head to the left and right 30 times on each side (Figure 46-1). This exercise can help resolve blood stasis in the body and relieve neck pain.

［操作要领与注意事项］右手放于腰部，以助命门精血生化；左右扭头可活血化瘀，行气止痛。

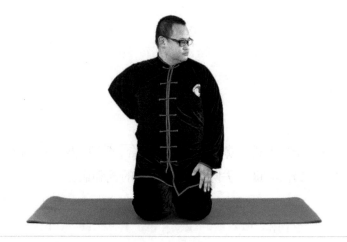

图46-1　Figure 46-1

[Tips and notes] Place the right hand on the waist to help with the generation of essence and blood at the gate of life (*Ming Men*). Turning the head left and right can promote blood circulation, resolve blood stasis, and alleviate pain by circulating qi.

（4）站式、坐式。两手托按腰部，两手手指相对（图46-2），尽力做到极势，前后振摇14次（图46-3，图46-4）。有助于去除云门穴、腰部、腋部的血气闭塞不通。

(4) Take a standing or sitting position. Place both hands on the waist, with the fingers facing each other (Figure 46–2), and shake back and forth 14 times, trying to reach the maximum range of motion (Figure 46–3 and Figure 46–4). This exercise can help promote the circulation of qi and blood in the point Yunmen (LU 2), lower back and armpits.

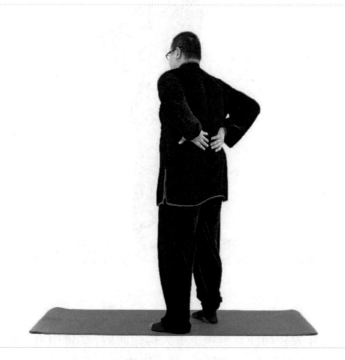

图46-2　Figure 46-2

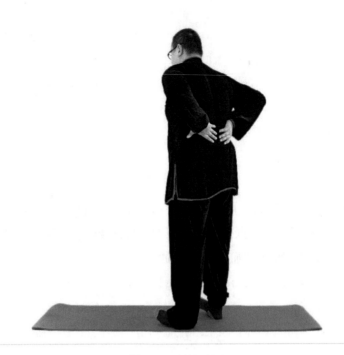

图46-3　　Figure 46-3

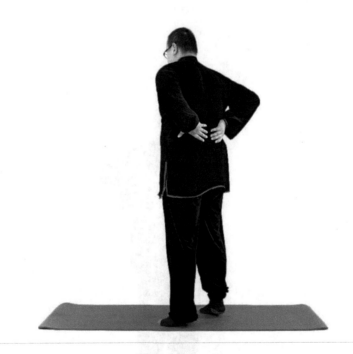

图46-4　　Figure 46-4

　　[操作要领与注意事项] 手大拇指向后，尽量用力，前后振摇14次；手不移动，上下揉动，尽可能让气向下走。

[Tips and notes] Use the thumbs to push backwards, and shake forward and backward 14 times. Do not move the hands, but rub up and down to circulate qi downward.

四十七、无子候提要
Daoyin Exercise for Infertility

本节论述无子候的导引术。妇人不能生育，大多由于伤及血气，冷热失调，感受风寒，风寒客于子宫，以致胞内生病，或月经涩滞不通、或血崩、或带下，使阴阳之气不和，所以不能生育。

This chapter introduces the daoyin exercise for infertility. In females, the damage of blood and qi coupled with the invasion of pathogenic wind and cold into the uterus may lead to such disorders as menstrual blockage, metrorrhagia and leucorrhea. These disorders can disrupt the harmony between yin and yang and subsequently result in infertility.

站式（立正）。吸收月亮的精华，在月亮初升，太阳将落尽时候，面向月亮站立，不呼不吸8次。仰头面向月亮吸收月光的精华，（因循着月光）咽下，8次（图47-1）。可以增长人的阴气，妇人吸收月亮精华，阴气更加旺盛，可使子道通畅。阴气增长可以益精补脑。

Follow the rules of the sun, moon, stars, and the yin-yang of the human body. For example, take an upright standing posture. Stand facing the moon when it rises at the beginning of the moon phase and the sun is about to set, and passively hold the breath 8 times. Look up and absorb the moonlight essence by swallowing it, and do this 8 times. Legend goes that this can increase a person's yin qi, and for females, absorbing

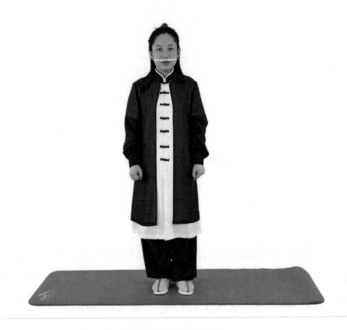

图47-1　Figure 47-1

the essence of the moon can make their yin qi more vigorous, which can promote conception. Increasing yin energy can also nourish the essence and improve brain function.

［操作要领与注意事项］遵循中医天人相应的规律，吸收月亮之精华以养精气。

[Tips and notes] Follow the principle of man-nature correspondence in TCM, and absorb the essence of the moon to nourish the essence and qi.

四十八、乳结核候提要
Daoyin Exercise for Breast Nodules

本节论述乳结核候的导引术。足阳明经行于乳房。如果经脉虚弱又受风寒，血气郁滞，则成结肿。结肿热化，变败成脓；

结肿寒化,则成结核,不易消散。

This chapter introduces the daoyin exercise for breast nodules. The stomach meridian of foot-Yangming runs through the breasts. Weakness of the meridians coupled with pathogenic wind and cold may lead to qi stagnation and blood stasis, and subsequently result in nodules. Nodules that become inflamed can develop into abscesses, while those further affected by pathogenic cold are difficult to treat.

坐式(跽踞)。两个手从弯曲的大腿内伸入,然后手放在地上,弯曲的大腿放于手上,把臀部举起来,做12次(图41-1)。这个动作可以用来行气。适用于瘰疬、乳房疼痛。

Take a cross-legged sitting position. Insert both hands into the bent legs, then place both hands on the ground, place the thighs on the hands, and lift the buttocks with the hands (Figure 41-1). This exercise can circulate qi and help treat scrofula and breast pain.

[操作要领与注意事项] 此动作可舒解改善胸胁部气血运行。此动作难度大,易受伤。初学者完成此动作时忌幅度大、速度快,宜循序渐进。

[Tips and notes] This exercise can improve the circulation of qi and blood in the chest and sub-costal region. This exercise is difficult and can easily cause injury. Beginners should start slowly and gradually increase the range of motion.

Application

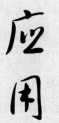

应

用

一、中风后遗症

Sequelae of Apoplexy

（一）概述

Introduction

"中风后遗症"指中风后经过救治，神志清醒后，遗留的以半身不遂、麻木不仁、语言不利、口眼歪斜为主要表现的一类病症。有关中风的记载，始见于《黄帝内经》，根据其症状及发病不同阶段有着不同的记载。中医古籍对"仆击""大厥""薄厥""偏枯""偏风""偏身不用""口喎""痱风"的描述可找到相关论述。《灵枢·刺节真邪》曰："虚邪偏客于身半，其入深，内居荣卫，荣卫稍衰，则真气去，邪气独留，发为偏枯。"后世医家对中风的论述大致分为两个阶段，唐宋以前多以"内虚邪中"立论，唐宋以后多以"内风"立论。中风病因主要包括素体气血亏虚、饮食不节、情志所伤、气虚中邪。中风病机较为复杂，但不外乎气血逆乱。

Sequelae of apoplexy refers to a group of symptoms that persist after treatment for apoplexy when consciousness has been restored, including hemiplegia, numbness, insensitivity, slurred speech, and deviation of the mouth and eyes. The earliest records of apoplexy can be found in *Huang Di Nei Jing*. This book recorded the corresponding symptoms of apoplexy at different stages. In addition, disease descriptions similar to the symptoms of apoplexy can also be found in other ancient Chinese medical books, for example, flopping syncope

(*Bo Jue*). *Ling Shu Ci Jie Zhen Xie* (Chapter 75 of the Spiritual Pivot) states, "When deficiency pathogens have settled in one side of the body and enter into the depth, where the *Ying*-nutrients and *Wei*-defence reside, the *Ying*-nutrients and *Wei*-defence will decrease and weaken, and as a result the true qi leaves, and only the evil qi remains and causes a unilateral paralysis." The discourse of later generations of medical practitioners on apoplexy can be broadly divided into two stages. Prior to the Tang and Song dynasties, most of them believed that apoplexy was primarily caused by "internal deficiency coupled with the invasion of pathogenic factors." During and after the Tang and Song dynasties, the prevailing belief shifted to considering "internal wind" as the main cause of apoplexy. The causative factors of apoplexy mainly include constitutional deficiency of qi and blood, an improper diet, emotional disturbances, and qi deficiency coupled with the invasion of pathogenic factors. Although the pathogenesis of apoplexy is complicated, it primarily involves the disorder of qi and blood.

根据中风后遗症的临床表现，主要见于西医学的脑卒中后遗症。脑卒中为脑血管疾病的主要类型，包括缺血性和出血性卒中两种类型，主要特征是突然的局限或弥散性的脑功能缺损。研究报告显示，脑卒中存活患者病情稳定后多伴有不同程度的运动功能障碍、认知功能障碍、语言功能障碍、中枢性面瘫、吞咽障碍、二便障碍、抑郁等后遗症。本节所论中风后遗症的辨证论治，脑卒中后遗症期的运动功能障碍、言语功能障碍、中枢性面瘫可参照本篇内容辨证论治。

Apoplexy is the main type of cerebrovascular diseases, including ischemic stroke and hemorrhagic stroke. Its main feature is the sudden localized or diffuse brain dysfunction.

Research reports have shown that stroke survivors often experience varying degrees of motor dysfunction, cognitive impairment, language impairment, facial paralysis, dysphagia, bladder/bowel incontinence, depression, and other sequelae after their conditions are stabilized. The pattern identification and treatment for sequelae of apoplexy discussed in this section applies to motor dysfunction, language impairment, and facial paralysis.

（二）辨证论治
Treatment Based on Pattern Identification

中风病机细分主要包含六端：虚（阴虚、气虚）、火（肝火、心火）、风（肝风、外风）、痰（风痰、湿痰）、气（气逆）、血（血瘀）。病之根本在于肝肾阴虚；病之标为风火相煽，痰湿壅盛，瘀血阻滞，导致经络闭阻，气血逆乱，蒙蔽清窍。病性多为本虚标实，上盛下虚。中风后遗症的辨证论治，总以扶正补虚为主，标本兼顾；并根据后遗症的主要症状及其证候特点，相应采用益气养阴、养血活血、熄风通络、祛风化痰、补肾利窍的治法。

The pathogenesis of stroke can be divided into six categories: deficiency (yin deficiency or/and qi deficiency), fire (liver fire or/and heart fire), wind (liver wind or/and external wind), phlegm (wind-phlegm or/and damp-phlegm), qi (counterflow of qi), and blood (blood stasis). The root of the disorder lies in yin deficiency of the liver and kidney, while the tip of the disorder involves the interplay of excess wind and fire, accumulation of phlegm and dampness, and blood stasis, leading to blocked meridians, disordered qi and blood, and clouded clear orifices. The disorder is usually present as a combination of deficiency at the root and excess at the tip, with the upper part of the body being in excess and the lower part in deficiency. In the treatment of sequelae of apoplexy, the primary focus is on reinforcing healthy qi to strengthen the body while considering both the tip and root. Based on the main symptoms and the characteristics of the syndrome, corresponding treatments are adopted, such as supplementing qi and nourishing yin, circulating and nourishing blood, extinguishing wind and unblocking collaterals, removing wind and resolving phlegm, or tonifying the kidney qi and unblocking the orifices.

中药、导引方皆适用于中风后遗症,临证不仅需掌握其辨证常规,亦需根据不同的后遗症表现灵活施治。对于中风后遗症的康复治疗,需提醒患者及其家属注意气候变化防止外邪诱发、调畅情志以免七情引动、薄滋味以杜生痰之源。若患者年迈体衰,肾气亏损,则恢复较慢,临证不可忽视耐心鼓励给予其信心。

Both Chinese medicines and daoyin exercises can be applied to treat sequelae of apoplexy. In clinical practice, it is essential not only to identify the pattern correctly but also to apply flexible treatments tailored to different manifestations. For the rehabilitation of post-stroke patients, it is necessary to remind them and also their families to pay attention to weather changes to prevent external pathogenic factors. In addition, the patients should prevent emotional disturbances, and maintain a light diet to prevent the generation of phlegm. For the elderly with physical weakness due to aging and kidney qi deficiency, the recovery may be slower. It is crucial to provide the patient with confidence and support during the treatment.

1. 半身不遂

1. Hemiplegia

（1）气虚血滞，脉络瘀阻

(1) Qi deficiency with blood stasis obstructing meridians

［症状］半身不遂，肢软无力，并伴有患侧手足浮肿，语言艰涩，口眼歪斜，面色萎黄，或暗淡无华，苔薄白，舌淡紫，或舌体不正，脉细涩无力。

[Symptoms] Hemiplegia with limb weakness, accompanied by edema on the affected side of the limbs, slurred speech, deviation of the mouth and eyes, a sallow or lusterless facial complexion, thin white tongue coating, pale purple tongue, or irregular tongue shape, and a thready and hesitant pulse.

［治法］通经活络。

[Treatment method] Unblock meridians.

［《诸病源候论》导引方 Daoyin Exercises in *Zhu Bing Yuan Hou Lun*］

1）调心

1) Mind regulation

站式、坐式、卧式。自膝部以下有病，当观想脐下有红光，红光里外相连周遍全身。自膝部以上至腰部有病，当观想脾有黄光。从腰部以上至头部有病，当观想心中有红光。病在皮肤有寒热，当观想肝内有青绿光。上述都要观想（各色）光里外相连周遍全身，同时通过闭气来收敛光芒向内照（病所）（图15-11）。

Take a standing, sitting or lying position. For disorders below the knees, visualize a red light below the navel. For disorders between the knees and the waist, visualize a yellow light in the spleen. For disorders between the waist and the head, visualize a red light in the heart. For skin disorders accompanied by cold or heat symptoms, visualize a green light in the liver. In all cases, visualize the respective colored light illuminating the entire body, while simultaneously holding the breath to draw the radiance inward towards the affected area (Figure 15–11).

站式、坐式、卧式。观想心气散布于身体上下，正赤色光芒四射通彻天地，自身高大（图36-2）。做这样的观想，可令人气力倍增、发白复黑、齿落再生。

Take a standing, sitting or lying position. Visualize that the heart qi is spreading throughout the body, emitting a bright red light that penetrates the sky and earth, and correspondingly, the body is becoming tall and huge (Figure 36–2). Legend goes that this visualization exercise can make the person full of vigor and vitality, increase physical strength, make the grey hair turn into black, and promote tooth regeneration.

2）调息、调身
2) Breath regulation and body regulation

站式、坐式（立正或正坐）。靠墙，不呼不吸，行气，从头至脚（图1-1）。适用于疽、疝、大风、偏枯以及由风邪引起的各种痹证。立正或正坐。背靠墙，伸展两脚，舒展脚趾，把心安静下来，不呼不吸，行气，从头引气到十个脚趾和脚心，这样的引气做21次，等待脚心有得气的感觉就可以停止了。

Take a standing or sitting position. Stand straight or sit upright. Lean against a wall, passively hold the breath, and circulate qi from the head to the feet (Figure 1–1). This exercise can help treat ulcers, hernia, blood deficiency stirring wind, hemiplegia, and varying *Bi*-impediment patterns caused by pathogenic wind. Stand straight or sit upright against a wall with the legs extended and the toes stretched out. Calm the mind, passively hold the breath, and circulate the qi from the head to the ten toes and two soles. Repeat this circulation 21 times until you feel the qi sensations in the soles.

站式。一脚踏地，另一脚向旁侧打开（成丁字步）（图1-5）。身体旋转侧身，一手从上往下，使两手并拢，尽力做到最大幅度（图1-6），然后两手快速收回，左右手脚互换做上述动作，各14次。适用于脊柱中的风冷，以及半身偏枯导致的气血不能畅通和濡养的病症。

Take a standing position. Take a step to the side with one foot (T-shape stance) (Figure 1–5). Turn the upper body to the side, fully lift and put down the hands one by one, and put them together (Figure 1–6). Quickly retract the hands and repeat the movements on the other side, 14 times on each side. This movement can dispel wind and cold in the spine, and deal with the obstruction and malnutrition of qi and blood caused by hemiplegia.

（2）肝阳上亢，脉络瘀阻

(2) Hyperactivity of liver yang with blocked meridians

［症状］患侧僵硬拘挛，兼见头疼头晕，面赤耳鸣，舌红绛，苔薄黄，脉弦硬有力。

[Symptoms] Stiffness and contracture on the affected side, accompanied by headache, dizziness, a red face, and tinnitus. The tongue is deep red with a thin yellow coating, and the pulse is wiry and tense.

［治法］熄风通络。

[Treatment methods] Remove wind and resolve phlegm.

［《诸病源候论》导引方 Daoyin Exercises in *Zhu Bing Yuan Hou Lun*]

1）调心

1) Mind regulation

站式、坐式、卧式。自膝部以下有病，当观想脐下有红光，红光里外相连周遍全身。自膝部以上至腰部有病，当观想脾有黄光。从腰部以上至头部有病，当观想心中有红光。病在皮肤有寒热，当观想肝内有青绿光。上述都要观想（各色）光里外相连周遍全身，同时通过闭气来收敛光芒向内照（病所）（图15-11）。

Take a standing, sitting or lying position. For disorders below the knees, visualize a red light below the navel. For disorders between the knees and the waist, visualize a yellow light in the spleen. For disorders between the waist and the head, visualize a red light in the heart. For skin disorders accompanied by cold or heat symptoms, visualize a green light in the liver. In all cases, visualize the respective colored light illuminating the entire body, while simultaneously holding the breath to draw the radiance inward towards the affected area (Figure 15–11).

站式（立正）。吸收月亮的精华，在月亮初升，太阳将落尽时候，面向月亮站立，不呼不吸8次。仰头面向月亮吸收月光的精华，（因循着月光）咽下，8次（图47-1）。可以增长人的阴气，妇人吸收月亮精华，阴气更加旺盛，可使子道通畅。阴气增长可以益精补脑。

Follow the rules of the sun, moon, stars, and the yin-yang of the human body. For example, take an upright standing posture. Stand facing the moon when it rises at the beginning of the moon phase and the sun is about to set, and passively hold the breath 8 times. Look up and absorb the moonlight essence by swallowing it, and do this 8 times. Legend goes that this can increase a person's yin qi, and for females, absorbing the essence of the moon can make their yin qi more vigorous, which can promote conception. Increasing yin energy can also nourish the essence and improve brain function.

2）调息、调身

2）Breath regulation and body regulation

站式、坐式、卧式。有肝病的人，容易忧愁不快乐，有悲伤、思虑、不满、恼怒的情绪，也会有头晕眼痛的症状。用"呵"字音出气，病就可以痊愈（图15-1）。

Take a standing, sitting or lying position. People with a liver disorder are prone to feeling unhappy and have emotional symptoms such as sadness, worry, dissatisfaction and anger, as well as symptoms such as dizziness and eye pain. Exhale with the sound "he" to recover from the disorder (Figure 15–1).

坐式(踞坐)。伸出右脚,两手抱住左膝,鼻纳气,腰部自然舒展,做7次这样的呼吸,同时向外侧舒展右脚(图1–10)。适用于腿脚难以完成屈伸和跪站动作的症状,以及小腿疼痛和痿软的病症。

Take a sitting position. Sit with the knees raised and the feet on the ground. Stretch out the right foot, hold the left knee with both hands, extend the waist naturally, breathe through the nose 7 times, and stretch the right foot outward at the same time (Figure 1–10). This exercise can help treat the difficulty of the legs and feet in flexion, extension, kneeling and standing, and can also treat pain and flaccidity in the lower legs.

2. 语言不利
2. Slurred Speech

(1) 风痰阻络
(1) Wind phlegm entering the meridians

[症状] 舌强语蹇或不语,肢体麻木,头晕目眩,舌歪,舌暗淡,苔白腻,脉弦滑。

[Symptoms] A stiff tongue, difficulty or inability to speak, numbness in the limbs, dizziness and vertigo, tongue deviation, a dark tongue with a greasy white coating, and a wiry and slippery pulse.

［治法］祛风化痰。

[Treatment methods] Remove wind and resolve phlegm.

［《诸病源候论》导引方 Daoyin Exercises in *Zhu Bing Yuan Hou Lun*］

1）调心

1) Mind regulation

站式、坐式、卧式。自膝部以下有病，当观想脐下有红光，红光里外相连周遍全身。自膝部以上至腰部有病，当观想脾有黄光。从腰部以上至头部有病，当观想心中有红光。病在皮肤有寒热，当观想肝内有青绿光。上述都要观想（各色）光里外相连周遍全身，同时通过闭气来收敛光芒向内照（病所）（图15-11）。

Take a standing, sitting or lying position. For disorders below the knees, visualize a red light below the navel. For disorders between the knees and the waist, visualize a yellow light in the spleen. For disorders between the waist and the head, visualize a red light in the heart. For skin disorders accompanied by cold or heat symptoms, visualize a green light in the liver. In all cases, visualize the respective colored light illuminating the entire body, while simultaneously holding the breath to draw the radiance inward towards the affected area (Figure 15–11).

站式、坐式、卧式。观想心气散布于身体上下，正赤色光芒四射通彻天地，自身高大（图36-2）。做这样的观想，可令人气力倍增、发白复黑、齿落再生。

Take a standing, sitting or lying position. Visualize that the heart qi is spreading throughout the body, emitting a bright red light that penetrates the sky and earth, and correspondingly, the body is becoming tall and huge (Figure 36–2). Legend goes that this visualization exercise can make the person full of vigor and vitality, increase physical strength, make the grey hair turn into black, and promote tooth regeneration.

2）调息、调身
2) Breath regulation and body regulation

站式、坐式。鹜行气。低头靠墙，不吸不呼12次，心意放松，浊气自然下降。痰饮和宿食向下排出就能痊愈。鹜行气时，身正（脊柱正），头颈部如鸭子一般上下伸缩运动，气向下行排出，做12次（图22-3）。适用于宿食。长期练此动作，不需要借助另外的通塞方法。

Take a standing or sitting position. Assume the posture of a duck to circulate qi. Lower the head, lean against a wall, passively hold the breath 12 times, relax the mind and descend turbid qi naturally. To treat phlegm-fluid retention and food retention, it is important to expel them downward. When assuming the posture of a duck to circulate qi, keep the body upright, and move the head and neck up and down like a duck, allowing qi to flow downward and out. Repeat this exercise 12 times (Figure 22–3). This exercise can help treat food retention.

卧式。仰卧，以右脚跟勾住左脚拇指，鼻纳气，至满，做7次这样的呼吸。适用于风痹（图1-30）。

Take a lying position. Take a supine position. Hook the

right heel around the left big toe, inhale through the nose deeply, and repeat this type of breathing 7 times. This exercise can eliminate wind *Bi*-impediment (Figure 1-30).

（2）肾虚精亏
(2) Kidney essence deficiency

［症状］音喑失语，心悸，气短，耳鸣耳聋，健忘恍惚，腰膝酸软，动作迟缓，舌淡，脉细弱。

[Symptoms] Hoarseness or loss of voice, palpitations, shortness of breath, tinnitus or hearing loss, forgetfulness and confusion, soreness and weakness in the lower back and knees, slow movements, a pale tongue, and a thready and weak pulse.

［治法］补肾利窍。

[Treatment method] Tonify kidney qi to unblock the orifices.

［《诸病源候论》导引方 Daoyin Exercises in *Zhu Bing Yuan Hou Lun*］

1）调心
1) Mind regulation

站式、坐式、卧式。自膝部以下有病，当观想脐下有红光，红光里外相连周遍全身。自膝部以上至腰部有病，当观想脾有黄光。从腰部以上至头部有病，当观想心中有红光。病在皮肤有寒热,当观想肝内有青绿光。上述都要观想(各色)光里外相连周遍全身,同时通过闭气来收敛光芒向内照(病所)(图15-11)。

Take a standing, sitting or lying position. For disorders below the knees, visualize a red light below the navel. For disorders between the knees and the waist, visualize a yellow light in the spleen. For disorders between the waist and the head, visualize a red light in the heart. For skin disorders accompanied by cold or heat symptoms, visualize a green light in the liver. In all cases, visualize the respective colored light illuminating the entire body, while simultaneously holding the breath to draw the radiance inward towards the affected area (Figure 15–11).

站式(立正)。吸收月亮的精华,在月亮初升,太阳将落尽时候,面向月亮站立,不呼不吸8次。仰头面向月亮吸收月光的精华,(因循着月光)咽下,8次(图47-1)。可以增长人的阴气,妇人吸收月亮精华,阴气更加旺盛,可使子道通畅。阴气增长可以益精补脑。

Follow the rules of the sun, moon, stars, and the yin-yang of the human body. For example, take an upright standing posture. Stand facing the moon when it rises at the beginning of the moon phase and the sun is about to set, and passively hold the breath 8 times. Look up and absorb the moonlight essence by swallowing it, and do this 8 times. Legend goes that this can increase a person's yin qi, and for females, absorbing the essence of the moon can make their yin qi more vigorous, which can promote conception. Increasing yin energy can also nourish the essence and improve brain function.

2) 调息、调身

2) Breath regulation and body regulation

卧式。治疗四肢疼闷、行动不便、腹中胀气。可以采用下面的方法：床席平稳，仰卧，松解衣带，枕高三寸，两手握固，伸展两手，各距离身体五寸（图1-16）。安心定意，调和气息，不想杂事，专注气息，慢慢地漱醴泉。所谓漱醴泉，即是用舌在口唇齿间转动（图1-17），使津液满口，而后缓缓咽下，然后徐徐以口吐气，再以鼻纳气。这些动作都须轻且慢，不要匆促硬做。调和呼吸，渐至自己听不到呼吸声后，以心行气，引气至脚趾端而出。每吸5或6次，呼1次，为一息。初学，由一息渐做到十息，以后慢慢增加到一百息、二百息，病就能好了。治疗期勿食生的蔬菜、鱼、肥肉。过饱和喜怒忧忿时都不可行气。在凌晨清静时候行气最好，能治疗各种疾病。

Take a supine position. To treat oppressive pain in the limbs, difficulty in movement, and abdominal distension, lie on a flat bed, wear loose clothes, use a pillow with 3 *cun* high, make fists with the hands, and stretch the arms outwards, with each hand being about 5 *cun* away from the body (Figure 1–16). Keep a peaceful mind, regulate and focus on the breath, close the mouth, and slowly rotate the tongue to make saliva fill the mouth, then slowly swallow, then slowly exhale through the mouth, and inhale through the nose (Figure 1–17). These movements should be done gently and slowly. Regulate the breath and gradually make it so quiet that you cannot hear it. Then focus the mind on guiding qi to the tips of the toes. Inhale 5 or 6 times and exhale once to complete a breath cycle. For beginners, start with 1 breath cycle and gradually increase to 10, and then slowly increase to 100 or 200 breath cycles. This exercise can help cure the disorder. During the treatment period, avoid eating uncooked vegetables, fish, or fatty meat. Do not circulate qi when you are overly full or emotional. The best time to circulate qi is in the early morning, which can help treat various disorders.

站式。两手交叉放于下颌，身体松沉到极点，可补肺气，治疗突然气逆咳嗽。两手放于下颌，轻抚两侧颈动脉（图10-3），以下颌尽力向胸中勾，极速牵拉至喉骨，尽力做3次，补气充足（图10-4）。适用于暴气上气、失音等病。令气息调和匀长，声音洪亮。

Take a standing position. Cross the hands, place them under the jaw, and totally relax the body. This exercise can supplement lung qi and treat sudden coughing induced by counterflow of qi. Place the hands under the chin, gently massage the carotid arteries on both sides (Figure 10–3), fully bring the chin close to the chest, and repeat 3 times to tonify qi (Figure 10–4). This exercise can help treat disorders such as counterflow of qi and aphonia. It can regulate the breath and make the voice loud and clear.

（3）痰邪阻窍
(3) Phlegm obstructing the orifices

［症状］舌强语蹇或不语，头重如蒙，胸闷恶心，舌歪，舌暗淡，苔白腻，脉濡滑。

[Symptoms] A stiff tongue, difficulty or inability to speak, heavy head and clouded mind, chest tightness, tongue deviation, a dark tongue with a greasy white coating, and a soft and slippery pulse.

［治法］化痰开窍。

[Treatment methods] Resolve phlegm and unblock the orifices.

［《诸病源候论》导引方 Daoyin Exercises in *Zhu Bing Yuan Hou Lun*］

1）调心

1) Mind regulation

站式、坐式、卧式。自膝部以下有病，当观想脐下有红光，红光里外相连周遍全身。自膝部以上至腰部有病，当观想脾有黄光。从腰部以上至头部有病，当观想心中有红光。病在皮肤有寒热，当观想肝内有青绿光。上述都要观想（各色）光里外相连周遍全身，同时通过闭气来收敛光芒向内照（病所）（图15-11）。

Take a standing, sitting or lying position. For disorders below the knees, visualize a red light below the navel. For disorders between the knees and the waist, visualize a yellow light in the spleen. For disorders between the waist and the head, visualize a red light in the heart. For skin disorders accompanied by cold or heat symptoms, visualize a green light in the liver. In all cases, visualize the respective colored light illuminating the entire body, while simultaneously holding the breath to draw the radiance inward towards the affected area (Figure 15-11).

站式、坐式、卧式。观想心气散布于身体上下，正赤色光芒四射通彻天地，自身高大（图36-2）。做这样的观想，可令人气力倍增、发白复黑、齿落再生。

Take a standing, sitting or lying position. Visualize that the heart qi is spreading throughout the body, emitting a bright red light that penetrates the sky and earth, and correspondingly, the body is becoming tall and huge (Figure 36–2). Legend goes that this visualization exercise can make the person full of vigor and vitality, increase physical strength, make the grey hair turn into black, and promote tooth regeneration.

2) 调息、调身
2) Breath regulation and body regulation

站式、坐式。鸯行气。低头靠墙,不吸不呼12次,心意放松,浊气自然下降。痰饮和宿食向下排出就能痊愈。鸯行气时,身正(脊柱正),头颈部如鸭子一般上下伸缩运动,气向下行排出,做12次(图22-3)。适用于宿食。长期练此动作,不需要借助另外的通塞方法。

Take a standing or sitting position. Assume the posture of a duck to circulate qi. Lower the head, lean against a wall, passively hold the breath 12 times, relax the mind and descend turbid qi naturally. To treat phlegm-fluid retention and food retention, it is important to expel them downward. When assuming the posture of a duck to circulate qi, keep the body upright, and move the head and neck up and down like a duck, allowing qi to flow downward and out. Repeat this exercise 12 times (Figure 22–3). This exercise can help treat food retention.

卧式(侧卧)。不吸不呼12次。适用于痰饮不消。右侧有痰饮,则右侧着地(图22-1),左侧有痰饮,则左侧着地(图22-2)。如果还有痰饮没有消除的情况,可用调整呼吸的方法来排除痰饮。不呼不吸12次,适用于痰饮。

Take a side-lying position. Passively hold the breath 12 times. This exercise can help treat disorders induced by phlegm-fluid retention. For phlegm-fluid retention on the right side, lie on the right side (Figure 22–1). For phlegm-fluid retention on the left side, lie on the left side (Figure 22–2). For phlegm-fluid retention after doing the exercise, adjust the breathing to help with expectoration. Passively holding the breath 12 times can help treat phlegm-fluid retention.

3. 口眼歪斜
3. Deviation of the mouth and eyes

［治法］祛风、除痰、通络。

[Treatment methods] Remove wind, resolve phlegm and unblock collaterals.

［《诸病源候论》导引方 Daoyin Exercises in *Zhu Bing Yuan Hou Lun*］

1）调心
1) Mind regulation

站式、坐式、卧式。自膝部以下有病，当观想脐下有红光，红光里外相连周遍全身。自膝部以上至腰部有病，当观想脾有黄光。从腰部以上至头部有病，当观想心中有红光。病在皮肤有寒热，当观想肝内有青绿光。上述都要观想（各色）光里外相连周遍全身，同时通过闭气来收敛光芒向内照（病所）（图15–11）。

Take a standing, sitting or lying position. For disorders below the knees, visualize a red light below the navel. For disorders between the knees and the waist, visualize a yellow light in the spleen. For disorders between the waist and the head, visualize a red light in the heart. For skin disorders accompanied by cold or heat symptoms, visualize a green light in the liver. In all cases, visualize the respective colored light illuminating the entire body, while simultaneously holding the breath to draw the radiance inward towards the affected area (Figure 15–11).

站式、坐式、卧式。观想心气散布于身体上下，正赤色光芒四射通彻天地，自身高大（图36-2）。做这样的观想，可令人气力倍增、发白复黑、齿落再生。

Take a standing, sitting or lying position. Visualize that the heart qi is spreading throughout the body, emitting a bright red light that penetrates the sky and earth, and correspondingly, the body is becoming tall and huge (Figure 36–2). Legend goes that this visualization exercise can make the person full of vigor and vitality, increase physical strength, make the grey hair turn into black, and promote tooth regeneration.

2）调息、调身
2) Breath regulation and body regulation

站式、坐式（立正或正坐）。靠墙，不呼不吸，行气（图1-3），从口部把气引至头部（图1-4）。适用于痈疽、风痹、大风病、偏枯等。

Take a standing or sitting position. Stand straight or sit upright. Lean against a wall, passively hold the breath, and circulate qi (Figure 1–3) from the mouth to the head (Figure

1–4). This exercise can help treat abscesses, wind *Bi*-impediment, blood deficiency stirring wind, and hemiplegia.

站式、坐式。有人觉得脊背僵紧不舒憋闷，无论什么时节，可以缩咽于肩（图1-36），仰面，肩胛骨上抬，头顺着左右两个方向移动，做21次（图1-37），然后稍停，待气血平复再做下一次。开始时要慢做再逐渐加快，不能先快后慢。如果是无病之人，可以在清晨3点至5点、中午11点至13点、下午17点至19点三个时间段操作，每个时段做14次。适用于寒热病、脊腰颈项痛、风痹、口内生疮、牙齿风、头眩。

Standing or sitting position. For back rigidity, tuck in the throat (Figure 1–36), raise the head and scapula, and rotate the head to both sides 21 times (Figure 1–37). Then take a break to calm down qi and blood and do it again. Begin slowly and gradually increase speed. Avoid starting fast and then slowing down. People in good health can do this exercise 14 times during each of the three time periods: 3–5 am, 11 am–1 pm, and 5–7 pm. This exercise can help treat chills, fever, and pain in the lower back, neck and shoulders, and can also treat wind *Bi*-impediment, mouth ulcer, toothache, and dizziness.

二、肺胀
Lung Distension

（一）概述
Introduction

"肺胀"是多种慢性肺系疾患反复发作迁延不愈，导致肺气胀满，不能敛降的一种病症。中医对肺胀病因病机的认识可追溯至《灵枢·胀论》："肺胀者，虚满而喘咳。"《金匮要略·肺痿肺痈咳嗽上气病》指出"咳而上气，此为肺胀，其人喘，目如脱状"为本病主症。《诸病源候论·咳逆短气候》记载"肺虚为微寒所伤则咳嗽，嗽则气还于肺间则肺胀，肺胀则气逆。而肺本虚，气为不足，复为邪所乘，壅痞不能宣畅，故咳逆短气也"。后世医家对肺胀不断加深认识，并在漫长的临床实践中积累了较丰富的治疗经验。肺胀的发生，多因内伤久咳、支饮、哮喘等肺系慢性疾患迁延失治，痰浊潴留，气还肺间，日久导致肺虚，成为发病基础。肺虚卫外不固，外淫六邪反复侵袭诱使病情发作加剧。病变首先在肺，继而影响脾、肾，后期病及心。

Lung distension is a chronic lung disorder characterized by recurrent attacks that result in chest stuffiness and an inability of lung qi to astringe and descend. The understanding of lung distension in TCM can be traced back to *Ling Shu Zhang Lun* (Chapter 35 of the Spiritual Pivot), which describes that "In the case of a lung distention, the lung is deficient but the patient has a feeling of fullness in the lung. Subsequently, the patient pants and coughs." *Jin Gui Yao Lüe* (Essentials from the Golden Cabinet) notes that "Cough with panting is a manifestation of lung distension, with protrusion of the eyes due to severe panting and a superficial, surging pulse." *Zhu Bing Yuan Hou Lun* (Treatise on the Origins and Manifestations of Various Diseases) states that "Lung deficiency due to the damage by slight pathogenic cold may cause coughing. Coughing may return qi to the lung, and thus cause lung distension. Lung distension may further induce counterflow of qi. Deficiency of lung qi coupled with the invasion of pathogenic factors may lead to stagnation and retention of phlegm that cannot be dissipated, resulting in persistent coughing and shortness of breath." Later TCM practitioners continued to deepen their understanding towards lung distension and accumulated experience in their clinical practice. Lung distension is predominantly caused by internal dysfunction from prolonged coughing, phlegm retention, and asthma, resulting in chronic lung disorders that are difficult to treat. The stagnation of phlegm and fluid retention causes qi to stay in the lung for an extended period, which leads to lung deficiency and becomes the root cause of the disorder. The deficiency of the lung makes it susceptible to repeated external pathogenic invasions, which worsens the condition. Primarily, the disorder is located in the lung and then involves the spleen, kidney and even the heart in later stages.

根据肺胀的临床表现，主要见于西医学的慢性阻塞性肺疾病（慢阻肺）。慢阻肺主要症状包括慢性咳嗽、咳痰和呼吸困难。慢阻肺早期患者可以没有明显的症状，随病情进展症状日益显著，急性加重愈渐频繁。慢阻肺常见的合并症如心脏病、骨质疏松症、肺癌、焦虑/抑郁等，对疾病进展和病死率有显著影响。本节对肺胀的辨证论治，主要针对慢阻肺高危人群（指在尚未达到诊断标准，但存在呼吸系统症状、或气流受限的人群）及稳定期轻中度患者。

The clinical manifestations of lung distension are consistent with those of chronic obstructive pulmonary disease (COPD) in Western medicine. The main symptoms of COPD include chronic cough, expectoration, and difficulty in breathing. In the early stages of COPD, patients may have no obvious symptoms. As the condition progresses, symptoms become more prominent and quickly aggravated. Common complications of COPD include heart disease, osteoporosis, lung cancer, anxiety/depression, etc., which have a significant impact on disease progression and mortality. The pattern identification and treatment for lung distension discussed in this section applies to high-risk groups for COPD (referring to those who have not yet met the diagnostic criteria, but have respiratory symptoms or airflow limitation) and COPD patients in the stable stages.

（二）辨证论治
Treatment Based on Pattern Identification

肺胀辨证总属本虚标实。早期多属气虚、气阴两虚，由肺及脾、肾，晚期气虚及阳，以肺、肾、心为主，或阴阳两虚。治疗时标本兼顾，同时有侧重的选用祛邪、扶正治法。本虚者，宜补肺、益肾、健脾、养心；标实者，宜祛邪宣肺、降气化痰。中药、导引方皆适用于肺胀，临证需结合病史、症状，舌脉等表现，辨证施治。

Generally, the root of lung distension is deficiency while the tip is excess. In the early stages, the causative factors include qi deficiency, and deficiency of both qi and yin; the condition is located in the lung primarily, and then involves the spleen and kidney. In the later stages, the causative factors include damage of yang due to qi deficiency, and deficiency of both yin and yang; the condition is located in the lung, kidney, and heart. Prior to treatment, take both the root and tip into consideration, and adopt strengthening healthy qi or eliminating pathogenic factors according to the nature of the condition. For deficiency at the root, the treatment methods are to tonify the lung and kidney, strengthen the spleen, and nourish the heart. For excess at the tip, the treatment methods are to expel pathogens, disperse the lung, descend qi, and resolve phlegm. Both Chinese medicines and daoyin exercises can be used to treat lung distention. In clinical practice, treatment should be determined based on the patient's medical history and symptoms including

此外，对于肺胀的预防需提醒患者注意加强对感冒、咳嗽、哮病、喘病等肺系疾病的治疗，以免迁延不愈发展为本病。

To prevent palpitations, it is of great significance to treat such diseases involving the lung as common cold, cough, dyspnea and wheezing.

1. 虚证
1. Deficiency syndrome

（1）肺脾气虚
(1) Qi deficiency of the lung and spleen

［症状］咳嗽或喘息、气短乏力、自汗动则加重，畏风、易感冒，痰稀，胃脘纳呆，便溏，胃脘胀满或腹胀，舌胖或有齿痕，苔白，脉细弱。

[Symptoms] Coughing or panting, shortness of breath, spontaneous sweating that worsens upon physical exertion, aversion to wind, susceptibility to common colds, thin phlegm, stomach stuffiness, a poor appetite, loose stools, abdominal distension or fullness, an enlarged tongue with teeth marks and a white coating, and a thready and weak pulse.

［治法］补肺健脾益气。

[Treatment methods] Tonify lung qi and strengthen the spleen.

[《诸病源候论》导引方 Daoyin Exercises in *Zhu Bing Yuan Hou Lun*]

1）调心

1) Mind regulation

站式、坐式、卧式。《无生经》曰：治百病、邪鬼、蛊毒，当仰卧。闭眼闭气，内视丹田，鼻缓缓纳气，令腹部胀满至极点，以口缓缓吐气，不要听到气息声，吸气多吐气少，气息轻柔（图1-85）。内视五脏，看到五脏的形色，再内视胃中，令神光充盈，鲜活明晰洁白如丝绢。做到疲倦至极并且出汗就可以停止了，用粉轻扑于身上，按摩身体。汗未出但感到疲倦的，也可以停止。待第二天再做。

Take a standing, sitting or lying position. *Wu Sheng Jing* (Sutra of Imperishable) states that to treat varying disorders, evil spirits and schistosomiasis, take a supine position. Close the eyes, hold the breath, focus on the *Dantian*, and inhale slowly through the nose to make the abdomen full. Then exhale slowly through the mouth without making any sound. The inhalation should be longer than the exhalation, and the breathing should be gentle and soft. Look at the five zang organs, and observe their forms and colors. Then look at the stomach, and make it bright, lively, clear and white as silk. Continue until exhaustion and sweating are present, then stop, lightly apply powders to the body, and massage the body. If exhaustion is felt but sweating has not yet occurred, stop and repeat the practice the following day.

站式、坐式、卧式。观想心气散布于身体上下，正赤色光芒四射通彻天地, 自身高大(图36-2)。做这样的观想, 可令人气力倍增、发白复黑、齿落再生。

Take a standing, sitting or lying position. Visualize that the heart qi is spreading throughout the body, emitting a bright red light that penetrates the sky and earth, and correspondingly, the body is becoming tall and huge (Figure 36–2). Legend goes that this visualization exercise can make the person full of vigor and vitality, increase physical strength, make the grey hair turn into black, and promote tooth regeneration.

2) 调息、调身
2) Breath regulation and body regulation

卧式(仰卧)。仰起两脚两手, 鼻纳气, 至满, 做7次这样的呼吸(图16-3)。适用于腹中拘急剧痛。

Take a supine position. Lift both legs and arms up, inhale through the nose deeply, and repeat this breathing pattern 7 times (Figure 16–3). This exercise can relieve severe abdominal pain and contracture.

站式。一手尽力前托, 做到极势; 一手放于乳房处, 向后牵拉使胸部舒展。不能用僵力令胸口打开, (气)向下松沉, 两手互换再做上述动作21次(图1-65)。将两手攀住膝盖, 身体向后仰, 尽力做到极势做21次(图1-66)。适用于风热导致的烦闷疼痛, 使风府和云门的邪气散去。

Take a standing position. Fully stretch forward one hand, while placing the other hand on the breast to pull backward to stretch the chest. Do not use rigid force to open the chest. Sink qi and then change the position of the hands to repeat the movements 21 times (Figure 1–65). Hold the knees with the hands and fully lean backward 21 times (Figure 1–66). This exercise can relieve vexation and pain caused by wind and heat, and disperse pathogenic factors in the points Fengfu (GV 16) and Yunmen (LU 2).

（2）肺肾气虚
(2) Qi deficiency of the lung and kidney

［症状］咳嗽或喘息、气短乏力、自汗动则加重，畏风、易感冒，痰白如沫，腰膝酸软，耳鸣头晕，面目虚浮，小便频而清，或咳而遗溺，舌质淡、舌苔白，脉沉细。

[Symptoms] Coughing or panting, shortness of breath, fatigue and spontaneous sweating that worsen upon physical exertion, aversion to wind, susceptibility to common colds, thin and frothy phlegm, low back/knee soreness and weakness, dizziness and tinnitus, a pale facial complexion coupled with puffiness, frequent and clear urination, or coughing with urinary incontinence, a pale tongue with a white coating, and a deep and thready pulse.

［治法］补肺纳肾。
[Treatment method] Tonify the lung and kidney.

［《诸病源候论》导引方 Daoyin Exercises in *Zhu Bing Yuan Hou Lun*]

1）调心

1) Mind regulation

站式、坐式、卧式。延年益寿的方法，观想心气红色，肝气青色，肺气白色，脾气黄色，肾气黑色，在身体四周围绕并辟邪驱鬼（图7-1）。

Take a standing, sitting or lying position. To achieve longevity, visualize the red heart qi, green liver qi, white lung qi, yellow spleen qi, and black kidney qi surrounding the body and warding off pathogenic factors (Figure 7-1).

站式、坐式、卧式。观想心气散布于身体上下，正赤色光芒四射通彻天地，自身高大（图36-2）。做这样的观想，可令人气力倍增、发白复黑、齿落再生。

Take a standing, sitting or lying position. Visualize that the heart qi is spreading throughout the body, emitting a bright red light that penetrates the sky and earth, and correspondingly, the body is becoming tall and huge (Figure 36-2). Legend goes that this visualization exercise can make the person full of vigor and vitality, increase physical strength, make the grey hair turn into black, and promote tooth regeneration.

2）调息、调身

2) Breath regulation and body regulation

卧式（俯卧）。两手撑地伏身向下，口纳气，鼻出气（图15-7）。适用于胸中肺中诸病。

Take a prone position. Place both hands on the ground,

lower the body, inhale through the mouth and exhale through the nose (Figure 15-7). This exercise helps alleviate varying disorders involving the chest and lung.

坐式。虾蟆行气。正坐。摇动两手臂，不吸不呼12次（图2-20）。适用于五劳七伤和水肿病。

Take an upright sitting position. Assume the posture of a toad to circulate qi. Shake the arms and passively hold the breath 12 times (Figure 2-20). This exercise can help treat the five exhaustions (Long- time observation damages blood; long-time lying damages qi; long-time sitting damages muscles; long-time standing damages bones; and long-time walking damages sinews) and seven damages (Refers to seven pathogenic factors that lead to deficiency and consumption, including improper diet, anxiety, drink, sex, hunger, over-exertion, and damage to meridians, collaterals, *Ying*-nutrients, *Wei*-defense and qi) as well as oedema.

（3）气阴两虚

(3) Deficiency of qi and yin

［症状］咳嗽或喘息、气短乏力、自汗动则加重，易感冒，腰膝酸软，耳鸣头晕，咽干口燥，咳嗽夜剧，干咳少痰，盗汗颧红，手足心热，舌红少薄，或花剥、无苔，脉细数。

[Symptoms] Coughing or panting, shortness of breath, fatigue and spontaneous sweating that worsen upon physical exertion, susceptibility to common colds, low back/knee soreness and weakness, dizziness and tinnitus, dry throat and mouth, severe nighttime cough with little phlegm, night sweats

Zhu Bing Yuan Hou Lun Dao Yin Shu (Explanations for the Daoyin Exercises in Zhu Bing Yuan Hou Lun) · 《诸病源候论》导引术 · 应用 · Application

392

and red cheeks, feverish sensations in palms and soles, a red tongue with little coating or a peeled tongue without coating, and a thready and rapid pulse.

［治法］益气养阴。
[Treatment methods] Supplement qi and nourish yin.

［《诸病源候论》导引方 Daoyin Exercises in *Zhu Bing Yuan Hou Lun*］

1）调心
1) Mind regulation

站式、坐式、卧式。延年益寿的方法，观想心气红色，肝气青色，肺气白色，脾气黄色，肾气黑色，在身体四周围绕并辟邪驱鬼（图7-1）。

Take a standing, sitting or lying position. To achieve longevity, visualize the red heart qi, green liver qi, white lung qi, yellow spleen qi, and black kidney qi surrounding the body and warding off pathogenic factors (Figure 7–1).

站式（立正）。吸收月亮的精华，在月亮初升，太阳将落尽时候，面向月亮站立，不呼不吸8次。仰头面向月亮吸收月光的精华，（因循着月光）咽下，8次（图47-1）。可以增长人的阴气，妇人吸收月亮精华，阴气更加旺盛，可使子道通畅。阴气增长可以益精补脑。

Follow the rules of the sun, moon, stars, and the yin-yang

of the human body. For example, take an upright standing posture. Stand facing the moon when it rises at the beginning of the moon phase and the sun is about to set, and passively hold the breath 8 times. Look up and absorb the moonlight essence by swallowing it, and do this 8 times. Legend goes that this can increase a person's yin qi, and for females, absorbing the essence of the moon can make their yin qi more vigorous, which can promote conception. Increasing yin energy can also nourish the essence and improve brain function.

2）调息、调身
2) Breath regulation and body regulation

站式、坐式、卧式。有肾病的人，有咽喉阻塞、腹部胀满、耳聋不聪的症状，用"呬"字音出气（图15-8）。

Take a standing, sitting or lying position. For those with a kidney disorder experiencing such symptoms as a foreign body sensation in the throat, abdominal fullness, impaired hearing and even deafness, exhale with the sound "hei" (Figure 15–8).

卧式。治疗四肢疼闷、行动不便、腹中胀气。可以采用下面的方法：床席平稳，仰卧，松解衣带，枕高三寸，两手握固，伸展两手，各距离身体五寸（图1-16）。安心定意，调和气息，不想杂事，专注气息，慢慢地漱醴泉。所谓漱醴泉，即是用舌在口唇齿间转动（图1-17），使津液满口，而后缓缓咽下，然后徐徐以口吐气，再以鼻纳气。这些动作都须轻且慢，不要匆促硬做。调和呼吸，渐至自己听不到呼吸声后，以心行气，引气至脚趾端而出。每吸5或6次，呼1次，为一息。初学，由一息渐做到十息，以后慢慢增加到一百息、二百息，病就能好了。治疗期勿食生的蔬菜、鱼、肥肉。过饱和喜怒忧忿时都不可行气。在凌晨清静时候行气最好，能治疗各种疾病。

Take a supine position. To treat oppressive pain in the limbs, difficulty in movement, and abdominal distension, lie on a flat bed, wear loose clothes, use a pillow with 3 *cun* high, make fists with the hands, and stretch the arms outwards, with each hand being about 5 *cun* away from the body (Figure 1–16). Keep a peaceful mind, regulate and focus on the breath, close the mouth, and slowly rotate the tongue to make saliva fill the mouth, then slowly swallow, then slowly exhale through the mouth, and inhale through the nose (Figure 1–17). These movements should be done gently and slowly. Regulate the breath and gradually make it so quiet that you cannot hear it. Then focus the mind on guiding qi to the tips of the toes. Inhale 5 or 6 times and exhale once to complete a breath cycle. For beginners, start with 1 breath cycle and gradually increase to 10, and then slowly increase to 100 or 200 breath cycles. This exercise can help cure the disease. During the treatment period, avoid eating uncooked vegetables, fish, and fatty meat. Do not circulate qi when you are overly full or emotional. The best time to circulate qi is in the early morning, which can help treat various disorders.

2. 实证
2. Excess syndrome

（1）痰浊壅肺
(1) Turbid phlegm accumulating in the lung

［症状］咳嗽或喘息，痰多色白黏腻或呈泡沫状，气短、乏

力, 脘痞纳呆, 舌苔白腻, 脉滑。

[Symptoms] Coughing or panting, with white and sticky or foamy phlegm, shortness of breath and fatigue, stomach stuffiness, a poor appetite, a white and greasy tongue coating, and a slippery pulse.

［治法］益气泻肺涤痰。

[Treatment methods] Supplement qi, drain the lung and transform phlegm.

［《诸病源候论》导引方 Daoyin Exercises in *Zhu Bing Yuan Hou Lun*］

1）调心

1) Mind regulation

站式、坐式、卧式。存想巨雷闪电, 雷鸣电闪, 进入腹中。能这样坚持存想, 疾病就能自然消除。

Take a standing, sitting or lying position. Visualize great thunder and lightning, with thunderbolts and flashes entering into the abdomen. Persistent visualization can help keep a peaceful mind.

站式、坐式、卧式。观想心气散布于身体上下, 正赤色光芒四射通彻天地, 自身高大（图36-2）。做这样的观想, 可令人气力倍增、发白复黑、齿落再生。

Take a standing, sitting or lying position. Visualize that the heart qi is spreading throughout the body, emitting a bright red light that penetrates the sky and earth, and correspondingly, the body is becoming tall and huge (Figure 36–2). Legend goes that this visualization exercise can make the person full of vigor and vitality, increase physical strength, make the grey hair turn into black, and promote tooth regeneration.

2）调息、调身

2) Breath regulation and body regulation

站式、坐式、卧式。有肾病的人，有咽喉阻塞、腹部胀满、耳聋不聪的症状，用"呬"字音出气（图15-8）。

Take a standing, sitting or lying position. For those with a kidney disorder experiencing such symptoms as a foreign body sensation in the throat, abdominal fullness, impaired hearing and even deafness, exhale with the sound "hei" (Figure 15–8).

站式、坐式。鹜行气。低头靠墙，不吸不呼12次，心意放松，浊气自然下降。痰饮和宿食向下排出就能痊愈。鹜行气时，身正（脊柱正），头颈部如鸭子一般上下伸缩运动，气向下行排出，做12次（图22-3）。适用于宿食。长期练此动作，不需要借助另外的通塞方法。

Take a standing or sitting position. Assume the posture of a duck to circulate qi. Lower the head, lean against a wall, passively hold the breath 12 times, relax the mind and descend turbid qi naturally. To treat phlegm-fluid retention and food retention, it is important to expel them downward. When assuming the posture of a duck to circulate qi, keep the body upright, and move the head and neck up and down like a duck, allowing qi to flow downward and out. Repeat this exercise 12 times (Figure 22–3). This exercise can help treat food retention.

（2）痰热郁肺
(2) Phlegm heat accumulating in the lung

[症状] 咳嗽或喘息,烦躁,胸满气粗,痰黄或白,黏稠难咯,或发热微恶寒,汗出,溲黄便干,口渴,舌质暗红,苔黄腻,脉滑数。

[Symptoms] Coughing or panting, restlessness, chest fullness with rapid breathing, yellow or white phlegm that is sticky and difficult to expectorate, or fever with mild aversion to cold, sweating, yellow urine, dry stools, thirst, a dark red tongue with a greasy and yellow coating, and a slippery and rapid pulse.

[治法] 益气清肺祛痰。
[Treatment methods] Supplement qi, clear lung heat and resolve phlegm.

[《诸病源候论》导引方 Daoyin Exercises in *Zhu Bing Yuan Hou Lun*]

1）调心
1) Mind regulation

站式、坐式、卧式。《无生经》曰：治百病、邪鬼、蛊毒，当

仰卧。闭眼闭气，内视丹田，鼻缓缓纳气，令腹部胀满至极点，以口缓缓吐气，不要听到气息声，吸气多吐气少，气息轻柔（图1-85）。内视五脏，看到五脏的形色，再内视胃中，令神光充盈，鲜活明晰洁白如丝绢。做到疲倦至极并且出汗就可以停止了，用粉轻扑于身上，按摩身体。汗未出但感到疲倦的，也可以停止。待第二天再做。

Take a standing, sitting or lying position. *Wu Sheng Jing* (Sutra of Imperishable) states that to treat varying disorders, evil spirits and schistosomiasis, take a supine position. Close the eyes, hold the breath, focus on the *Dantian*, and inhale slowly through the nose to make the abdomen full. Then exhale slowly through the mouth without making any sound. The inhalation should be longer than the exhalation, and the breathing should be gentle and soft (Figure 1–85). Look at the five zang organs, and observe their forms and colors. Then look at the stomach, and make it bright, lively, clear and white as silk. Continue until exhaustion and sweating are present, then stop, lightly apply powders to the body, and massage the body. If exhaustion is felt but sweating has not yet occurred, stop and repeat the practice the following day.

站式、坐式、卧式。观想心气散布于身体上下，正赤色光芒四射通彻天地，自身高大（图36-2）。做这样的观想，可令人气力倍增、发白复黑、齿落再生。

Take a standing, sitting or lying position. Visualize that the heart qi is spreading throughout the body, emitting a bright red light that penetrates the sky and earth, and correspondingly, the body is becoming tall and huge (Figure 36–2). Legend goes that this visualization exercise can make the person full of vigor and vitality, increase physical strength, make the grey hair turn into black, and promote tooth regeneration.

2）调息、调身

2）Breath regulation and body regulation

站式、坐式、卧式。有肾病的人，有咽喉阻塞、腹部胀满、耳聋不聪的症状，用"呬"字音出气（图15-8）。

Take a standing, sitting or lying position. For those with a kidney disorder experiencing such symptoms as a foreign body sensation in the throat, abdominal fullness, impaired hearing and even deafness, exhale with the sound "hei" (Figure 15–8).

站式、坐式。鹜行气。低头靠墙，不吸不呼12次，心意放松，浊气自然下降。痰饮和宿食向下排出就能痊愈。鹜行气时，身正（脊柱正），头颈部如鸭子一般上下伸缩运动，气向下行排出，做12次（图22-3）。适用于宿食。长期练此动作，不需要借助另外的通塞方法。

Take a standing or sitting position. Assume the posture of a duck to circulate qi. Lower the head, lean against a wall, passively hold the breath 12 times, relax the mind and descend turbid qi naturally. To treat phlegm-fluid retention and food retention, it is important to expel them downward. When assuming the posture of a duck to circulate qi, keep the body upright, and move the head and neck up and down like a duck, allowing qi to flow downward and out. Repeat this exercise 12 times (Figure 22–3). This exercise can help treat food retention.

三、郁证

Depression

（一）概述

Introduction

"郁证"是由于情志不舒，气机郁滞所引起的一类病症。主要临床表现为心情低落、情绪不宁、易悲易怒善哭、胸胁胀痛、咽中如有异物梗阻、失眠等。中医对"郁证"的认识最早可追溯至《黄帝内经》。首先，《黄帝内经》提出五脏与情志关系密切，情志失调将伤及脏腑，脏腑虚实盛衰变化也会直接影响情志稳定。《素问·阴阳应象大论》载："人有五脏化五气，以生喜怒悲忧恐。"《灵枢·寿夭刚柔》："忧恐忿怒伤气；气伤脏，乃病脏。"《灵枢·本神》："肝藏血，血舍魂，肝气虚则恐，实则怒……心藏脉，脉舍神，心气虚则悲，实则笑不休。"其次，《黄帝内经》认为气机紊乱是情志失调的主要原因。《素问·举痛论》指出："余知百病生于气也，怒则气上，喜则气缓，悲则气消，恐则气下。"再次，《黄帝内经》提出"郁"的相关理论与调畅气机为基本治则，如《素问·六元正纪大论》载："木郁达之，火郁发之，土郁夺之，金郁泄之，水郁折之，然调其气……"此后，历代中医在《黄帝内经》的基础上发挥和演绎郁证的理论和治疗。郁证有"六郁"之说，即气郁、血郁、痰郁、湿郁、热郁、食郁，其中以气郁为先。

Depression is a type of disorder caused by emotional frustration or stress and qi stagnation. Its clinical manifestations include depressed mood, restlessness, chest fullness or oppression and distending pain in the sub-costal region, irritability, crying spells for no apparent reason, insomnia, or the sensation of a foreign body stuck in the throat. The understanding of depression in TCM can be traced back to

Huang Di Nei Jing. Firstly, *Huang Di Nei Jing* proposes that the five zang organs are closely related to emotions. Emotional disturbances may impair the zang-fu organs, and the imbalance of deficiency and excess in the zang-fu organs will also affect emotions. *Su Wen Yin Yang Ying Xiang Da Lun* (Chapter 5 of the Basic Questions) states, "In the human body, there are the five zang organs that produce five kinds of qi, respectively responsible for the five emotional activities of joy, anger, grief, excessive thinking, and fear." *Ling Shu Shou Yao Gang Rou* (Chapter 6 of the Spiritual Pivot) states, "Fear and anger impair qi. Impairment of qi eventually affects the organs and leads to disorders." *Ling Shu Ben Shen* (Chapter 8 of the Spiritual Pivot) states, "The liver stores blood, and blood houses the ethereal soul. Deficiency of liver qi causes fear while excess of liver qi causes anger... The heart controls blood vessels, and the vessels house the spirit. Deficiency of heart qi will cause sorrow while excess of heart qi will cause uncontrollable laughter." Secondly, *Huang Di Nei Jing* believes that the disorder of qi is the main cause of emotional imbalance. *Su Wen Ju Tong Lun* (Chapter 39 of the Basic Questions) points out, "All diseases are caused by qi disorders. Anger causes qi to ascend, joy causes qi to slow down, sorrow causes qi to disperse, fear causes qi to disorder, and worry causes qi to stagnate." Thirdly, *Huang Di Nei Jing* puts forward the theory of depression and regards regulating qi circulation as the basic treatment principle for depression. *Su Wen Liu Yuan Zheng Ji Da Lun* (Chapter 71 of the Basic Questions) states, "For depression caused by disorder of wood qi, open its way; for depression caused by disorder of fire qi, effuse it; for depression caused by disorder of earth qi, take it away; for depression caused by disorder of metal qi, drain it; for depression caused by disorder of water qi, break it. These are the ways to regulate qi..." Subsequently, generations of TCM practitioners have developed and interpreted the theory and treatment methods of depression based on *Huang Di Nei Jing*. In TCM, depression includes the following six stagnations: qi stagnation, blood stagnation, phlegm stagnation, dampness stagnation, fire stagnation, and food stagnation. These six stagnations often result from qi stagnation of the liver and spleen.

根据郁证的临床表现，主要见于西医学的抑郁障碍、焦虑障碍、混合性抑郁焦虑障碍。抑郁障碍临床以显著而持久的心境低落为主要特征，临床表现可以从闷闷不乐到悲痛欲绝，部分患者会出现明显的焦虑和运动性激越，严重者可以出现幻觉、妄想等精神病性症状，更有甚者出现自伤、自杀行为。广泛性焦虑障碍的关键临床特点是对于各种情境持久、过度、难以控制的焦虑和担忧，常见临床症状还包括紧张、烦躁、注意力不集中、易激惹、坐立不安、易疲乏、肌肉紧张、睡眠紊乱等。临床一部分患者为混合性抑郁焦虑障碍，临床特征是同时出现焦虑和抑郁的症状，但两组症状的严重程度、发作次数或持续时间都不足以成为诊断为抑郁障碍或焦虑障碍。治疗后大部分抑郁症状和焦虑症状可缓解或减轻，但20%～35%患者会有残留症状和社会功能损害。本节对郁证的辨证论治，以气郁为主，轻中度抑郁障碍、轻中度广泛性焦虑障碍、轻中度混合性抑郁焦虑障碍、抑郁焦虑状态可参照本篇内容辨证论治。

The manifestations of depression mainly correspond to depressive disorder, anxiety disorder, and mixed anxiety and depressive disorder in Western medicine. Depressive disorder is manifested as significant and persistent depressed mood, ranging from melancholy to extreme sadness. Some patients may experience evident anxiety and restlessness. In severe cases, psychotic symptoms like hallucinations and delusions may occur. In addition, the patient may hurt himself/herself and even commit suicide. The clinical characteristic of generalized anxiety disorder is persistent, excessive, and uncontrollable anxiety and worry in various situations. Common symptoms also include anxiety, restlessness, inattention, irritability, fatigue, muscle tension, and sleep disorders. Some patients in clinical settings may have mixed anxiety and depressive disorder, where symptoms of both anxiety and depression coexist. However, the severity, frequency, and duration of both sets of symptoms are insufficient to diagnose either depressive disorder or anxiety disorder independently. After treatment, most symptoms can be alleviated or reduced, but 20% to 35% of patients may experience residual symptoms and impaired social function. The pattern identification and treatment for depression, mainly for qi stagnation, discussed in this section applies to depressive disorder, generalized anxiety, mixed anxiety and depressive disorder, or depression and anxiety state in mild/moderate stages.

（二）辨证论治
Treatment Based on Pattern Identification

郁证的发生多由忧思、郁怒、悲愁、恐惧等七情所伤，进而气机失调而致郁。病位首先在肝，继而使脾、心受累。因此，疏畅气机为郁证总的治则。临证时亦需明辨虚实：郁证初起，因气滞而挟痰、挟湿、挟食、兼瘀、兼火，多属实证，以理气为主，配以化痰、祛湿、消食、祛瘀、清火；郁证日久，抑脾气、伤心神、耗津液，由实转虚，以益气养血扶正为主，配以健脾、养心、滋阴。

Emotional disturbances including excessive worry, excessive thinking, anger, sadness and fear, may cause qi disorders, and subsequently result in depression. Primarily, this condition is located in the liver, and gradually involves the spleen and heart. The general treatment principle is to regulate the qi activity. It is also important to differentiate between deficiency and excess for diagnosis. The nature of depression in the early stages is mostly excess, present with qi stagnation accompanied by phlegm stagnation, dampness stagnation, food stagnation, fire stagnation, or blood stasis. The specific treatment principle is to regulate qi, accompanied by resolving phlegm, eliminating dampness, promoting digestion, removing blood stasis, and clearing fire. Over time, both spleen qi and heart spirit may be damaged, body fluids are consumed, and subsequently the nature of depression goes into deficiency. Correspondingly, the specific treatment principle is to tonify qi, nourish blood, and support healthy qi, accompanied by strengthening the spleen, nourishing the heart, and nourishing yin.

中药、导引方皆适用于郁证, 关键在于中医思维的灵活应用。临证需结合病史、症状, 舌脉等表现, 辨证施治。同时需提醒患者重视生活调摄, 避免劳逸无度、饮食不节。此外, 给予患者适当的心理安慰亦十分重要。

Both Chinese medicines and daoyin exercises can be utilized to treat depression. Prior to pattern identification and treatment, take the patient's medical history, symptoms, tongue manifestations and pulse manifestations into consideration. It is also important to tell patients to pay attention to lifestyle modifications, avoid overexertion, both physically and mentally, and maintain a balanced diet. Moreover, providing appropriate emotional support and comfort to patients is also significant.

1. 实证

1. Excess syndrome

（1）肝气郁结

(1) Liver qi stagnation

［症状］精神抑郁，情绪不宁，善太息，胸胁胀痛，痛无定处，腹胀纳呆，或呕吐，大便失常，女子月事不调，苔薄腻，脉弦。

[Symptoms] Mental depression, emotional restlessness, frequent sighing, migratory distending pain in the chest and sub-costal region, abdominal distension and poor appetite, vomiting, irregular bowel movements, irregular menstrual cycles in women, a thin and greasy tongue coating, and a wiry pulse.

［治法］疏肝理气解郁。

[Treatment methods] Soothe the liver and regulate qi to relieve depression.

［《诸病源候论》导引方 Daoyin Exercises in *Zhu Bing Yuan Hou Lun*]

1）调心

1) Mind regulation

站式、坐式、卧式。《无生经》曰：治百病、邪鬼、蛊毒，当

仰卧。闭眼闭气，内视丹田，鼻缓缓纳气，令腹部胀满至极点，以口缓缓吐气，不要听到气息声，吸气多吐气少，气息轻柔（图1-85）。内视五脏，看到五脏的形色，再内视胃中，令神光充盈，鲜活明晰洁白如丝绢。做到疲倦至极并且出汗就可以停止了，用粉轻扑于身上，按摩身体。汗未出但感到疲倦的，也可以停止。待第二天再做。

Take a standing, sitting or lying position. *Wu Sheng Jing* (Sutra of Imperishable) states that to treat varying disorders, evil spirits and schistosomiasis, take a supine position. Close the eyes, hold the breath, focus on the *Dantian*, and inhale slowly through the nose to make the abdomen full. Then exhale slowly through the mouth without making any sound. The inhalation should be longer than the exhalation, and the breathing should be gentle and soft (Figure 1-85). Look at the five zang organs, and observe their forms and colors. Then look at the stomach, and make it bright, lively, clear and white as silk. Continue until exhaustion and sweating are present, then stop, lightly apply powders to the body, and massage the body. If exhaustion is felt but sweating has not yet occurred, stop and repeat the practice the following day.

站式、坐式、卧式。观想心气散布于身体上下，正赤色光芒四射通彻天地，自身高大（图36-2）。做这样的观想，可令人气力倍增、发白复黑、齿落再生。

Take a standing, sitting or lying position. Visualize that the heart qi is spreading throughout the body, emitting a bright red light that penetrates the sky and earth, and correspondingly, the body is becoming tall and huge (Figure 36-2). Legend goes that this visualization exercise can make the person full of vigor and vitality, increase physical strength, make the grey hair turn into black, and promote tooth regeneration.

2）调息、调身

2) Breath regulation and body regulation

站式、坐式、卧式。有肺病的人，躯体、胸背有疼痛胀满的症状，四肢感到烦闷不适，用"嘘"字音出气（图 15-6）。

Take a standing, sitting or lying position. People with a lung disorder may experience distending pain in the upper body and discomfort in the limbs. To alleviate these symptoms, exhale with the sound "xu" (Figure 15–6).

站式。举左手，用左脚踩地，仰掌向上，持续到鼻纳气 40 次为止（图 5-2）。适用于身体发热，脊背疼痛。

Take a standing position. Raise the left hand, stomp the left foot, turn the palm upward, and inhale through the nose 40 times (Figure 5–2). This exercise can alleviate feverish sensations in the body, and back pain.

（2）气郁化火

(2) Qi depression transforming into fire

［症状］性情急躁易怒，胸闷胁胀，嘈杂吞酸，口干而苦，大便秘结，或头痛、目赤、耳鸣，舌质红，苔黄，脉弦数。

[Symptoms] Restlessness, irritability, chest tightness and sub-costal region distension, burning stomachache, acid reflux, a dry and bitter mouth, constipation, and possibly headache, red eyes, and tinnitus. The tongue appears red with a yellow coating, and the pulse is wiry and rapid.

［治法］清肝泻火，解郁和胃。

［Treatment methods］Clear liver fire, relieve depression and harmonize the stomach.

［《诸病源候论》导引方 Daoyin Exercises in *Zhu Bing Yuan Hou Lun*］

1）调心

1）Mind regulation

站式、坐式、卧式。想要辟邪驱鬼，应当常常诚意观想心（气）炎火如斗，煌煌光明。这样各种邪气就不敢侵犯，可以进入瘟疫地区之中（图7-1）。

Take a standing, sitting or lying position. To expel pathogenic factors, visualize the heart (qi) as a blazing fire. In this way, all kinds of pathogenic factors will not dare to invade the body, and one can enter areas affected by epidemics with confidence (Figure 7-1).

站式（立正）。吸收月亮的精华，在月亮初升，太阳将落尽时候，面向月亮站立，不呼不吸8次。仰头面向月亮吸收月光的精华，（因循着月光）咽下，8次（图47-1）。可以增长人的阴气，妇人吸收月亮精华，阴气更加旺盛，可使子道通畅。阴气增长可以益精补脑。

Follow the rules of the sun, moon, stars, and the yin-yang of the human body. For example, take an upright standing posture. Stand facing the moon when it rises at the beginning of the moon phase and the sun is about to set, and passively hold the breath 8 times. Look up and absorb the moonlight essence by swallowing it, and do this 8 times (Figure 47–1). Legend goes that this can increase a person's yin qi, and for females, absorbing the essence of the moon can make their yin qi more vigorous, which can promote conception. Increasing yin energy can also nourish the essence and improve brain function.

2）调息、调身
2) Breath regulation and body regulation

站式、坐式、卧式。有肝病的人，容易忧愁不快乐，有悲伤、思虑、不满、恼怒的情绪，也会有头晕眼痛的症状。用"呵"字音出气，病就可以痊愈（图 15–1）。

Take a standing, sitting or lying position. People with a liver disorder are prone to feeling unhappy and have emotional symptoms such as sadness, worry, dissatisfaction and anger, as well as symptoms such as dizziness and eye pain. Exhale with the sound "he" to recover from the disorder (Figure 15–1).

站式。举左手，用左脚跺地，仰掌向上，持续到鼻纳气 40 次为止（图 5–2）。适用于身体发热，脊背疼痛。

Take a standing position. Raise the left hand, stomp the left foot, turn the palm upward, and inhale through the nose 40 times (Figure 5–2). This exercise can alleviate feverish sensations in the body, and back pain.

（3）气滞痰郁

(3) Qi stagnation with phlegm retention

［症状］咽中不适，如有物梗阻，吐出不出，咽之不下，胸中窒闷，或兼胁痛，苔白腻，脉弦滑。

[Symptoms] Discomfort in the throat with a foreign body sensation, chest tightness, and possibly accompanied by pain in the sub-costal region. The tongue coating is white and greasy, and the pulse is wiry and slippery.

［治法］化痰理气解郁。

[Treatment methods] Resolve phlegm and regulate qi to relieve depression.

［《诸病源候论》导引方 Daoyin Exercises in *Zhu Bing Yuan Hou Lun*]

1）调心

1) Mind regulation

站式、坐式、卧式。《无生经》曰：治百病、邪鬼、蛊毒，当仰卧。闭眼闭气，内视丹田，鼻缓缓纳气，令腹部胀满至极点，以口缓缓吐气，不要听到气息声，吸气多吐气少，气息轻柔（图1-85）。内视五脏，看到五脏的形色，再内视胃中，令神光充盈，鲜活明晰洁白如丝绢。做到疲倦至极并且出汗就可以停止了，用粉轻扑于身上，按摩身体。汗未出但感到疲倦的，也可以停止。待第二天再做。

Take a standing, sitting or lying position. *Wu Sheng Jing* (Sutra of Imperishable) states that to treat varying disorders, evil spirits and schistosomiasis, take a supine position. Close the eyes, hold the breath, focus on the *Dantian*, and inhale slowly through the nose to make the abdomen full. Then exhale slowly through the mouth without making any sound. The inhalation should be longer than the exhalation, and the breathing should be gentle and soft (Figure 1–85). Look at the five zang organs, and observe their forms and colors. Then look at the stomach, and make it bright, lively, clear and white as silk. Continue until exhaustion and sweating are present, then stop, lightly apply powders to the body, and massage the body. If exhaustion is felt but sweating has not yet occurred, stop and repeat the practice the following day.

你站式、坐式、卧式。存想巨雷闪电，雷鸣电闪，进入腹中。能这样坚持存想，疾病就能自然消除。

Take a standing, sitting or lying position. Visualize great thunder and lightning, with thunderbolts and flashes entering into the abdomen. Persistent visualization can help keep a peaceful mind.

2）调息、调身

2) Breath regulation and body regulation

站式、坐式。鹜行气。低头靠墙，不吸不呼12次，心意放松，浊气自然下降。痰饮和宿食向下排出就能痊愈。鹜行气时，身正（脊柱正），头颈部如鸭子一般上下伸缩运动，气向下行排出，做12次（图22-3）。适用于宿食。长期练此动作，不需要借助另外的通塞方法。

Take a standing or sitting position. Assume the posture of a duck to circulate qi. Lower the head, lean against a wall, passively hold the breath 12 times, relax the mind and descend turbid qi naturally. To treat phlegm-fluid retention and food retention, it is important to expel them downward. When assuming the posture of a duck to circulate qi, keep the body upright, and move the head and neck up and down like a duck, allowing qi to flow downward and out. Repeat this exercise 12 times (Figure 22–3). This exercise can help treat food retention.

坐式。两手交叉，反向撑地，身体慢慢向后仰。这个过程中脐腹自然用力，腰部向前散气，尽力做到极势时放松。上下来回做14次（图9-6）。适用于脐下寒冷、脚疼、五脏六腑不和。

Take a sitting position. Cross both hands to support the body, and slowly and fully lean backward. During this process, exert force with the abdomen, and dissipate qi with the waist. Repeat this exercise 14 times (Figure 9–6). This exercise can help alleviate cold in the lower abdomen, foot pain, and disharmony between the zang organs and fu organs.

2. 虚证
2. Deficiency syndrome

（1）忧郁伤神
(1) Depression damaging the spirit

［症状］精神恍惚，心神不宁，悲忧善哭，时时欠伸，舌质淡，

苔薄白, 脉弦细。

[Symptoms] Mind wandering, a tendency to feel sad and cry easily, frequent yawning, a pale tongue with a thin white coating, and a thready and wiry pulse.

[治法] 养心安神。

[Treatment methods] Nourish the heart and calm the mind.

[《诸病源候论》导引方 Daoyin Exercises in *Zhu Bing Yuan Hou Lun*]

1) 调心

1) Mind regulation

站式、坐式、卧式。观想心气散布于身体上下, 正赤色光芒四射通彻天地, 自身高大(图36-2)。做这样的观想, 可令人气力倍增、发白复黑、齿落再生。

Take a standing, sitting or lying position. Visualize that the heart qi is spreading throughout the body, emitting a bright red light that penetrates the sky and earth, and correspondingly, the body is becoming tall and huge (Figure 36–2). Legend goes that this visualization exercise can make the person full of vigor and vitality, increase physical strength, make the grey hair turn into black, and promote tooth regeneration.

站式(立正)。吸收月亮的精华, 在月亮初升, 太阳将落尽时候, 面向月亮站立, 不呼不吸8次。仰头面向月亮吸收月光的精华,(因循着月光)咽下,8次(图47-1)。可以增长人的阴气,妇人吸收月亮精华,阴气更加旺盛,可使子道通畅。阴气增长可以益精补脑。

Follow the rules of the sun, moon, stars, and the yin-yang of the human body. For example, take an upright standing posture. Stand facing the moon when it rises at the beginning of the moon phase and the sun is about to set, and passively hold the breath 8 times. Look up and absorb the moonlight essence by swallowing it, and do this 8 times (Figure 47–1). Legend goes that this can increase a person's yin qi, and for females, absorbing the essence of the moon can make their yin qi more vigorous, which can promote conception. Increasing yin energy can also nourish the essence and improve brain function.

2）调息、调身
2) Breath regulation and body regulation

站式、坐式、卧式。有肝病的人,容易忧愁不快乐,有悲伤、思虑、不满、恼怒的情绪,也会有头晕眼痛的症状。用"呵"字音出气,病就可以痊愈(图15-1)。

Take a standing, sitting or lying position. People with a liver disorder are prone to feeling unhappy and have emotional symptoms such as sadness, worry, dissatisfaction and anger, as well as symptoms such as dizziness and eye pain. Exhale with the sound "he" to recover from the disorder (Figure 15–1).

坐式(端坐)。患心下积聚之病,舒展腰部,仰头面向太阳,以口缓缓纳气,因循着阳光咽下,超过30次就可以停止,睁开眼睛(图19-2)。

Take an upright sitting position. For abdominal masses, stretch the waist, raise the head to face the sun, inhale slowly through the mouth, swallow qi 30 times, and open the eyes (Figure 19–2).

（2）心脾两虚
(2) Deficiency of the heart and spleen

［症状］多思善虑，心悸胆怯，少寐健忘，面色不华，头晕神疲，食欲不振，舌质淡，脉细弱。

[Symptoms] Excessive pensiveness, palpitations and timidity, insomnia and forgetfulness, a lusterless facial complexion, dizziness and fatigue, a poor appetite, a pale tongue, and a thready and weak pulse.

［治法］健脾养心，益气补血。

[Treatment methods] Strengthen the spleen, nourish the heart, supplement qi and tonify blood.

［《诸病源候论》导引方 Daoyin Exercises in *Zhu Bing Yuan Hou Lun*]

1）调心
1) Mind regulation

站式、坐式、卧式。《无生经》曰：治百病、邪鬼、蛊毒，当

仰卧。闭眼闭气，内视丹田，鼻缓缓纳气，令腹部胀满至极点，以口缓缓吐气，不要听到气息声，吸气多吐气少，气息轻柔（图1-85）。内视五脏，看到五脏的形色，再内视胃中，令神光充盈，鲜活明晰洁白如丝绢。做到疲倦至极并且出汗就可以停止了，用粉轻扑于身上，按摩身体。汗未出但感到疲倦的，也可以停止。待第二天再做。

Take a standing, sitting or lying position. *Wu Sheng Jing* (Sutra of Imperishable) states that to treat varying disorders, evil spirits and schistosomiasis, take a supine position. Close the eyes, hold the breath, focus on the *Dantian*, and inhale slowly through the nose to make the abdomen full. Then exhale slowly through the mouth without making any sound. The inhalation should be longer than the exhalation, and the breathing should be gentle and soft (Figure 1–85). Look at the five zang organs, and observe their forms and colors. Then look at the stomach, and make it bright, lively, clear and white as silk. Continue until exhaustion and sweating are present, then stop, lightly apply powders to the body, and massage the body. If exhaustion is felt but sweating has not yet occurred, stop and repeat the practice the following day.

站式、坐式、卧式。观想心气散布于身体上下，正赤色光芒四射通彻天地，自身高大（图36-2）。做这样的观想，可令人气力倍增、发白复黑、齿落再生。

Take a standing, sitting or lying position. Visualize that the heart qi is spreading throughout the body, emitting a bright red light that penetrates the sky and earth, and correspondingly, the body is becoming tall and huge (Figure 36–2). Legend goes that this visualization exercise can make the person full of vigor and vitality, increase physical strength, make the grey hair turn into black, and promote tooth regeneration.

2）调息、调身

2）Breath regulation and body regulation

卧式（仰卧）。口缓缓纳气，鼻出气（图2-25，图2-26）。适用于腹内拘急疼痛、饱食不消化。然后小咽气几十口，起到温中的效果。如果受寒邪，使人干呕腹痛，以口纳气70次，腹部充盈则可扶正祛邪。再小咽气几十口，两手掌摩擦，温热后摩腹，令气下行（图2-27）。

Take a supine position. Inhale slowly through the mouth and exhale through the nose (Figure 2–25 and Figure 2–26). This exercise can help treat abdominal cramps and pain, as well as indigestion. Then, swallow the air dozens of times to warm the stomach. For retching and abdominal pain caused by contraction of pathogenic cold, inhaling through the mouth 70 times to make the abdomen full can reinforce healthy qi to eliminate pathogenic factors. Then, swallow the air dozens of times, rub the hands to generate warmth and knead the abdomen in order to promote downward movement of qi (Figure 2–27).

卧式、坐式。蛇行气。先曲身侧卧（图2-18），然后翻身仰卧，再起身踞坐（图2-19）。闭眼，身体随着内在气机缓缓自然流动运行，不吸不呼12次。少食，肠胃才可以畅通。服气为食，舌抵上腭，津液自生，如琼浆般饮下。适时养生，春天适合活动升发，冬天适宜收敛封藏。不宜过分贪求财富，不宜过分贪求安逸。这样才能治疗五劳七伤。

Take a lying or sitting position. Assume the posture of a snake to circulate qi. First, lie down on the side with the body bent (Figure 2–18), then lie on the back, and sit with the knees raised and the feet on the ground (Figure 2–19). Close the eyes, perceive qi movements within the body and passively hold the breath 12 times. Eat less food and ingest qi. Press the tongue against the palate to produce saliva and swallow it. Health preservation should follow the rules of nature. Spring is suitable for promoting the upward flow of qi, while winter is best for consolidating and preserving. Do not be excessively greedy for wealth or comfort. Only in this way can the five exhaustions and seven damages be treated.

（3）阴虚火旺
(3) Yin deficiency leading to fire hyperactivity

[症状] 眩晕,心悸,少寐,心烦易怒,或腰酸遗精,女子月事不调,舌质红,脉弦细而数。

[Symptoms] Dizziness, palpitations, insomnia, restlessness, or lower back pain and nocturnal emissions, irregular menstrual cycles in women, a red tongue, and a wiry, thready, and rapid pulse.

[治法] 滋阴清热,镇心安神。

[Treatment methods] Nourish yin, clear heat, and tranquillize and calm the mind.

[《诸病源候论》导引方 Daoyin Exercises in *Zhu Bing Yuan Hou Lun*]

1）调心
1) Mind regulation

站式、坐式、卧式。延年益寿的方法,观想心气红色,肝气青色,肺气白色,脾气黄色,肾气黑色,在身体四周围绕并辟邪驱鬼（图7-1）。

Take a standing, sitting or lying position. To achieve longevity, visualize the red heart qi, green liver qi, white lung qi, yellow spleen qi, and black kidney qi surrounding the body and warding off pathogenic factors (Figure 7-1).

站式（立正）。吸收月亮的精华,在月亮初升,太阳将落尽时候,面向月亮站立,不呼不吸8次。仰头面向月亮吸收月光的精华,（因循着月光）咽下,8次（图47-1）。可以增长人的阴气,妇人吸收月亮精华,阴气更加旺盛,可使子道通畅。阴气增长可以益精补脑。

Follow the rules of the sun, moon, stars, and the yin-yang of the human body. For example, take an upright standing posture. Stand facing the moon when it rises at the beginning of the moon phase and the sun is about to set, and passively hold the breath 8 times. Look up and absorb the moonlight essence by swallowing it, and do this 8 times. Legend goes that this can increase a person's yin qi, and for females, absorbing the essence of the moon can make their yin qi more vigorous, which can promote conception. Increasing yin energy can also nourish the essence and improve brain function.

2）调息、调身
2) Breath regulation and body regulation

卧式。治疗四肢疼闷、行动不便、腹中胀气。可以采用下面的方法：床席平稳,仰卧,松解衣带,枕高三寸,两手握固,伸展两手,各距离身体五寸（图1-16）。安心定意,调和气息,不想杂事，专注气息，慢慢地漱醴泉。所谓漱醴泉，即是用舌在口唇齿间转动（图1-17），使津液满口，而后缓缓咽下，然后徐徐以口吐气，再以鼻纳气。这些动作都须轻且慢，不要匆促硬做。调和呼吸，渐至自己听不到呼吸声后，以心行气，引气至脚趾端而出。每吸5次或6次，呼1次，为一息。初学，由一息渐做到十息，以后慢慢增加到一百息、二百息，病就能好了。治疗期勿食生的蔬菜、鱼、肥肉。过饱和喜怒忧恚时都不可行气。在凌晨清静时候行气最好，能治疗各种疾病。

Take a supine position. To treat oppressive pain in the limbs, difficulty in movement, and abdominal distension, lie on a flat bed, wear loose clothes, use a pillow with 3 *cun* high, make fists with the hands, and stretch the arms outwards, with each hand being about 5 *cun* away from the body (Figure 1–16). Keep a peaceful mind, regulate and focus on the breath, close the mouth, and slowly rotate the tongue to make saliva fill the mouth, then slowly swallow, then slowly exhale through the mouth, and inhale through the nose (Figure 1–17). These movements should be done gently and slowly. Regulate the breath and gradually make it so quiet that you cannot hear it. Then focus the mind on guiding qi to the tips of the toes. Inhale 5 or 6 times and exhale once to complete a breath cycle. For beginners, start with 1 breath cycle and gradually increase to 10, and then slowly increase to 100 or 200 breath cycles. This exercise can help cure the disease. During the treatment period, avoid eating uncooked vegetables, fish, and fatty meat. Do not circulate qi when you are overly full or emotional. The best time to circulate qi is in the early morning, which can help treat various disorders.

跪式（跪伏）。龙行气。叩头，额头着地，眼睛向下看，不呼不吸12次（图44-1）。适用于风疠、恶疮，可使热邪不进入体内。

Take a kneeling position. Assume the posture of a dragon to circulate qi. Place the forehead on the ground, look downward, and passively hold the breath 12 times (Figure 44–1). This exercise can help treat scabies and intractable ulcers, and prevent the invasion of pathogenic heat into the body.

四、虚劳
Consumptive Conditions

（一）概述
Introduction

"虚劳"又称虚损，是由于禀赋薄弱、后天失养、外感、内伤等多种原因引起的，以脏腑功能衰退、气血阴阳亏损，日久不复为主要病机的，以五脏虚证为主要临床表现的多种慢性虚弱症候的总称。历代医籍对虚劳的认识以"虚"为其核心病机。《素问·通评虚实论》"精气夺则虚"可视为虚证的提纲。《素问·调经论》所谓"阳虚则外寒，阴虚则内热"则进一步说明虚证有阴虚、阳虚的区别，并指明阴虚、阳虚的主要特点。虚劳涉及的疾病范围较广，与内科其他病证的虚症证型有较多相似之处。

"Consumptive conditions" is a collective term for a group of chronic consumptive conditions. The causative factors of consumptive conditions include congenital weakness, postnatal malnutrition, contraction of external pathogenic factors, and internal injuries. Decreased zang-fu functions may consume qi, blood, yin and yang, and subsequently lead to chronic disease duration. This is the pathogenesis of consumptive conditions and the core is deficiency. The main clinical manifestations are

　　根据虚劳的临床表现，主要见于西医学的慢性疲劳综合征。慢性疲劳综合征是一种躯体、精神的虚弱状态，指以持续6个月以上的慢性、反复发作性疲劳为主要特征，常伴随低热、淋巴结肿痛、肌肉疼痛、关节疼痛、头痛、咽痛、睡眠障碍、记忆力下降、注意力不集中等多种躯体和神经精神症状，且不能通过休息或睡眠得到缓解的临床综合征。国内外学者对其病因和发病机制进行广泛的研究，但目前尚不十分明确，主要涉及病毒感染、免疫功能异常、神经内分泌功能紊乱、心理障碍、遗传等因素。本节讨论的虚劳，以精气不足的症状为主要特征，病程较长，病势延绵。慢性疲劳综合征可参照本篇内容辨证论治。

The clinical manifestations of consumptive conditions in TCM closely resemble chronic fatigue syndrome (CFS) in Western medicine. CFS is a state of physical and mental fatigue, defined by chronic, recurrent fatigue lasting for more than six months. It is typically accompanied by various physical and neuropsychiatric symptoms such as low fever, swollen lymph nodes, muscle pain, joint pain, headache, sore throat, sleep disorders, memory decrease, and inattention. These symptoms cannot be alleviated by rest or sleep. Scholars worldwide have conducted extensive research on its causative factors and pathogenesis, but current understanding remains somewhat unclear, involving factors such as viral infection, abnormal immune function, neuroendocrine dysfunction, psychological disorders, and genetics. The consumptive disorders discussed in this section are primarily characterized by insufficient essence qi, with chronic disease duration. The pattern identification and treatment discussed in this section applies to CFS.

（二）辨证论治
Treatment Based on Pattern Identification

虚劳的辨证论治以气血阴阳为纲，五脏虚证为目。在虚劳的共有特征基础上，气虚者主要表现为面色萎黄、神疲体倦、懒言声低、自汗、脉细；血虚者主要表现为面色不华、唇甲淡白、头晕眼花、脉细；阴虚者主要表现为口干舌燥、五心烦热、盗汗、舌红苔少、脉细数；阳虚损者主要表现为面色苍白、形寒肢冷、舌质淡胖有齿印、脉沉细。气虚含肺气虚、心气虚、脾气虚、肾气虚；血虚含心血虚、脾血虚、肝血虚；阴虚含肺阴虚、心阴虚、脾胃阴虚、肝阴虚、肾阴虚；阳虚含心阳虚、脾阳虚、肾阳虚。

The pattern identification of consumptive disorders mainly focuses on identifying the conditions of qi, blood, yin, and yang, accompanied by identifying the conditions of the five zang organs. In addition to the common manifestations of consumptive conditions, the manifestations of qi deficiency include a sallow facial complexion, fatigue, lassitude, reluctance to talk, low voice, spontaneous sweating, and a thready pulse; the manifestations of blood deficiency include a lusterless facial complexion, pale lips and nails, dizziness, blurred vision, and a thready pulse; the manifestations of yin deficiency include dry mouth and tongue, feverish sensations in palms, soles and chest, night sweats, a red tongue with little coating, and a thready, rapid pulse; the manifestations of yang deficiency include a pale facial complexion, cold body and limbs, a pale, enlarged tongue with teeth marks, and a deep, thready pulse. Qi deficiency includes lung qi deficiency, heart qi deficiency, spleen qi deficiency, and kidney qi deficiency; blood deficiency includes heart blood deficiency, spleen blood deficiency, and liver blood deficiency; yin deficiency includes lung yin deficiency, heart yin deficiency, spleen-stomach yin deficiency, liver yin deficiency, and kidney yin deficiency; yang deficiency includes heart yang deficiency, spleen yang deficiency, and kidney yang deficiency.

中药、导引方皆适用于虚劳，补益为治疗的基本原则。临证需根据病理属性不同，分别采用益气、养血、滋阴、温阳；且要密切结合五脏病位的不同而选方，以加强治疗的针对性。

Both Chinese medicines and daoyin methods can be used to treat consumptive conditions. The general treatment principle is to reinforce. The specific treatment principles include tonifying qi, nourishing blood, nourishing yin and warming yang, which can be selected according to the nature of the disorder. In addition, pay attention to the location of the disorder in order to enhance the efficacy of the treatment.

1. 气虚
1. Qi deficiency

（1）肺气虚
(1) Lung qi deficiency

［症状］短气自汗，声音低怯，时寒时热，平素易于感冒，面白，舌质淡，脉弱。

[Symptoms] Shortness of breath, spontaneous sweating, a low and timid voice, alternating feelings of cold and heat, susceptibility to common colds, a pale facial complexion, a pale tongue, and a weak pulse.

［治法］补益肺气。

[Treatment method] Tonify lung qi.

［《诸病源候论》导引方 Daoyin Exercises in *Zhu Bing Yuan Hou Lun*]

1）调心

1) Mind regulation

站式、坐式、卧式。观想心气散布于身体上下，正赤色光芒四射通彻天地，自身高大（图36-2）。做这样的观想，可令人气力倍增、发白复黑、齿落再生。

Take a standing, sitting or lying position. Visualize that the heart qi is spreading throughout the body, emitting a bright red light that penetrates the sky and earth, and correspondingly, the body is becoming tall and huge (Figure 36-2). Legend goes that this visualization exercise can make the person full of vigor and vitality, increase physical strength, make the grey hair turn into black, and promote tooth regeneration.

站式、坐式、卧式。延年益寿的方法，观想心气红色，肝气青色，肺气白色，脾气黄色，肾气黑色，在身体四周围绕并辟邪驱鬼（图7-1）。

Take a standing, sitting or lying position. To achieve longevity, visualize the red heart qi, green liver qi, white lung qi, yellow spleen qi, and black kidney qi surrounding the body and warding off pathogenic factors (Figure 7-1).

2）调息、调身

2）Breath regulation and body regulation

站式、坐式、卧式。有肺病的人，躯体、胸背有疼痛胀满的症状，四肢感到烦闷不适，用"嘘"字音出气（图15-6）。

Take a standing, sitting or lying position. People with a lung disorder may experience distending pain in the upper body and discomfort in the limbs. To alleviate these symptoms, exhale with the sound "xu" (Figure 15–6).

站式。两手交叉放于下颌，身体松沉到极点，可补肺气，治疗突然气逆咳嗽。两手放于下颌，轻抚两侧颈动脉（图10-3），以下颌尽力向胸中勾，极速牵拉至喉骨，尽力做3次，补气充足（图10-4）。适用于暴气上气、失音等病。令气息调和匀长，声音洪亮。

Take a standing position. Cross the hands, place them under the jaw, and totally relax the body. This exercise can supplement lung qi and treat sudden coughing induced by the counterflow of qi. Place the hands under the chin, gently massage the carotid arteries on both sides (Figure 10–3), fully bring the chin close to the chest, and repeat 3 times to tonify qi (Figure 10–4). This exercise can help treat disorders such as counterflow of qi and aphonia. It can regulate the breath and make the voice loud and clear.

（2）心气虚

(2) Heart qi deficiency

［症状］心悸，气短，劳则尤甚，神疲体倦，自汗，舌质淡，脉弱。

[Symptoms] Palpitations and shortness of breath that

worsen upon physical exertion, fatigue, lassitude, spontaneous sweating, a pale tongue, and a weak pulse.

［治法］益气养心。

[Treatment methods] Supplement qi and nourish the heart.

［《诸病源候论》导引方 Daoyin Exercises in *Zhu Bing Yuan Hou Lun*］

1）调心

1) Mind regulation

站式、坐式、卧式。观想心气散布于身体上下，正赤色光芒四射通彻天地，自身高大（图36-2）。做这样的观想，可令人气力倍增、发白复黑、齿落再生。

Take a standing, sitting or lying position. Visualize that the heart qi is spreading throughout the body, emitting a bright red light that penetrates the sky and earth, and correspondingly, the body is becoming tall and huge (Figure 36-2). Legend goes that this visualization exercise can make the person full of vigor and vitality, increase physical strength, make the grey hair turn into black, and promote tooth regeneration.

2）调息、调身

2) Breath regulation and body regulation

站式、坐式、卧式。有心病的人，身体有发冷发热的症状。

如果身体发冷，用"呼"字音吸气（图15-2）；如果发热，用"吹"字音出气（图15-3）。

Take a standing, sitting or lying position. People with a heart disorder may experience symptoms such as chills and fever. For chills, inhale with the sound "hu". For fever, exhale with the sound "ci" (Figure 15–3).

蹲式（蹲踞）。雁行气。低下胳臂推着膝盖，用绳捆绑左臂与左膝，低头，不呼不吸12次（图27-7）。可消化积食、轻健身体、增长精神，使恶气不得侵犯，各种病邪得以去除。

Take a squatting position. Assume the posture of a wild goose to circulate qi. Push the knees with the arms, tie the left arm and left knee with a rope, lower the head, and passively hold the breath 12 times (Figure 27–7). This exercise can help treat food retention, strengthen the body, enhance mental spirit, and prevent pathogenic qi from invading the body.

（3）脾气虚

(3) Spleen qi deficiency

［症状］饮食减少，食后胃脘不舒，倦怠乏力，大便溏薄，面色萎黄，舌淡苔薄，脉弱。

[Symptoms] A decreased appetite, stomach discomfort after meals, fatigue, lassitude, loose stools, a sallow facial complexion, a pale tongue with a thin coating, and a weak pulse.

［治法］健脾益气。

[Treatment methods]　Strengthen the spleen and supplement qi.

[《诸病源候论》导引方 Daoyin Exercises in *Zhu Bing Yuan Hou Lun*]

1）调心

1) Mind regulation

站式、坐式、卧式。《无生经》曰：治百病、邪鬼、蛊毒，当仰卧。闭眼闭气，内视丹田，鼻缓缓纳气，令腹部胀满至极点，以口缓缓吐气，不要听到气息声，吸气多吐气少，气息轻柔（图1-85）。内视五脏，看到五脏的形色，再内视胃中，令神光充盈，鲜活明晰洁白如丝绢。做到疲倦至极并且出汗就可以停止了，用粉轻扑于身上，按摩身体。汗未出但感到疲倦的，也可以停止。待第二天再做。

Take a standing, sitting or lying position. *Wu Sheng Jing* (Sutra of Imperishable) states that to treat varying disorders, evil spirits and schistosomiasis, take a supine position. Close the eyes, hold the breath, focus on the *Dantian*, and inhale slowly through the nose to make the abdomen full. Then exhale slowly through the mouth without making any sound. The inhalation should be longer than the exhalation, and the breathing should be gentle and soft (Figure 1–85). Look at the five zang organs, and observe their forms and colors. Then look at the stomach, and make it bright, lively, clear and white as silk. Continue until exhaustion and sweating are present, then stop, lightly apply powders to the body, and massage the body. If exhaustion is felt but sweating has not yet occurred, stop and repeat the practice the following day.

2）调息、调身

2）Breath regulation and body regulation

站式、坐式、卧式。腹中苦于发胀且有寒气，用"呼"字音出气，做30次（图16-6）。

Take a standing, sitting or lying position. For abdominal distention, and cold in the abdomen, exhale with the sound "hu" 30 times (Figure 16–6).

站式、坐式。鹜行气。低头靠墙，不吸不呼12次，心意放松，浊气自然下降。痰饮和宿食向下排出就能痊愈。鹜行气时，身正（脊柱正），头颈部如鸭子一般上下伸缩运动，气向下行排出，做12次（图22-3）。适用于宿食。长期练此动作，不需要借助另外的通塞方法。

Take a standing or sitting position. Assume the posture of a duck to circulate qi. Lower the head, lean against a wall, passively hold the breath 12 times, relax the mind and descend turbid qi naturally. To treat phlegm-fluid retention and food retention, it is important to expel them downward. When assuming the posture of a duck to circulate qi, keep the body upright, and move the head and neck up and down like a duck, allowing qi to flow downward and out. Repeat this exercise 12 times (Figure 22–3). This exercise can help treat food retention.

（4）肾气虚

（4）Kidney qi deficiency

［症状］神疲乏力，腰膝酸软，小便频数而清，白带清稀，舌

质淡,脉弱。

[Symptoms] Fatigue, weakness, low back/knee soreness and weakness, frequent and clear urination, clear and watery vaginal discharge, a pale tongue and a weak pulse.

[治法] 益气补肾。
[Treatment method] Tonify kidney qi.

[《诸病源候论》导引方 Daoyin Exercises in *Zhu Bing Yuan Hou Lun*]

调心
Mind regulation

站式、坐式、卧式。观想心气散布于身体上下,正赤色光芒四射通彻天地,自身高大(图36-2)。做这样的观想,可令人气力倍增、发白复黑、齿落再生。

Take a standing, sitting or lying position. Visualize that the heart qi is spreading throughout the body, emitting a bright red light that penetrates the sky and earth, and correspondingly, the body is becoming tall and huge (Figure 36-2). Legend goes that this visualization exercise can make the person full of vigor and vitality, increase physical strength, make the grey hair turn into black, and promote tooth regeneration.

站式、坐式、卧式。有肾病的人,有咽喉阻塞、腹部胀满、耳聋不聪的症状,用"呬"字音出气(图15-8)。

Take a standing, sitting or lying position. For those with a kidney disorder experiencing such symptoms as a foreign body sensation in the throat, abdominal fullness, impaired hearing and even deafness, exhale with the sound "hei" (Figure 15–8).

坐式。虾蟆行气。正坐。摇动两手臂, 不吸不呼12次（图2-20）。适用于五劳七伤和水肿病。

Take an upright sitting position. Assume the posture of a toad to circulate qi. Shake the arms and passively hold the breath 12 times (Figure 2–20). This exercise can help treat the five exhaustions (Long-time observation damages blood; long-time lying damages qi; long-time sitting damages muscles; long-time standing damages bones; and long-time walking damages sinews) and seven damages (Refers to seven pathogenic factors that lead to deficiency and consumption, including improper diet, anxiety, drink, sex, hunger, over-exertion, and damage to meridians, collaterals, *Ying*-nutrients, *Wei*-defense and qi) as well as oedema.

2. 血虚
2. Blood deficiency

（1）心血虚
(1) Heart blood deficiency

[症状] 心悸怔忡, 健忘, 失眠, 多梦, 面色不华, 舌质淡, 脉细或结代。

[Symptoms] Mild or severe palpitations, dizziness, forgetfulness, insomnia, dream-disturbed sleep, a lusterless facial complexion, a pale tongue, and a threadly, knotted or regularly intermittent pulse.

[治法]养血宁心。

[Treatment methods] Nourish blood and calm the heart.

[《诸病源候论》导引方 Daoyin Exercises in *Zhu Bing Yuan Hou Lun*]

1）调心

1) Mind regulation

站式、坐式、卧式。观想心气散布于身体上下，正赤色光芒四射通彻天地，自身高大（图36-2）。做这样的观想，可令人气力倍增、发白复黑、齿落再生。

Take a standing, sitting or lying position. Visualize that the heart qi is spreading throughout the body, emitting a bright red light that penetrates the sky and earth, and correspondingly, the body is becoming tall and huge (Figure 36-2). Legend goes that this visualization exercise can make the person full of vigor and vitality, increase physical strength, make the grey hair turn into black, and promote tooth regeneration.

2）调息、调身

2) Breath regulation and body regulation

站式、坐式、卧式。有心病的人，身体有发冷发热的症状。

如果身体发冷，用"呼"字音吸气（图15-2）；如果发热，用"吹"字音出气（图15-3）。

Take a standing, sitting or lying position. People with a heart disorder may experience symptoms such as chills and fever. For chills, inhale with the sound "hu". For fever, exhale with the sound "ci" (Figure 15–3).

卧式（侧卧）。左胁着地，伸直手脚，口纳气，鼻出气，周而复始不断练习（图15-4），适用于积聚和心下不适。

Take a side-lying position. Place the left flank on the ground, stretch out the arms and legs, inhale through the mouth and exhale through the nose. Regular practice (Figure 15–4) can remove accumulation and discomfort in the chest.

站式。一脚踏地，另一脚向旁侧打开（成丁字步）（图1-5）。身体旋转侧身，一手从上往下，使两手并拢，尽力做到最大幅度（图1-6），然后两手快速收回，左右手脚互换做上述动作，各14次。适用于脊柱中的风冷，以及半身偏枯导致的气血不能畅通和濡养的病症。

Take a standing position. Take a step to the side with one foot (T-shape stance) (Figure 1–5). Turn the upper body to the side, fully lift and put down the hands one by one, and put them together (Figure 1–6). Quickly retract the hands and repeat the movements on the other side, 14 times on each side. This movement can dispel wind and cold in the spine, and deal with the obstruction and malnutrition of qi and blood caused by hemiplegia.

（2）脾血虚

(2) Spleen blood deficiency

［症状］体倦乏力，纳差食少，心悸气短，健忘，失眠，面色萎黄，舌质淡，苔白薄，脉细缓。

[Symptoms] Fatigue, a poor appetite, palpitations, shortness of breath, forgetfulness, insomnia, a sallow facial complexion, a pale tongue with a thin, white coating, and a thready and slowdown pulse.

［治法］补脾养血。

[Treatment methods] Tonify the spleen and nourish blood.

［《诸病源候论》导引方 Daoyin Exercises in *Zhu Bing Yuan Hou Lun*]

1）调心

1) Mind regulation

站式、坐式、卧式。《无生经》曰：治百病、邪鬼、蛊毒，当仰卧。闭眼闭气，内视丹田，鼻缓缓纳气，令腹部胀满至极点，以口缓缓吐气，不要听到气息声，吸气多吐气少，气息轻柔（图1-85）。内视五脏，看到五脏的形色，再内视胃中，令神光充盈，鲜活明晰洁白如丝绢。做到疲倦至极并且出汗就可以停止了，用粉轻扑于身上，按摩身体。汗未出但感到疲倦的，也可以停止。待第二天再做。

Take a standing, sitting or lying position. *Wu Sheng Jing*

(Sutra of Imperishable) states that to treat varying disorders, evil spirits and schistosomiasis, take a supine position. Close the eyes, hold the breath, focus on the *Dantian*, and inhale slowly through the nose to make the abdomen full. Then exhale slowly through the mouth without making any sound. The inhalation should be longer than the exhalation, and the breathing should be gentle and soft (Figure 1–85). Look at the five zang organs, and observe their forms and colors. Then look at the stomach, and make it bright, lively, clear and white as silk. Continue until exhaustion and sweating are present, then stop, lightly apply powders to the body, and massage the body. If exhaustion is felt but sweating has not yet occurred, stop and repeat the practice the following day.

2）调息、调身
2) Breath regulation and body regulation

卧式（仰卧）。口缓缓纳气，鼻出气（图2-25，图2-26）。适用于腹内拘急疼痛、饱食不消化。然后小咽气几十口，起到温中的效果。如果受寒邪，使人干呕腹痛，以口纳气70次，腹部充盈则可扶正祛邪。再小咽气几十口，两手掌摩擦，温热后摩腹，令气下行（图2-27）。

Take a supine position. Inhale slowly through the mouth and exhale through the nose (Figure 2–25 and Figure 2–26). This exercise can help treat abdominal cramps and pain, as well as indigestion. Then, swallow the air dozens of times to warm the stomach. For retching and abdominal pain caused by contraction of pathogenic cold, inhaling through the mouth 70 times to make the abdomen full can reinforce healthy qi to eliminate pathogenic factors. Then, swallow the air dozens of times, rub the hands to generate warmth and knead the abdomen in order to promote downward movement of qi (Figure 2–27).

站式。两手向后托腰，尽力缩紧两肩，左右转身，来回做21次（图9-7）。适用于腹肚脐冷、肩胛发紧、胸部和腋下不适。

Take a standing position. Place both hands on the lower back to hold it, fully close the shoulders, rotate the body left and right, and repeat 21 times (Figure 9–7). This exercise can help alleviate cold in the abdomen, tightness in the shoulders and scapula, and discomfort in the chest and armpits.

（3）肝血虚
(3) Liver blood deficiency

［症状］头晕，目眩，胁痛，肢体麻木，筋脉拘急，或筋惕肉瞤，妇女月经不调甚则闭经，面色不华，舌质淡，脉弦细或细涩。

[Symptoms] Dizziness, blurred vision, pain in the sub-costal region, numbness in the limbs, stiffness and rigidity of the tendons and muscles, or spasms and twitching of the muscles. In women, it can cause irregular menstruation and even amenorrhea. The facial complexion appears lusterless, the tongue is pale, and the pulse is wiry and thready, or thready and hesitant.

［治法］补血养肝。
[Treatment methods] Tonify blood and nourish the liver.

［《诸病源候论》导引方 Daoyin Exercises in *Zhu Bing Yuan Hou Lun*]

1）调心

1) Mind regulation

站式、坐式、卧式。观想心气散布于身体上下，正赤色光芒四射通彻天地，自身高大（图36-2）。做这样的观想，可令人气力倍增、发白复黑、齿落再生。

Take a standing, sitting or lying position. Visualize that the heart qi is spreading throughout the body, emitting a bright red light that penetrates the sky and earth, and correspondingly, the body is becoming tall and huge (Figure 36-2). Legend goes that this visualization exercise can make the person full of vigor and vitality, increase physical strength, make the grey hair turn into black, and promote tooth regeneration.

站式、坐式、卧式。延年益寿的方法，观想心气红色，肝气青色，肺气白色，脾气黄色，肾气黑色，在身体四周围绕并辟邪驱鬼（图7-1）。

Take a standing, sitting or lying position. To achieve longevity, visualize the red heart qi, green liver qi, white lung qi, yellow spleen qi, and black kidney qi surrounding the body and warding off pathogenic factors (Figure 7-1).

2）调息、调身

2) Breath regulation and body regulation

站式、坐式、卧式。有肝病的人，容易忧愁不快乐，有悲伤、思虑、不满、恼怒的情绪，也会有头晕眼痛的症状。用"呵"字音出气，病就可以痊愈（图15-1）。

Take a standing, sitting or lying position. People with a liver disorder are prone to feeling unhappy and have emotional symptoms such as sadness, worry, dissatisfaction and anger, as well as symptoms such as dizziness and eye pain. Exhale with the sound "he" to recover from the disorder (Figure 15–1).

站式。一脚踏地，另一脚向旁侧打开（成丁字步）（图1-5）。身体旋转侧身，一手从上往下，使两手并拢，尽力做到最大幅度（图1-6），然后两手快速收回，左右手脚互换做上述动作，各14次。适用于脊柱中的风冷，以及半身偏枯导致的气血不能畅通和濡养的病症。

Take a standing position. Take a step to the side with one foot (T-shape stance) (Figure 1–5). Turn the upper body to the side, fully lift and put down the hands one by one, and put them together (Figure 1–6). Quickly retract the hands and repeat the movements on the other side, 14 times on each side. This movement can dispel wind and cold in the spine, and deal with the obstruction and malnutrition of qi and blood caused by hemiplegia.

3. 阴虚
3. Yin deficiency

（1）肺阴虚
(1) Lung yin deficiency

［症状］干咳，咽燥，甚或失音，咯血，潮热，盗汗，面色潮红，舌红少津，脉细数。

[Symptoms] Dry cough, a dry throat, and, in severe cases, loss of voice, hemoptysis, tidal fever, night sweats, a flushed complexion, a red tongue with little moisture, and a thready and rapid pulse.

［治法］养阴润肺。

[Treatment methods] Nourish yin and moisten the lung.

［《诸病源候论》导引方 Daoyin Exercises in *Zhu Bing Yuan Hou Lun*]

1）调心

1) Mind regulation

站式（立正）。吸收月亮的精华，在月亮初升，太阳将落尽时候，面向月亮站立，不呼不吸8次。仰头面向月亮吸收月光的精华，（因循着月光）咽下，8次（图47-1）。可以增长人的阴气，妇人吸收月亮精华，阴气更加旺盛，可使子道通畅。阴气增长可以益精补脑。

Follow the rules of the sun, moon, stars, and the yin-yang of the human body. For example, take an upright standing posture. Stand facing the moon when it rises at the beginning of the moon phase and the sun is about to set, and passively hold the breath 8 times. Look up and absorb the moonlight essence by swallowing it, and do this 8 times. Legend goes that this can increase a person's yin qi, and for females, absorbing the essence of the moon can make their yin qi more vigorous, which can promote conception. Increasing yin energy can also nourish the essence and improve brain function.

2）调息、调身
2) Breath regulation and body regulation

卧式（俯卧）。去掉枕头，竖起两脚，鼻纳气40多次，再以鼻
呼出。要令吸入鼻中的气极其微细，以至鼻子无法觉察的程度
（图9-1）。适用于身中发热、脊背痛。

Take a prone position. Remove the pillow, raise both feet, subtly inhale through the nose more than 40 times, and then subtly exhale through the nose (Figure 9–1). This exercise can alleviate feverish sensations in the body and relieve back pain.

站式。一手尽力前托，做到极势；一手放于乳房处，向后牵
拉使胸部舒展。不能用僵力令胸口打开，（气）向下松沉，两手
互换再做上述动作21次（图1-65）。将两手攀住膝盖，身体向
后仰，尽力做到极势做21次（图1-66）。适用于风热导致的烦
闷疼痛，使风府和云门的邪气散去。

Take a standing position. Fully stretch forward one hand, while placing the other hand on the breast to pull backward to stretch the chest. Do not use rigid force to open the chest, sink qi and then change the position of the hands to repeat the movements 21 times (Figure 1–65). Hold the knees with the hands and fully lean backward 21 times (Figure 1–66). This exercise can relieve vexation and pain caused by wind and heat, and disperse pathogenic factors in the points Fengfu (GV 16) and Yunmen (LU 2).

（2）心阴虚

（2）Heart yin deficiency

［症状］心悸，失眠，烦躁，潮热，盗汗，或口舌生疮，面色潮红，舌红少津，脉细数。

[Symptoms] Palpitations, insomnia, restlessness, tidal fever, night sweats, or mouth/tongue ulcerations, a flushed complexion, a red tongue with little moisture, and a thready and rapid pulse.

［治法］滋阴养心。

[Treatment methods] Nourish heart yin and calm the mind.

［《诸病源候论》导引方 Daoyin Exercises in *Zhu Bing Yuan Hou Lun*］

1）调心

1）Mind regulation

站式（立正）。吸收月亮的精华，在月亮初升，太阳将落尽时候，面向月亮站立，不呼不吸8次。仰头面向月亮吸收月光的精华，（因循着月光）咽下，8次（图47-1）。可以增长人的阴气，妇人吸收月亮精华，阴气更加旺盛，可使子道通畅。阴气增长可以益精补脑。

Follow the rules of the sun, moon, stars, and the yin-yang of the human body. For example, take an upright standing posture. Stand facing the moon when it rises at the beginning of the moon phase and the sun is about to set, and passively hold the breath 8 times. Look up and absorb the moonlight essence by swallowing it, and do this 8 times. Legend goes that this can increase a person's yin qi, and for females, absorbing the essence of the moon can make their yin qi more vigorous, which can promote conception. Increasing yin energy can also nourish the essence and improve brain function.

2）调息、调身
2) Breath regulation and body regulation

卧式。治疗四肢疼闷、行动不便、腹中胀气。可以采用下面的方法：床席平稳，仰卧，松解衣带，枕高三寸，两手握固，伸展两手，各距离身体五寸（图1–16）。安心定意，调和气息，不想杂事，专注气息，慢慢地漱醴泉。所谓漱醴泉，即是用舌在口唇齿间转动（图1–17），使津液满口，而后缓缓咽下，然后徐徐以口吐气，再以鼻纳气。这些动作都须轻且慢，不要匆促硬做。调和呼吸，渐至自己听不到呼吸声后，以心行气，引气至脚趾端而出。每吸5或6次，呼1次，为一息。初学，由一息渐做到十息，以后慢慢增加到一百息、二百息，病就能好了。治疗期勿食生的蔬菜、鱼、肥肉。过饱和喜怒忧忿时都不可行气。在凌晨清静时候行气最好，能治疗各种疾病。

Take a supine position. To treat oppressive pain in the limbs, difficulty in movement, and abdominal distension, lie on a flat bed, wear loose clothes, use a pillow with 3 *cun* high, make fists with the hands, and stretch the arms outwards, with each hand being about 5 *cun* away from the body (Figure 1–16). Keep a peaceful mind, regulate and focus on the breath, close the mouth, and slowly rotate the tongue to make saliva fill the mouth, then slowly swallow, then slowly exhale through the mouth, and inhale through the nose (Figure 1–17). These movements should be done gently and slowly. Regulate the breath and gradually make it so quiet that you cannot hear it. Then focus the mind on guiding qi to the tips of the toes. Inhale 5 or 6 times and exhale once to complete a breath cycle. For beginners, start with 1 breath cycle and gradually increase to 10, and then slowly increase to 100 or 200 breath cycles. This exercise can help cure the disease. During the treatment period, avoid eating uncooked vegetables, fish, and fatty meat. Do not circulate qi when you are overly full or emotional. The best time to circulate qi is in the early morning, which can help treat various disorders.

站式。两手向同一侧伸展，身体同向侧转，尽力做到极势；头顶好像悬挂起来，使气自然散下，如同腐烂的东西从上往下松解散开，十指舒展伸直（图16-8）。左右两个方向都做上述导引动作，21次。然后正身直立，前后转动肩部和腰部，7次（图16-9）。适用于腹肚胀满、膀胱腰脊手臂寒冷、血脉拘急强硬、心悸。

Take a standing position. Stretch both hands to the same side, fully turn the upper body in the same direction, imagine that the top of your head is being suspended, descend qi naturally as if the decaying things are loosening and dissolving from top to bottom, and extend all fingers (Figure 16–8). Perform the above movements on both sides (left and right), and repeat 21 times on each side. Then stand straight and swing the shoulders and waist back and forth 7 times (Figure 16–9). This exercise can relieve abdominal distension, treat cold in the bladder, lower back, spine and arms, and also relieve muscle/tendon spasm and stiffness, as well as palpitations.

（3）脾胃阴虚

(3) Yin deficiency of the spleen and stomach

［症状］口干唇燥，不思饮食，大便燥结，甚则干呕，呃逆，面色潮红，舌干，苔少或无苔，脉细数。

[Symptoms] Dry mouth and lips, loss of appetite, constipation with dry stools, and in severe cases, retching and hiccups. The facial complexion is flushed, the tongue is dry with little or no coating, and the pulse is thready and rapid.

［治法］养阴和胃。

[Treatment methods] Nourish yin and benefit the stomach.

［《诸病源候论》导引方 Daoyin Exercises in *Zhu Bing Yuan Hou Lun*］

1）调心

1) Mind regulation

站式（立正）。吸收月亮的精华，在月亮初升，太阳将落尽时候，面向月亮站立，不呼不吸8次。仰头面向月亮吸收月光的精华，（因循着月光）咽下，8次（图47-1）。可以增长人的阴气，妇人吸收月亮精华，阴气更加旺盛，可使子道通畅。阴气增长可以益精补脑。

Follow the rules of the sun, moon, stars, and the yin-yang of the human body. For example, take an upright standing posture. Stand facing the moon when it rises at the beginning of the moon phase and the sun is about to set, and passively hold

Zhu Bing Yuan Hou Lun Dao Yin Shu (Explanations for the Daoyin Exercises in *Zhu Bing Yuan Hou Lun*) · 《诸病源候论》导引术 · 应用 · Application

445

the breath 8 times. Look up and absorb the moonlight essence by swallowing it, and do this 8 times (Figure 47-1). Legend goes that this can increase a person's yin qi, and for females, absorbing the essence of the moon can make their yin qi more vigorous, which can promote conception. Increasing yin energy can also nourish the essence and improve brain function.

2）调息、调身
2) Breath regulation and body regulation

卧式、坐式。蛇行气。先曲身侧卧（图2-18），然后翻身仰卧，再起身踞坐（图2-19）。闭眼，身体随着内在气机缓缓自然流动运行，不吸不呼12次。少食，肠胃才可以畅通。服气为食，舌抵上腭，津液自生，如琼浆般饮下。适时养生，春天适合活动升发，冬天适宜收敛封藏。不宜过分贪求财富，不宜过分贪求安逸。这样才能治疗五劳七伤。

Take a lying or sitting position. Assume the posture of a snake to circulate qi. First, lie down on the side with the body bent (Figure 2-18), then lie on the back, and sit with the knees raised and the feet on the ground (Figure 2-19). Close the eyes, perceive qi movements within the body and passively hold the breath 12 times. Eat less food and ingest qi. Press the tongue against the palate to produce saliva and swallow it. Health preservation should follow the rules of nature. Spring is suitable for promoting the upward flow of qi, while winter is best for consolidating and preserving. Do not be excessively greedy for wealth or comfort. Only in this way can the five exhaustions and seven damages be treated.

站式、坐式、卧式。不宜随意吐津液，应当随有随咽，如同经常含着一颗枣核一般，口内产生津液，而后咽下（图2-24）。要爱惜精气、津液，这是养生的关键。

Take a standing, sitting or lying position. Swallow the saliva, imagine holding a jujube pit in the mouth to produce saliva and then swallow it (Figure 2–24).

（4）肝阴虚
(4) Liver yin deficiency

［症状］头痛，眩晕，耳鸣，目干畏光，视物不明，急躁易怒，或肢体麻木，筋惕肉瞤，面潮红，舌干红，脉弦细数。

[Symptoms] Headache, dizziness, tinnitus, dry eyes with sensitivity to light, blurred vision, restlessness, irritability, or numbness in the limbs, muscle spasms and twitches. The facial complexion is flushed, the tongue is dry and red, and the pulse is wiry, thready, and rapid.

［治法］养肝补阴。

[Treatment methods] Nourish and supplement liver yin.

［《诸病源候论》导引方 Daoyin Exercises in *Zhu Bing Yuan Hou Lun*］

1）调心
1) Mind regulation

站式（立正）。吸收月亮的精华，在月亮初升，太阳将落尽时候，面向月亮站立，不呼不吸8次。仰头面向月亮吸收月光的精华，（因循着月光）咽下，8次（图47-1）。可以增长人的阴气，妇人吸收月亮精华，阴气更加旺盛，可使子道通畅。阴气增长可以益精补脑。

Follow the rules of the sun, moon, stars, and the yin-yang of the human body. For example, take an upright standing posture. Stand facing the moon when it rises at the beginning of the moon phase and the sun is about to set, and passively hold the breath 8 times. Look up and absorb the moonlight essence by swallowing it, and do this 8 times (Figure 47–1). Legend goes that this can increase a person's yin qi, and for females, absorbing the essence of the moon can make their yin qi more vigorous, which can promote conception. Increasing yin energy can also nourish the essence and improve brain function.

站式、坐式、卧式。延年益寿的方法，观想心气红色，肝气青色，肺气白色，脾气黄色，肾气黑色，在身体四周围绕并辟邪驱鬼（图7-1）。

Take a standing, sitting or lying position. To achieve longevity, visualize the red heart qi, green liver qi, white lung qi, yellow spleen qi, and black kidney qi surrounding the body and warding off pathogenic factors (Figure 7–1).

2）调息、调身
2）Breath regulation and body regulation

坐式（端坐）。舒展腰部，向右转头，两眼看右方，口缓缓纳气，咽气30口。适用于左胁区疼痛，使眼睛明亮（图3-9）。

Take an upright sitting position. Stretch the waist, turn the head to the right, look to the right, slowly inhale through the mouth, and swallow qi 30 times. This exercise can help relieve pain in the left side of the sub-costal region and brighten the eyes (Figure 3–9).

卧式。践行养生大道，常常根据日月星辰运行的规律。在凌晨1～3点间内心清净纯澈，身体安卧，漱液满口分3次咽下（图16–10）。可以调和五脏，杀虫虫，令人长寿，也能治心腹痛。

Take a lying position. To practice health preservation, it is important to follow the rules of the movement of the sun, moon, and stars. Between 1 am and 3 am, with a clear and calm mind and a relaxed body, produce some saliva in the mouth and swallow it in 3 times (Figure 16–10). This exercise can regulate the five zang organs, treat schistosomiasis, promote longevity, and also alleviate abdominal pain.

（5）肾阴虚
(5) Kidney yin deficiency

［症状］腰酸，遗精，两足痿弱，眩晕，耳鸣，甚则耳聋，口干，咽痛，颧红，舌红，少津，脉沉细。

[Symptoms] Low back soreness, nocturnal emissions, weakness and flaccidity of both legs, dizziness, tinnitus, and in severe cases, hearing loss; a dry mouth, a sore throat, flushed cheeks, a red tongue with little moisture, and a deep, thready pulse.

［治法］滋阴补肾。
[Treatment methods] Nourish and supplement kidney yin.

[《诸病源候论》导引方 Daoyin Exercises in *Zhu Bing Yuan Hou Lun*]

1）调心

1) Mind regulation

站式（立正）。吸收月亮的精华，在月亮初升，太阳将落尽时候，面向月亮站立，不呼不吸8次。仰头面向月亮吸收月光的精华，（因循着月光）咽下，8次（图47-1）。可以增长人的阴气，妇人吸收月亮精华，阴气更加旺盛，可使子道通畅。阴气增长可以益精补脑。

Follow the rules of the sun, moon, stars, and the yin-yang of the human body. For example, take an upright standing position. Stand facing the moon when it rises at the beginning of the moon phase and the sun is about to set, and passively hold the breath 8 times. Look up and absorb the moonlight essence by swallowing it, and do this 8 times (Figure 47–1). Legend goes that this can increase a person's yin qi, and for females, absorbing the essence of the moon can make their yin qi more vigorous, which can promote conception. Increasing yin energy can also nourish the essence and improve brain function.

2）调息、调身

2) Breath regulation and body regulation

卧式（仰卧）。松解衣服，松静自然，舒展腰部，做5次自然呼吸，使少腹抬起（图4-2）。引动肾气，适用于消渴，通利阴阳。

Take a supine position. Loosen the clothes, relax the body, stretch the waist, and breathe naturally 5 times to lift the lower abdomen (Figure 4-2). This exercise can stimulate kidney qi, treat wasting and thirst disorders and improve the balance of yin and yang.

卧式（跪伏）。侧身以耳贴地，不呼不吸6次（图1-82）。适用于耳聋目眩。以耳聋侧伏卧，两膝并拢，耳紧贴地，专心用力贴住至极限。长期练此动作可改善听力，耳闻十方；也可使头倒转向下时不觉眩晕，也可以用于一些难治的疾病。

Take a lying position. Lie on the side with the ear touching the ground, and passively hold the breath 6 times (Figure 1-82). This exercise can help treat deafness and blurred vision. Lie on the side with the deaf ear, bring both knees together, and press the ear firmly against the ground. Regular practice can improve hearing and also help relieve blurred vision when the head is inverted. In addition, this exercise can be used to treat certain intractable diseases.

4. 阳虚
4. Yang deficiency

（1）心阳虚
(1) Heart yang deficiency

［症状］心悸，自汗，神倦嗜卧，心胸憋闷疼痛，形寒肢冷，面色苍白，舌质淡或紫暗，脉细弱或沉迟。

[Symptoms] Palpitations, spontaneous sweating, fatigue,

lassitude, chest tightness and pain, cold limbs, a pale facial complexion, a pale or dark purple tongue, and a thready, weak, or deep and slow pulse.

［治法］益气温阳。

[Treatment methods] Supplement qi and warm yang.

［《诸病源候论》导引方 Daoyin Exercises in *Zhu Bing Yuan Hou Lun*］

1）调心

1) Mind regulation

站式、坐式、卧式。想要辟邪驱鬼，应当常常诚意观想心（气）炎火如斗，煌煌光明。这样各种邪气就不敢侵犯，可以进入瘟疫地区之中（图 7-1）。

Take a standing, sitting or lying position. To expel pathogenic factors, visualize the heart (qi) as a blazing fire. In this way, all kinds of pathogenic factors will not dare to invade the body, and one can enter areas affected by epidemics with confidence (Figure 7-1).

2）调息、调身

2) Breath regulation and body regulation

坐式（端坐）。患心下积聚之病，舒展腰部，仰头面向太阳，以口缓缓纳气，因循着阳光咽下，超过30次就可以停止，睁开眼睛（图19-2）。

Take an upright sitting position. For abdominal masses, stretch the waist, raise the head to face the sun, inhale slowly through the mouth, swallow qi 30 times, and open the eyes (Figure 19–2).

站式、坐式、卧式。有心病的人，身体有发冷发热的症状。如果身体发冷，用"呼"字音吸气（图15-2）；如果发热，用"吹"字音出气（图15-3）。

Take a standing, sitting or lying position. People with a heart disorder may experience symptoms such as chills and fever. For chills, inhale with the sound "hu". For fever, exhale with the sound "ci" (Figure 15–3).

站式（立正）。两手托按整个腰部，使身体正直，骨节筋膜肌肉放松，气自然向下到达它该去的地方，脚前后振摇49次；双脚并拢，与头部朝两个方向振摇14次；头上下摇动，同时缩咽后仰，使两肩胛自然上抬，使脊背柔和，这样做7次。可使冷气消散，脏腑之气向涌泉穴通彻。

Take an upright standing position. Place both hands on the waist, hold and press the waist to straighten the body, relax the joints, tendons, fascia and muscles, sink down qi, and shake the feet back and forth 49 times (Figure 2–51). Bring the feet together and shake the feet in the opposite direction of the head 14 times (Figure 2–52). Move the head up and down while tucking in the throat to lift the scapulae and soften the back, and repeat 7 times (Figure 2–53). This exercise can disperse cold qi and facilitate the flow of qi in the zang-fu organs towards the point Yongquan (KI 1).

坐式。两脚对踏，脚掌合拢，向会阴侧做快速的轻微收缩，两手捧膝头，朝两个方向用力到极致，按捺14次（图2-6）。然后身体尽力向两侧活动14次（图2-7），腰部前后活动7次（图2-8）。适用于心劳、痔病、膝冷。调理虚劳未完全恢复时，须谨言慎语、不怒不喜。

Take a sitting position. Bring the soles together, quickly and slightly contract the pelvic muscles, hold both knees with both hands and pull the knees 14 times (Figure 2–6). Then fully bend the body to both sides 14 times (Figure 2–7), and move the waist forward and backward 7 times (Figure 2–8). This exercise can help treat heart deficiency, hemorrhoids, and cold in the knees. To treat consumptive conditions, talk less and keep a peaceful mind.

（2）脾阳虚
(2) Spleen yang deficiency

［症状］面色萎黄，食少，形寒，神倦乏力，少气懒言，大便溏薄，肠鸣腹痛，每因受寒或饮食不慎而加剧，舌质淡，苔白，脉弱。

[Symptoms] A sallow facial complexion, a low food intake, cold limbs, fatigue, reluctance to talk, loose stools, bowel sounds, and abdominal pain that worsens with exposure to cold or an improper diet. The tongue appears pale with a white coating, and the pulse is weak.

［治法］温中健脾。
[Treatment methods] Warm the middle jiao and strengthen the spleen.

[《诸病源候论》导引方 Daoyin Exercises in *Zhu Bing Yuan Hou Lun*]

1）调心
1) Mind regulation

站式、坐式、卧式。存想巨雷闪电，雷鸣电闪，进入腹中。能这样坚持存想，疾病就能自然消除。

Take a standing, sitting or lying position. Visualize great thunder and lightning, with thunderbolts and flashes entering into the abdomen. Persistent visualization can help keep a peaceful mind.

2）调息、调身
2) Breath regulation and body regulation

卧式（仰卧）。闭眼，不吸不呼12次，适用于饮食不消化。

Take a supine position. Close the eyes and passively hold the breath 12 times. This exercise can help treat indigestion.

坐式。两手交叉，反向撑地，身体慢慢向后仰。这个过程中脐腹自然用力，腰部向前散气，尽力做到极势时放松。上下来回做14次（图9-6）。适用于脐下寒冷、脚疼、五脏六腑不和。

Take a sitting position. Cross both hands to support the body, and slowly and fully lean backward. During this process, exert force with the abdomen, and dissipate qi with the waist. Repeat this exercise 14 times (Figure 9-6). This exercise can help alleviate cold in the lower abdomen, foot pain, and disharmony between the zang organs and fu organs.

（3）肾阳虚
(3) Kidney yang deficiency

［症状］腰背酸痛，遗精，阳痿，多尿或不禁，面色苍白，畏寒肢冷，下利清谷或五更腹泻，舌质淡胖，有齿痕，苔白，脉沉迟。

[Symptoms] Low back soreness, nocturnal emissions, impotence, frequent urination or incontinence, a pale facial complexion, aversion to cold with cold limbs, diarrhea with clear or watery stools, or nocturnal diarrhea, a swollen and tooth-marked tongue with a white coating, and a deep and slow pulse.

［治法］温补肾阳。

[Treatment methods] Warm and tonify kidney yang.

［《诸病源候论》导引方 Daoyin Exercises in *Zhu Bing Yuan Hou Lun*］

1）调心
1) Mind regulation

站式、坐式、卧式。自膝部以下有病，当观想脐下有红光，红光里外相连周遍全身。自膝部以上至腰部有病，当观想脾有黄光。从腰部以上至头部有病，当观想心中有红光。病在皮肤有寒热，当观想肝内有青绿光。上述都要观想（各色）光里外相连周遍全身，同时通过闭气来收敛光芒向内照（病所）（图15-11）。

Take a standing, sitting or lying position. For disorders below the knees, visualize a red light below the navel. For disorders between the knees and the waist, visualize a yellow light in the spleen. For disorders between the waist and the head, visualize a red light in the heart. For skin disorders accompanied by cold or heat symptoms, visualize a green light in the liver. In all cases, visualize the respective colored light illuminating the entire body, while simultaneously holding the breath to draw the radiance inward towards the affected area (Figure 15–11).

2）调息、调身
2) Breath regulation and body regulation

坐式。虾蟆行气。正坐。摇动两手臂，不吸不呼12次（图2-20）。适用于五劳七伤和水肿病。

Take an upright sitting position. Assume the posture of a toad to circulate qi. Shake the arms and passively hold the breath 12 times (Figure 2–20). This exercise can help treat the five exhaustions (Long- time observation damages blood; long-time lying damages qi; long-time sitting damages muscles; long-time standing damages bones; and long-time walking damages sinews) and seven damages (Refers to seven pathogenic factors that lead to deficiency and consumption, including improper diet, anxiety, drink, sex, hunger, over-exertion, and damage to meridians, collaterals, *Ying*-nutrients, *Wei*-defense and qi) as well as oedema.

坐式。脚放于头上,不呼不吸12次(图1-80)。适用于身体大寒感觉不到暖热,顽固性冷疾、耳聋目眩。长期练此动作就能有效,每次做30次,不能改变。

Take a sitting position. Place the feet on the top of the head and passively hold the breath 12 times (Figure 1–80). Persistent exercise can help treat extreme cold sensations in the body, intractable cold-related disorders, deafness and blurred vision. Do this exercise 30 times per session.

参考文献
References

[1] 张伯臾.中医内科学[M].上海：上海科学技术出版社，2005.

Zhang B Y. Chinese Internal Medicine[M]. Shanghai: Shanghai Scientific & Technical Publishers, 2005.

[2] 乔文彪，孙理军.《诸病源候论》版本流传考[J].时珍国医国药，2007(11)：2843-2844.

Qiao W B, Sun L J. Transmission and Study of *Zhu Bing Yuan Hou Lun* in Its Various Editions [J]. Lishizhen Medicine and Materia Medica Research, 2007(11): 2843-2844.

[3] 南京中医学院.诸病源候论校释（下）（第二版）[M].北京：人民卫生出版社，2009.

Nanjing University of Chinese Medicine. Annotated Edition of *Zhu Bing Yuan Hou Lun* (Part 2) (2nd Edition) [M]. Beijing: People's Medical Publishing House, 2009.

[4] 丁光迪.诸病源候论养生方导引法研究（第6辑）[M].北京：人民卫生出版社，2010.

Ding G D. Research on the Daoyin Methods in *Zhu Bing Yuan Hou Lun* (Volume 6) [M]. Beijing: People's Medical Publishing House, 2010.

459

[5] 刘峰,刘天君.《诸病源候论》导引术还原[M].北京：人民军医出版社,2012.

Liu F, Liu T J. Restoration of the Daoyin Methods in *Zhu Bing Yuan Hou Lun* [M]. Beijing: People's Military Medical Press, 2012.

[6] 丁光迪.中医古籍整理丛书重刊诸病源候论校注[M].北京：人民卫生出版社,2013.

Ding G D. Revised and Republished Series on Compilation of Ancient Chinese Medical Classics: Annotations on *Zhu Bing Yuan Hou Lun* [M]. Beijing: People's Medical Publishing House, 2013.

[7] 李凌江.中国抑郁障碍防治指南（第二版）[M/CD].北京：中华医学电子音像出版社,2015.

Li L J. Guidelines on the Prevention and Treatment of Depression in China (2nd Edition) [M/CD]. Beijing: Chinese Medical Multimedia Press, 2015.

[8] 周仲瑛,于文明.中医古籍珍本集成（综合卷）巢氏诸病源候论[M].长沙：湖南科学技术出版社,2016.

Zhou Z Y, Yu W M. Comprehensive Collection of Rare Ancient Chinese Medical Literature (Comprehensive Volume): *Zhu Bing Yuan Hou Lun* [M]. Changsha: Hunan Science & Technology Press, 2016.

[9] 柳长华.珍本中医古籍精校丛书诸病源候论[M].北京：北京科学技术出版社,2016.

Liu C H. Exquisite Edition Series of Precious Ancient Chinese Medical Classics: *Zhu Bing Yuan Hou Lun* [M]. Beijing: Beijing Science & Technology Press, 2016.

[10] 林志诚,薛偕华,江一静,等.中医康复临床实践指南·脑卒中[J].康复学报,2019,29(06):6-9,15.
Lin Z C, Xue X H, Jiang Y J, et al. Clinical Practice Guidelines for Stroke of Chinese Medicine Rehabilitation [J]. Rehabilitation Medicine, 2019, 29(06): 6-9, 15.

[11] 南京中医学院.诸病源候论校释(上)(第二版)[M].北京:人民卫生出版社,2020.
Nanjing University of Chinese Medicine. Annotated Edition of *Zhu Bing Yuan Hou Lun* (Part 1) (2nd Edition) [M]. Beijing: People's Medical Publishing House, 2020.

[12] 樊长征,苗青,樊茂蓉等.慢性阻塞性肺疾病稳定期中医临床实践指南(征求意见稿)[J].中国中药杂志,2020,45(22):5309-5322.
Fan C Z, Miao Q, Fan M R, et al. Clinical Practice Guideline for Stable Chronic Obstructive Pulmonary Disease with Traditional Chinese Medicine (Draft Version for Comments) [J]. China Journal of Chinese Materia Medica, 2020, 45(22): 5309-5322.

[13] 中华人民共和国国家卫生健康委员会.中国脑卒中防治指导规范(2021年)[OL].[2021-12-25].http://www.nhc.gov.cn/yzygj/s3593/202108/50c4071a86df4bfd9666e9ac2aaac605.shtml.

National Health Commission of the People's Republic of China. Guidelines on Prevention and Treatment of Stroke in China (2021) [OL]. [2021–12–25]. http://www.nhc.gov.cn/yzygj/s3593/202108/50c4071a86df4bfd9666e9ac2aaac605.shtml.

[14] 中华医学会呼吸病学分会慢性阻塞性肺疾病学组, 中国医师协会呼吸医师分会慢性阻塞性肺疾病工作委员会. 慢性阻塞性肺疾病诊治指南(2021年修订版)[J]. 中华结核和呼吸杂志, 2021, 44(03): 170–205.
Chronic Obstructive Pulmonary Disease Study Group of Chinese Thoracic Society, Chronic Obstructive Pulmonary Disease Working Committee of Chinese Association of Chest Physicians. Guidelines on the Diagnosis and Treatment of Chronic Obstructive Pulmonary Disease (Revised Edition 2021) [J]. Chinese Journal of Tuberculosis and Respiratory Diseases, 2021, 44(03): 170–205.

[15] 李匡时, 邹忆怀, 李宗衡, 等. 慢性疲劳综合征病机及辨证治疗研究进展[J]. 现代中西医结合杂志, 2021, 30(11): 1245–1249.
Li K S, Zou Y H, Li Z H, et al. Research Progress on Pathogenesis and Treatment Based on Pattern Identification of Chronic Fatigue Syndrome [J]. Modern Journal of Integrated Traditional Chinese and Western Medicine, 2021, 30(11): 1245–1249.

[16] 张兆晖, 李立华. 中医治疗慢性疲劳综合征的新进展[J]. 世界中医药, 2021, 16(06): 991–995.
Zhang Z H, Li L H. New Progress of Traditional Chinese

Medicine in the Treatment of Chronic Fatigue Syndrome [J]. World Chinese Medicine, 2021, 16(06): 991–995.

[17] 谭丽, 冯兴中. 基于"虚气流滞"探析慢性疲劳综合征中医病机及治法[J]. 环球中医药, 2021, 14 (10): 1801–1804.
Tan L, Feng X Z. Analyzing the TCM Pathogenesis and Treatment of Chronic Fatigue Syndrome Based on the Concept of "Qi Deficiency with Stagnation" [J]. Global Traditional Chinese Medicine, 2021, 14(10): 1801–1804.

《 诸 病 源 候 论 》 导 引 术 • *Zhu Bing Yuan Hou Lun Dao Yin Shu* (Explanations for the Daoyin Exercises in *Zhu Bing Yuan Hou Lun*)

The Meridian Charts

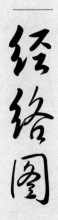

经 络 图 • The Meridian Charts

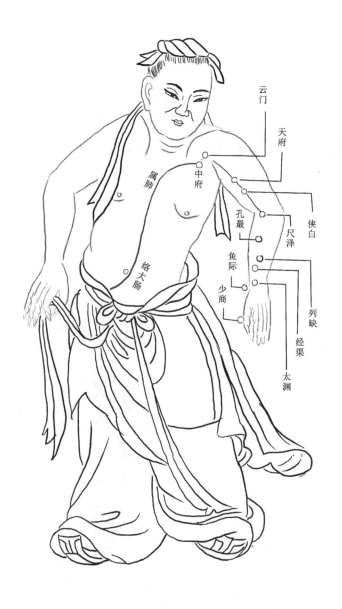

云门

天府

中府

属肺

侠白

孔最

尺泽

鱼际

络大肠

列缺

少商

经渠

太渊

手太阴肺经

Lung Meridian of Hand-Taiyin

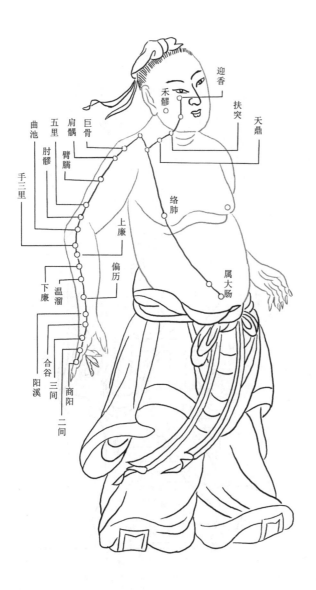

迎香

禾髎

扶突

天鼎

巨骨

肩髃

曲池

五里

臂臑

肘髎

络肺

手三里

上廉

属大肠

偏历

下廉

温溜

合谷

三间

商阳

阳溪

二间

手阳明大肠经

Large Intestine Meridian of Hand-Yangming

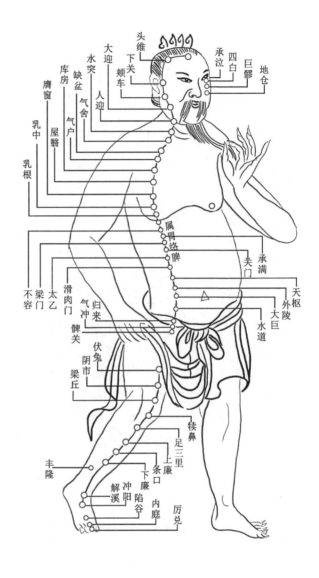

足阳明胃经

Stomach Meridian of Foot-Yangming

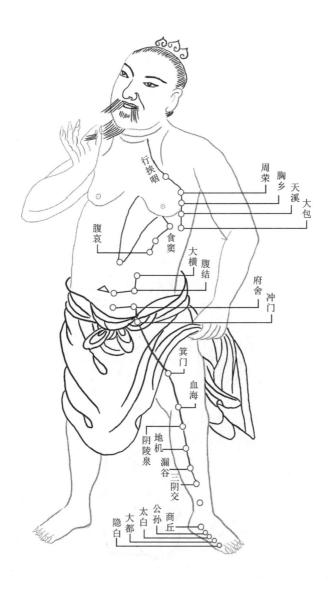

足太阴脾经

Spleen Meridian of Foot-Taiyin

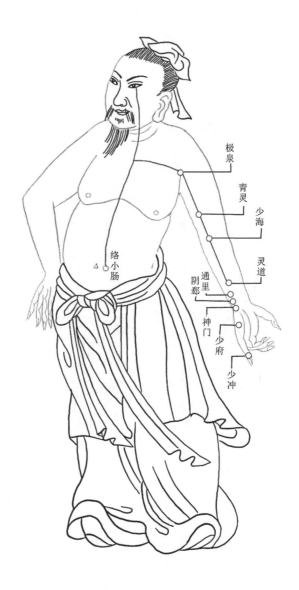

极泉
青灵
少海
灵道
通里
阴郄
神门
少府
少冲
络小肠

手少阴心经

Heart Meridian of Hand-Shaoyin

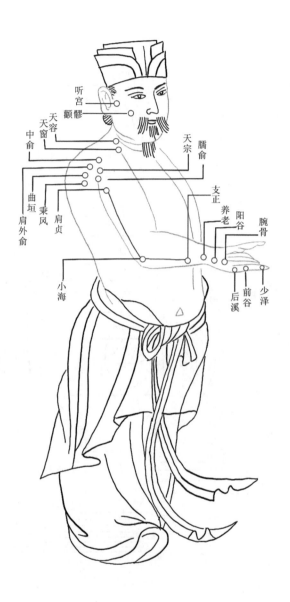

Zhu Bing Yuan Hou Lun Dao Yin Shu (Explanations
for the Daoyin Exercises in Zhu Bing Yuan Hou Lun)

·

《诸病源候论》导引术

471

经 络 图

·

The Meridian Charts

手太阳小肠经

Small Intestine Meridian of Hand-Taiyang

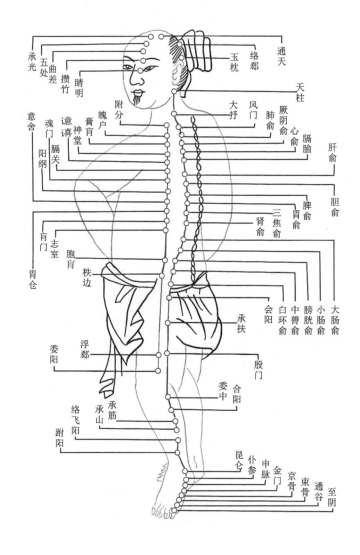

足太阳膀胱经

Bladder Meridian of Foot-Taiyang

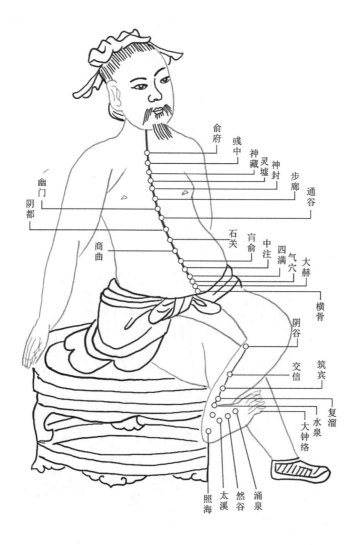

俞府
彧中
神藏
灵墟
神封
步廊
通谷
幽门
阴都
石关
肓俞
商曲
中注
四满
气穴
大赫
横骨
阴谷
交信
筑宾
复溜
水泉
大钟络
照海
太溪
然谷
涌泉

足少阴肾经

Kidney Meridian of Foot-Shaoyin

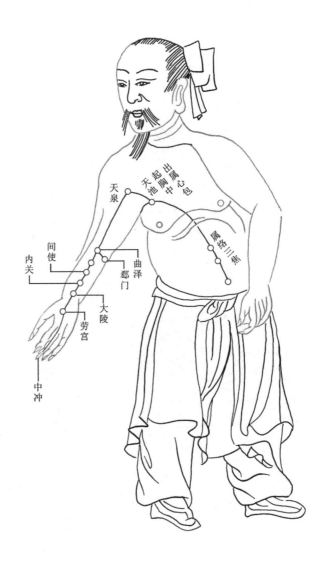

手厥阴心包经

Pericardium Meridian of Hand-Jueyin

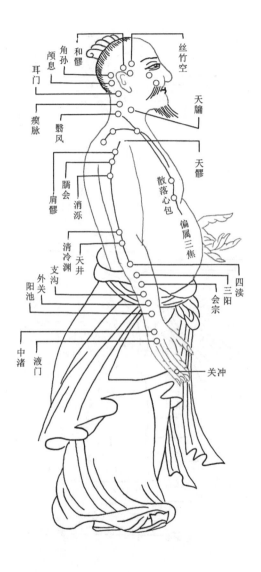

手少阳三焦经

Triple Energizer Meridian of Hand-Shaoyang

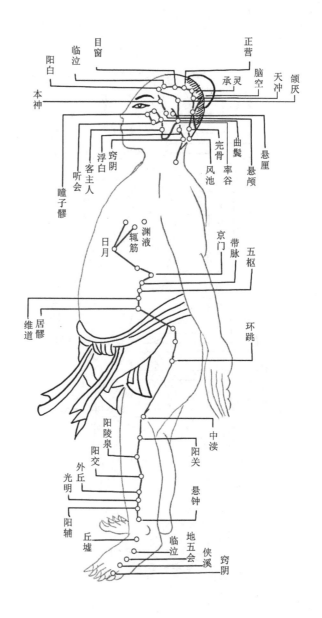

足少阳胆经

Gallbladder Meridian of Foot-Shaoyang

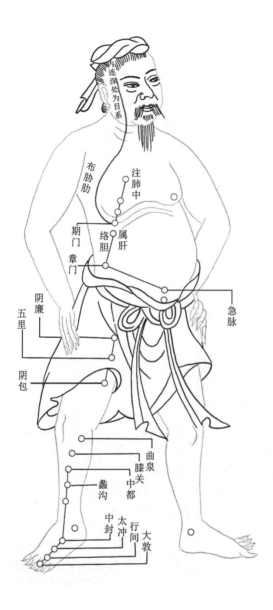

内连巅处为目系

布胁肋

注肺中

期门
络胆
章门
属肝

急脉

阴廉
五里

阴包

曲泉
膝关
中都
蠡沟

中封
太冲
行间
大敦

足厥阴肝经

Liver Meridian of Foot-Jueyin

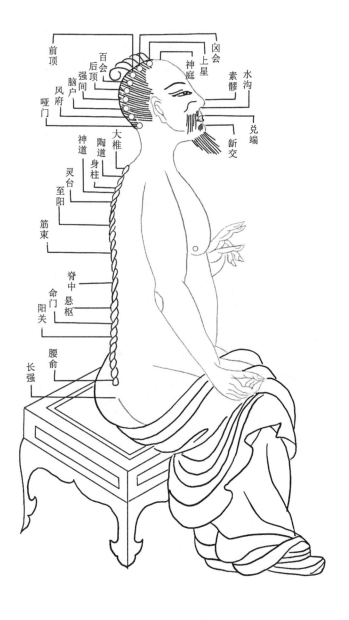

督脉

Governor Vessel (Du)

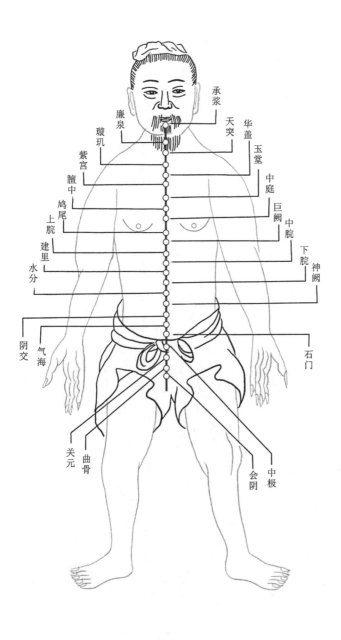

Zhu Bing Yuan Hou Lun Dao Yin Shu (Explanations
for the Daoyin Exercises in *Zhu Bing Yuan Hou Lun*) · 〈诸 病 源 候 论〉导 引 术

479

经 络 图 · The Meridian Charts

承浆
廉泉
璇玑
紫宫
膻中
鸠尾
上脘
建里
水分
阴交
气海
关元
曲骨
会阴
中极
石门
神阙
下脘
中脘
巨阙
中庭
玉堂
华盖
天突

任脉

Conception Vessel (Ren)

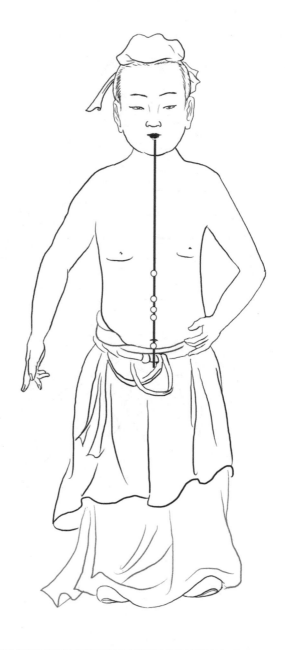
冲脉

Thoroughfare Vessel (Chong)

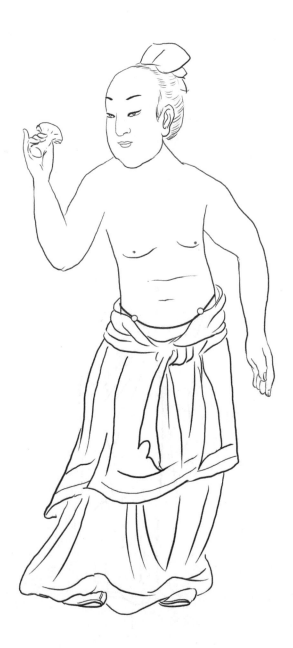

带脉

Belt Vessel (Dai)

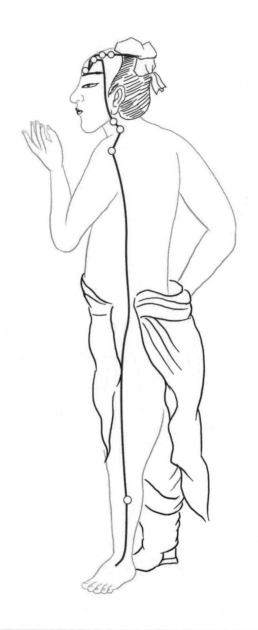

阳维脉

Yang Link Vessel (Yang Wei)

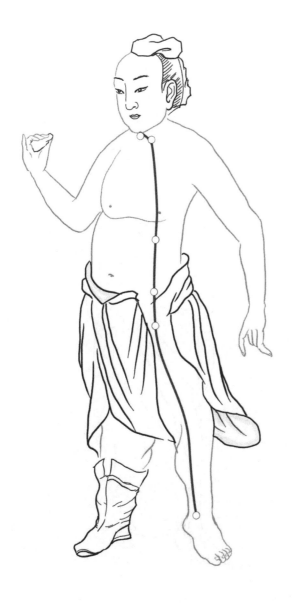

阴维脉

Yin Link Vessel (Yin Wei)

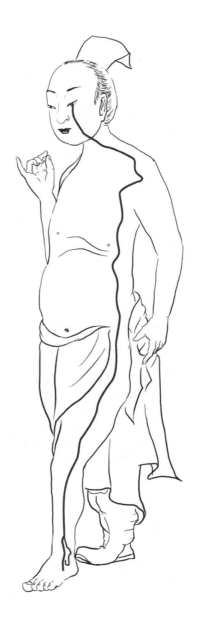

阳蹻脉

Yang Heel Vessel (Yang Qiao)

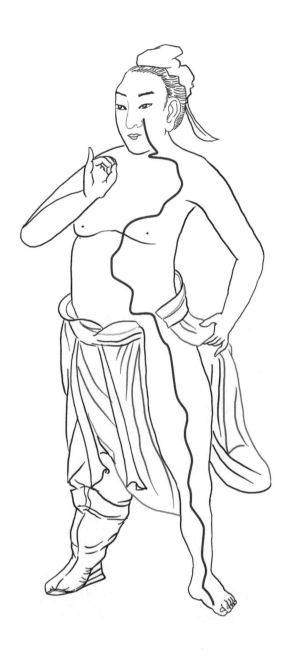

阴蹻脉

Yin Heel Vessel (Yin Qiao)